Medical Device Regulatory Practices

Medical Device Regulatory Practices

An International Perspective

Val Theisz

Pan Stanford Publishing

Published by

Pan Stanford Publishing Pte. Ltd.
Penthouse Level, Suntec Tower 3
8 Temasek Boulevard
Singapore 038988

Email: editorial@panstanford.com
Web: www.panstanford.com

British Library Cataloguing-in-Publication Data
A catalogue record for this book is available from the British Library.

Medical Device Regulatory Practices: An International Perspective

ISBN 978-981-4669-10-8 (Hardcover)
ISBN 978-981-4669-11-5 (eBook)

Printed in the USA

To my partner Günther Theisz, founder and CEO of Certification Body Australia, and my lovely daughter, Nadine

Contents

Preface

"This is a culture war." These comments by the Food and Drug Administration (FDA) consultant Steve Grossman, reported in a November 9, 2014, article by AP Health Writer Matthew Perrone, refer to the cultural divide between the highly regulated medical device industry and the Silicon Valley tech industry "used to just bringing their products straight to the market" and for whom "any regulatory scheme that involves scrutiny and delay is alien". The article tells the story of two Silicon Valley companies and their very different experiences with getting medical apps through the FDA regulatory hoops (1).

23andMe, a Mountain View, California, based company became the poster child for tech companies' dysfunctional relationship with the FDA in 2013, when the company was ordered to stop selling its medical app for genetic testing. In a warning letter, the FDA said that despite "hundreds of email exchanges" the Google-backed company failed to demonstrate the effectiveness of its saliva-based kit, which claimed to tell customers if they were at risk for more than 250 health conditions.

Since then, the article said, 23andMe has brought in four new executives with experience in the drug and medical testing fields and submitted an FDA application for the first in a series of genetic health tests. The company's CEO, Anne Wojcicki, compared the process of working in healthcare to doing business in a foreign country. "You need to understand that language and the way that they do business there almost in the same way you would going into China or India," she said.

On the other end of the spectrum is Alivercor, a San Francisco company selling a hand-held device that attaches to a smartphone to detect dangerous heart rhythms. Alivercor submitted its FDA application in August 2012 and received clearance four months later. The company's CEO, Euan Thomson, said tech industry people exaggerate the difficulties of regulation because they don't understand it.

But this is not just about Silicon Valley tech struggling in a highly regulated environment. It is also the story of medical technology start-ups striving to transition to financially viable businesses and that of big companies held back by ineffective internal systems and processes. Obtaining regulatory approvals in the United States and the European Union (EU), the two largest and most lucrative markets, is a sort of Darwinian make or break for developers of medical devices, including the latest medical apps for smart phones.

In my 20 years of experience working on both sides of the regulatory divide – as an EU notified body reviewer and auditor, as well as managing regulatory affairs in various medical device companies – I have seen this happening again and again. Some organizations struggle for many months trying to obtain marketing authorizations even for "me too", lower-risk products, while others manage to breeze through with innovative, complex, high-risk products. Whilst many companies find themselves in the former category, they all aspire to be in the latter. To get there, though, it takes a thorough understanding of the terminology and processes governing the healthcare product industry.

It is my hope that this book will demystify the "alien" world of medical device regulations and help organizations get to market faster and smoother.

I finished writing the book at the end of 2014, a year that saw the enactment of major reforms of medical device regulatory regimes in China and Japan and the introduction in Europe of unannounced audits by notified bodies in the aftermath of the Poly Implant Prothèse (PIP) scandal. For many years the French company PIP, one of the world's biggest suppliers of breast implants at the time, had fraudulently used industrial silicone instead of the approved medical-grade silicone in many of its breast implants that were marketed worldwide, and it concealed this fact during the pre-announced audits of it EU notified body. PIP breast implants were withdrawn from the market in 2010 after it came to light that they'd been deliberately manufactured with a much cheaper industrial-grade silicone and were far more prone to rupture than other breast implants.

Also in 2014, Frances Oldham Kelsey, the pharmacologist and FDA reviewer who famously refused to authorize thalidomide for the US market in 1960, celebrated her 100th birthday. Thalidomide had been used as a sedative and to reduce morning sickness in pregnant women in many countries since the late 1950s. Despite a constant and increasing pressure from the pharmaceutical company, Dr. Kelsey refused to approve the application for marketing authorization without adequate evidence that the drug was safe, a decision that prevented thousands of babies in the United States being born with crippling birth defects. In 1962 Dr. Kelsey received the President's Award for Distinguished Federal Civilian Service from President J. F. Kennedy in recognition of her "exceptional judgment in evaluating a new drug".

Such lessons are a reminder of why therapeutic goods are so highly regulated. The main role of regulatory agencies is to protect the health and well-being of patients, consumers, healthcare workers and the community at large. They strive to strike a balance between preventing unsafe or ineffective products from being distributed in the market and enabling fast access to innovative technologies that improve patients' health and quality of life.

I would like to express my gratitude to those who have reviewed and contributed valuable comments and content to sections of this book: Dr. Sean Williams, BE (Elec.) (Hons.), PhD, on design controls (Chapter 4) and configuration management (Chapter 6); Dr. Sylvia Roins, PhD Pharm., on combination products (Chapters 2 and 5); Ms. Kathy Wang, APAC Regulatory Affairs Expert, on China and Association of Southeast Asian Nations (ASEAN) regulations (Chapter 5); and Mr. Phillip Prather, BSc (Biology, Economics), MComm (Marketing), on the product launch process for medical devices (Chapter 6).

Also, this book has benefited from the many questions I had to find answers to and the challenges encountered during the course of my work, as well as from the expertise and insights of people I have worked with and learned from in the past 20 years – too many to mention here. My thanks and appreciation goes to all of you.

Val Theisz

Reference

1. Perrone, M., Associated Press. *Silicon Valley Struggles to Speak FDA's Language.* Thu, 09/11/2014, Washington: s.n., 2014.

Introduction

This book is intended to serve as a reference for professionals in the medical device industry, in particular those seeking to learn from practical examples and case studies. Medical devices, like pharmaceuticals, are highly regulated and the bar is raised constantly as patients and consumers expect the best-quality healthcare and safe and effective medical technologies. Obtaining marketing authorization is the first major hurdle that med techs need to overcome in their pursuit of commercial success. In today's competitive environment a few months delay in time to market can cost millions of dollars in missed opportunities.

Start-up companies in particular may find that bringing innovative medical technologies to market is daunting and fraught with difficulty. Growing and larger companies may also struggle to meet product launch deadlines and keep compliance costs under control. A product recall can tarnish the reputation of a medical device company within weeks. However, the cost of development and regulatory compliance can be significantly reduced, and delivery of new medical devices that are safe and effective to patients around the world can be accelerated, if sponsors and manufacturers understand the regulatory requirements and processes involved.

In addition to the expertise required to design and manufacture a medical device, a manufacturer needs to have an understanding of how to test and clinically evaluate medical devices, how to identify and address the root causes of adverse events and device malfunctions and, in general, how to apply regulatory requirements throughout the product life cycle.

Many problems faced by medical device manufacturers are a result of a lack of understanding of the intent rather than the letter of regulations, poor business processes or deficient implementation of regulatory controls. It is a common misconception, for instance, that to be compliant one must have lots of procedures, forms and templates. Nothing is further from the truth. Too much bureaucracy, overly complicated and opaque processes, a lack of structure, clarity and visibility throughout the business – all these have a negative impact on the ability to obtain marketing approvals quickly and to maintain regulatory compliance. Worse still, overly complicated systems and processes are prone to frequent non-conformities and are difficult, time-consuming and expensive to maintain. Robust regulatory controls co-exist a lot better with streamlined, agile and effective systems and processes.

Another frequently encountered issue is an insular approach to applications for marketing authorizations. Often regulatory professionals receive engineering documents full of technical jargon, which they then "translate" into submission documentation that an external reviewer can understand without requiring substantial prior product knowledge. This is then usually repeated for every country or region where marketing authorizations are sought. After going through multiple and exhausting cycles of questions and answers with the various authorities lessons learned are lost and mistakes repeated, efforts duplicated and deadlines missed. Regulatory requirements are taken out of context, misunderstood or misinterpreted, and bureaucracy takes over, sucking the life out of projects and bringing down teams' motivation and energy.

In this book the reader will find examples and practical recommendations on how to implement statutory requirements applicable throughout the life cycle of a medical device: design and development, clinical evaluation, manufacturing and the post-market phase. Although the case studies are fictional, they are based on real-world scenarios and depict common errors. The proposed solutions are pragmatic, tried and tested in both large and small medical device companies, but there is no intention to suggest they are the best or the only solutions.

The book has two parts:

Part 1, comprised of three chapters, gives an overview of the international regulatory framework for medical devices and introduces basic concepts and terminology (Chapter 1); covers compliance with requirements for safety and effectiveness of medical devices (Chapter 2); and provides recommendations for the content and structure of technical documentation required by regulations (Chapter 3).

Part 2, also comprised of three chapters, goes into more detail, outlying the regulatory controls applicable in each of the main phases of a medical device's life cycle: the pre-market phase (Chapter 4); regulatory submissions, approvals and registrations (Chapter 5); and the post-market phase (Chapter 6).

The major established markets – the European Union, the United States, Australia, Canada and Japan – have center stage, but significant developments in international harmonization and emerging markets such as China, ASEAN countries and Brazil are mentioned as well. Various national and regional regulations are presented as they apply to major topics such as compliance with safety and effectiveness requirements, and in alignment with the typical medical device life cycle: the pre-market phase, regulatory approvals and registrations, and the post-market phase. The reason behind choosing such a structure is that in reality this is how regulatory knowledge is used and applied (see Fig. I.1).

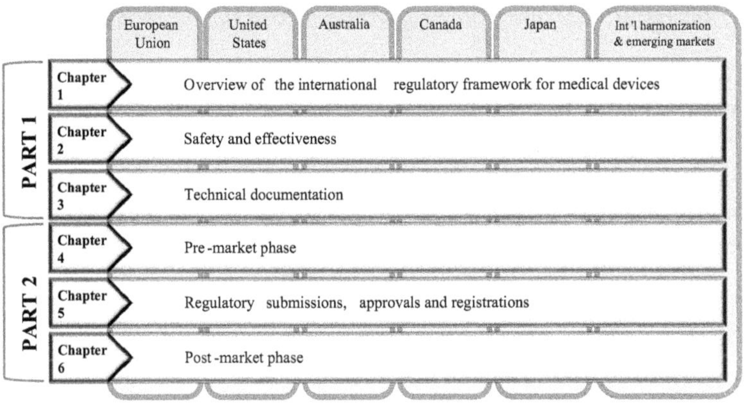

Figure I.1 This book's structure: rows represent chapters, and columns represent regulatory jurisdictions covered.

Table I.1 Orientation guide

Steps	What to do	Useful reading
Step 1	Confirm that the product is indeed a medical device.	Chapter 1, Section 1.4, "Medical Devices"; Section 1.6, "Components, Spare Parts, Accessories, Device Families, Kits, Systems and Procedure Packs"
Step 2	Determine the risk classification of the medical device.	Chapter 1, Section 1.5, "Risk-Based Classification"
Step 3	Identify the applicable regulatory controls in the target market(s).	Chapter 1, Section 1.7, "Risk-Based Approach for Regulatory Controls and Conformity Assessment"
Step 4	Implement regulatory controls during the pre-market phase.	Chapter 2, "Safety and Effectiveness"; Chapter 3, "Technical Documentation"; Chapter 4, "Pre-Market Phase"
Step 5	Submit regulatory application(s) and obtain marketing approval(s) in the target market(s).	Chapter 5, "Regulatory Submissions, Approvals and Registrations"
Step 6	Maintain compliance until product obsolescence.	Chapter 6, "Post-Market Phase"

Part 1 should be read by anyone involved in developing, manufacturing or marketing medical devices, and especially by novices in the regulatory affairs space, as it explains relevant terminology and the basics required to understand medical device regulations.

Part 2 chapters can be used as a reference according to the reader‘s needs. For instance, a company developing, manufacturing and marketing medical devices would need to know about the regulatory controls applicable in all phases of a product's life cycle, but an importer may only need to concentrate on the regulatory submission and post-market phases.

For those new to medical device regulations, asking the question, What do I need to do and where do I even start?, here is, in a nutshell, a quick orientation guide (Table I.1).

There was no intention to reproduce entire texts of regulations and guidelines in this book, as these are already publicly available from the official websites of relevant agencies, but some of the most important definitions and excerpts have been included for convenience, along with explanations and discussions.

Moreover, every effort has been made to ensure that the latest information is used in writing of this book; however, regulations and guidelines are often being revised and some information may be already outdated at the time of publishing. By providing detailed references the reader can refer directly to the information source to confirm the latest status.

Chapter 1

Overview of the International Regulatory Framework for Medical Devices

This chapter provides an overview of how medical devices are regulated worldwide. It also introduces fundamental concepts, definitions and terminology that the reader needs to become familiar with to be able to understand medical device regulations. Basic regulatory processes are introduced at a general level, before dealing with them in greater detail in later chapters.

1.1 Established and Emerging Markets

According to a 2012 report compiled jointly by the World Health Organization (WHO), the World Trade Organization (WTO) and the World Intellectual Property Organization (WIPO), the European Union, or EU (see Fig. 1.1), and the United States are the top two biggest importers and exporters of medical devices (1 pp. 192–193). They account for more than half of the global trade in medical devices.

Medical Device Regulatory Practices: An International Perspective
Val Theisz

ISBN 978-981-4669-10-8 (Hardcover), 978-981-4669-11-5 (eBook)
www.panstanford.com

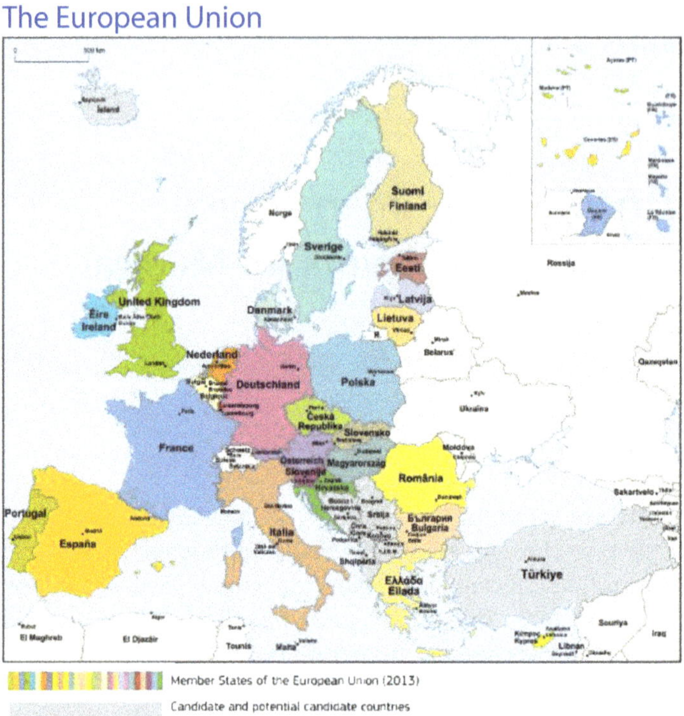

Figure 1.1 The European Union as of July 1, 2013. *Source*: European Commission official website.

It is not unusual for medical device companies to have a combined EU and US trade represent more than 70% of their business. No wonder then that having a significant share of the business in these two markets is a measure of a manufacturer's international commercial success.

This situation will most likely change in the future as the emerging economies of Brazil, Russia, India and China, the so-called BRIC nations, as well as of the 10 countries that make up the Association of Southeast Asian Nations, or ASEAN (see Fig. 1.2), continue to grow. It is expected that their large populations and rising middle class will lead to changes in consumer lifestyles, higher expectations for quality healthcare and increasing demand for the latest medical technologies.

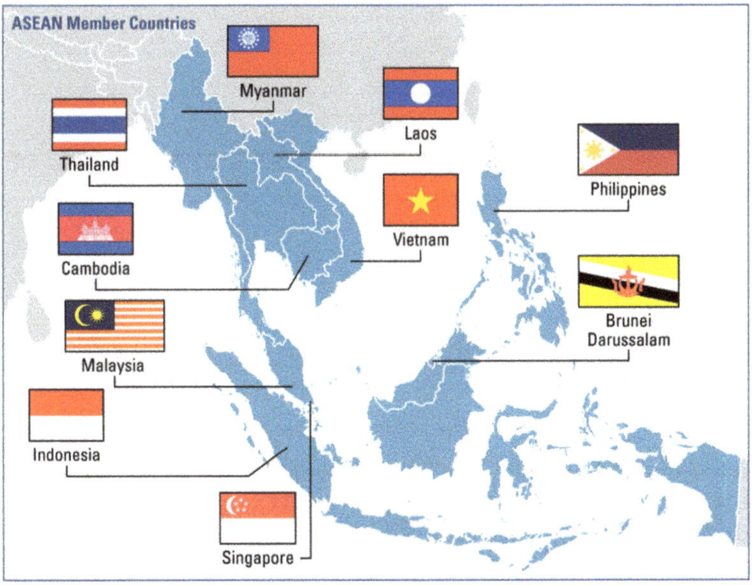

Figure 1.2 The ASEAN member states in 2013. *Source*: US Global Investors.

Currently, a start-up company would typically obtain the Conformité Européenne (CE) marking certification for the EU first and then apply for approval in the United States, which is arguably more difficult and takes longer to obtain. The revenue earned from EU sales would sustain the business until the US marketing approval is received. Access to the top two largest medical device markets would allow the company to grow and consolidate earnings, and then expand into emerging regions as well.

Once a company has reached a certain size, with a growing product portfolio, it would typically want to release its new products and upgrades in parallel in all markets according to an established cycle – let's say a new product every two years and one significant upgrade every year or twice a year. It would be very inefficient to generate *full sets* of technical dossiers separately for every regulatory submission and then maintain them in parallel or, worse, not maintain them and become non-compliant. A better and far more efficient way to manage multiple international marketing applications and ensure ongoing regulatory compliance in all

Table 1.1 Regulatory Authorities represented in the IMDRF

Country	Regulatory Authority
Australia	Therapeutic Goods Administration (TGA)
Brazil	National Health Surveillance Agency (ANVISA)
Canada	Health Canada (HC)
China	China Food and Drug Administration (CFDA)
European Union	European Commission Directorate General Health and Consumers (EC)
Japan	Pharmaceuticals and Medical Devices Agency (PMDA)
	Ministry of Health, Labour and Welfare (MHLW)
Russia	Russian Ministry of Health
United States	US Food and Drug Administration (FDA)

markets without duplication or rework is to generate and maintain one full set of product documentation that addresses regulatory requirements in the main markets, a sort of "one size fits most" approach. This requires a thorough knowledge and understanding of all relevant international regulatory requirements and very good upfront planning.

The EU, the United States, Australia, Canada and Japan have well-established, mature regulations and regulatory processes for healthcare products. Approvals issued by authorities in these countries are widely recognized and would usually enable obtaining marketing approvals in many countries in the emerging markets in Latin America and the Asia Pacific.

The Global Harmonization Taskforce (GHTF), which was founded in 1992 by the Regulatory Authorities (RAs) in EU, the United States, Australia, Canada and Japan to promote convergence between their national medical device regulatory systems, was replaced in 2012 by the International Medical Device Regulatory Forum (IMDRF) [2]. The IMDRF remains a voluntary forum just like the GHTF was, but extending its membership to Brazil, China and the Russian Federation represents the recognition of how important it is to align the regulatory regimes of the largest emerging economies with those in the established markets. The IMDRF Management Committee is comprised of representatives from the RAs listed in Table 1.1.

These RAs, with the exception of the European Commission (EC), issue approvals for medical devices in their own jurisdictions. In the EU, the national Competent Authorities and ministries of

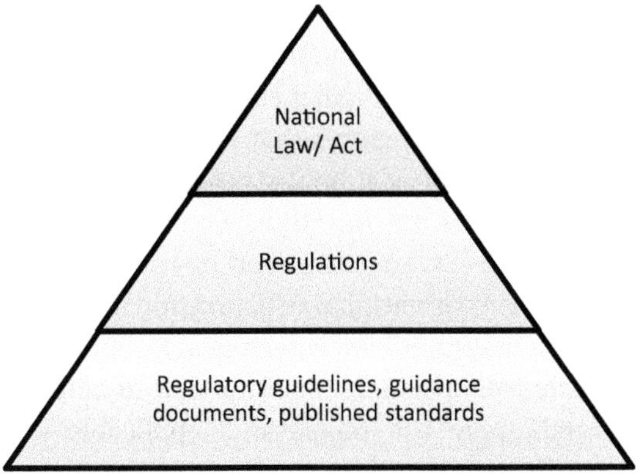

Figure 1.3 Typical hierarchy of regulatory requirements in established markets.

health in the member states enforce the medical device legislation. The Competent Authorities are responsible for the designation of national Conformity Assessment Bodies (CABs), called Notified Bodies, that carry out conformity assessments and issue certificates of approval for medical devices. The Competent Authorities notify the EC and other member states of the certification bodies they have accredited. Once a certification body has been officially notified to the EC it becomes an EU Notified Body.

In established markets, such as Australia, Canada and the United States, the hierarchy of regulatory requirements can be represented by the pyramid in Fig. 1.3.

At the top there is the law or the legislative act that sets out the legal requirements for the manufacture, distribution, import and export of medical devices in that particular jurisdiction. On the next level down there are the regulations that translate in a more accessible language and in more detail the legal requirements. At the base of the pyramid there are the guidelines and technical standards that provide guidance on how to apply the regulations. Although guidelines and standards are generally voluntary, complying with them usually provides a presumption of conformity in most situations.

In the United States, the federal Food, Drug, and Cosmetic Act (FD&C Act) is the law governing medical devices. *Code of Federal*

Regulations (CFR), in particular Parts 800 to 1299, covers various aspects of design, clinical evaluation, manufacturing, packaging, labeling and post-market surveillance of medical devices, as well as standards and product reports that apply to radiation-emitting products [3]. Food and Drug Administration (FDA) Good Guidance Practice (GGP) documents and Blue Book Memos, as well as Recognized Consensus Standards issued by various standard organizations such as the International Organization for Standardization (ISO) and the International Electrotechnical Commission (IEC) are non-binding technical specifications intended to help the industry to interpret and apply the regulations applicable to particular regulated products and certain procedures [4, 5].

Similarly in Australia, the Australian Therapeutic Goods Act is the law that governs medical devices (along with medicines and biological products). Regulations, Orders and Determinations provide details on aspects covered by the Act. Relevant to medical devices are the Therapeutic Goods (Medical devices) Regulations of 2002 [6]. *Australian Regulatory Guidelines for Medical Devices* (ARGMD) is a guide intended to assist the industry understand and apply the regulatory requirements [7]. In addition, non-mandatory medical device standards orders (MDSO) and conformity assessment standards orders (CASO) can be used to demonstrate compliance with the regulatory requirements [8].

In Canada, the Food and Drugs Act is the law governing medical devices. The Medical Devices Regulations represent the subordinate legislation that defines the application and enforcement of the Act [9]. Guidelines (also referred to as guidance documents or directives) are non-binding and their purpose is to assist in interpreting the legislation and regulations [10]. Also, the Therapeutic Products Directorate of Health Canada publishes a list of recognized national and international standards for medical devices that can be used to demonstrate conformity with mandatory regulatory requirements for safety and effectiveness [11].

Regulatory requirements in Japan have a similar hierarchical structure (refer to Fig. 1.4). The Act on Securing Quality, Efficacy and Safety of Pharmaceuticals, Medical Devices, Regenerative and Cellular Therapy Products, Gene Therapy Products and Cosmetics – or shortly, the Pharmaceutical and Medical Device (PMD) Act, which replaced the Japanese Pharmaceutical Affairs Law, or J-PAL,

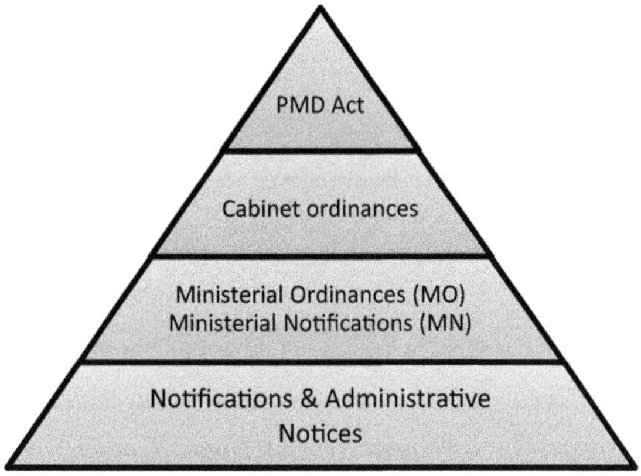

Figure 1.4 Hierarchy of regulatory requirements in Japan.

on November 25, 2014 – sits at the top. Cabinet Ordinances are on the next level down, and then Ministerial Ordinances and Ministerial Notifications enforcing law and Cabinet Ordinances. At the bottom of the pyramid there are notifications and administrative notices [12, 13].

Japan's Ministry of Health, Labor and Welfare (MHLW) specifies the review guidelines and the national (Japanese Industrial Standards, or JIS) and international standards (ISO, IEC) to be used for the conformity assessment of medical devices [14].

In the EU the situation is somewhat different (refer to Fig. 1.5). The main goal of the EU is to establish a single market with free movement of goods (including medical devices), people, money and services. By adhering to the Treaty on the Functioning of the European Union (TFEU), the EU member states cede part of their sovereignty and thus empower the EU institutions to adopt regulations, directives and decisions that take precedence over national laws and that are legally binding on national authorities [15].

The European directives, including those governing medical devices, become mandatory only after adoption into the national laws of the member states. Every member state is obliged to adapt its national laws to meet the end goals stipulated in the directives by a certain deadline, which is also specified in the directives [16]. There are three EU directives covering medical devices [17]:

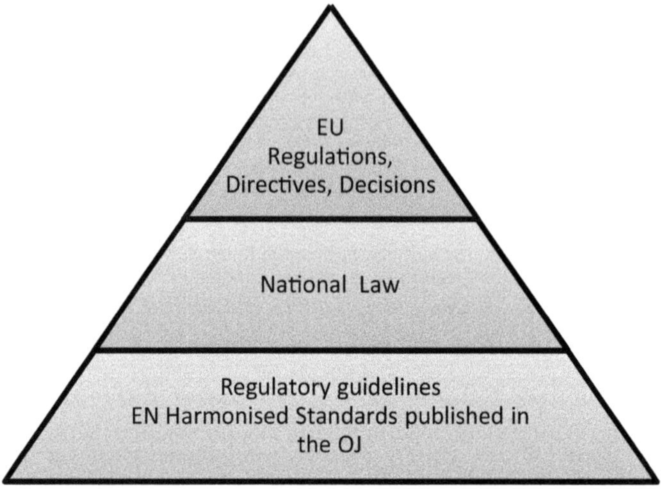

Figure 1.5 Hierarchy of regulatory requirements in the EU.

- Active Implantable Medical Device (AIMD) Directive, or AIMDD (Council Directive 90/385/EEC)
- Medical Device (MD) Directive, or MDD (Council Directive 93/42/EEC)
- In Vitro Diagnostics (IVD) Directive, or IVDD (Council Directive 98/79/EC)

In 2012 the EC adopted two proposals for new regulations [18]:

- The Proposal for a combined medical devices regulation intended to replace the current AIMD and the MD directives, and
- The Proposal on IVD medical devices, which is intended to replace the existing IVD directive

EU regulations become legally binding in all member states as soon as they are passed jointly by the EU Council and the European Parliament. They represent the most direct form of EU law, without the need for the member states to take action in order to implement them into national law [19].

There are also EU decisions, which, unlike EU regulations, apply in specific cases only, involving particular authorities or individuals.

They can be issued by the EU Council (sometimes jointly with the European Parliament) or by the EU Commission and are fully binding [20].

EU guidance documents such as Medical Devices (MEDDEV), Notified Bodies Medical Devices (NB-MED), Notified Body Operations Group Best Practice Guides (NBOG BPG) and consensus statements, interpretative documents and Harmonised Standards are not legally binding. They aim to promote a uniform interpretation of relevant regulatory requirements and a common conformity assessment approach throughout the EU [21].

Harmonised Standards are European Norms (EN) developed by European standardization organizations such as the European Committee for Standardization (CEN) and the European Committee for Electrotechnical Standardization (CENELEC), following a standardization request (mandate) from the EC. Their purpose is to provide detailed technical specifications in order to fulfill legally binding objectives set in relevant EU legislation. EN Harmonised Standards providing a presumption of conformity with the mandatory requirements for medical device safety and effectiveness are published in *Official Journal of the European Union* (*OJ*) [22].

In emerging markets, some countries have little or no regulations specific to medical devices and they either apply their existing national regulations for pharmaceuticals or rely on the regulatory approval from an established jurisdiction. Brazil, China and Russia have a testing and certification framework in place for the assessment and approval of medical devices.

In the last decade or so there have been efforts in some of the emerging markets to set up regional working parties with the aim of establishing and harmonizing existing regulations for medical devices and diagnostics (see Table 1.2).

In 2012, the ASEAN Medical Device Product Working Group (MDPWG) released the draft ASEAN Medical Devices Directive (AMDD) [23]. The AMDD, similar in content and structure with the EU medical devices directives, is a high-level, non-binding document that lays out a uniform set of rules for product pre-market registration and post-market surveillance. It has benefited from the input of ASEAN member countries, industry representatives, the GHTF and the WHO. At the time of going to print a number of

Table 1.2 Medical devices and diagnostics harmonization working parties in emerging markets

Harmonization working party	Year established	Member countries/organizations (status: 2014)
Asian Harmonization Working Party (AHWP)	1999	Abu Dhabi, Brunei Darussalam, Cambodia, Chile, China, Chinese Taipei, Hong Kong SAR, India, Indonesia, Jordan, Korea, Kuwait, Laos, Malaysia, Myanmar, Pakistan, Philippines, Saudi Arabia, Singapore, South Africa, Tanzania, Thailand, Vietnam and Yemen
ASEAN Medical Device Product Working Group (MDPWG)	2004	ASEAN member states participating in the ASEAN Consultative Committee on Standards and Quality (ACCSQ)
Pan African Harmonization Working Party on Medical Devices and Diagnostics (PAHWP)	2012	Regulatory Authorities, medical device and diagnostics industry representatives, regional economic communities (RECs), WHO, New Partnership for Africa's Development (NEPAD), the African Society for Laboratory Medicine (ASLM), German International Co-operation (EAC-GIZ) and the London School of Hygiene & Tropical Medicine (LSHTM)

ASEAN countries had expressed their commitment to implement the AMDD before the end of 2015. The Asian Harmonization Working Party (AHWP) developed a playbook to guide member economies in development of their medical device regulatory framework. The AHWP playbook is available from the AHWP official website (http://www.ahwp.info/index.php?q=node/497).

On January 1, 2012, Singapore's Health Sciences Authority (HSA) rolled out a state-of-the-art regulatory system for medical devices, making the small nation state the first ASEAN country to adopt the AMDD [24], which is not surprising considering that Singapore's economy is one of the most developed, not just in the ASEAN region, but also in the world.

1.2 Credibility and Authority of Approvals

Regulatory approvals are often supported by test reports and certificates of compliance issued by testing laboratories and certification bodies, both public and private. The proliferation of testing and certification providers in the past 20 years or so has emphasized the need for defining a set of standards for the operation of testing and certification schemes, in particular in regulated areas like medical devices, so that all interested parties can be confident that a certified product, process or service fulfils specified requirements.

The terms "certified", "accredited" and "recognized" are often employed interchangeably or simply misused. Each has a particular meaning and should be used in the right context.

Conformity assessment is demonstrating that a product, process, system, person or body (legal entity) fulfills specific requirements. An attestation is a formal statement, based on a decision following a review, that fulfilment of specified requirements has been demonstrated.

"Certification" and "to certify" originate from the Latin word "certus", meaning "certain" or "ascertained". In other words, certification is an attestation of compliance with requirements. For persons, being certified means holding officially recognized qualifications or competencies in a certain area, based on examinations that use objective criteria to measure competence and scoring. A certification body is an independent legal entity that certifies products, processes, services or persons against specified requirements.

"Accreditation" and "to accredit" originate from the Latin word "accreditus", meaning "to impart credibility to" or "to trust". In other words, accreditation is an attestation of a legal entity's competence, credibility, independence and integrity in carrying out specific tasks, such as testing, calibration, conformity assessment and certification. Accreditation reduces the risk for business and its customers by providing assurance that accredited laboratories and certification bodies are competent to carry out the work they undertake within their scope of accreditation. An accreditation body is typically a government authority or a statutory non-profit organization designated by the government to carry out accreditation functions.

Accreditation is granted for specified requirements or standards. For example, a laboratory claiming to be accredited to perform safety testing for electrical medical equipment to the IEC 60601-1 standard should have this standard listed in its scope of accreditation. Accreditation bodies make publicly available lists of accredited organizations and what they are accredited for.

Laboratories or certification bodies may issue test reports or certificates but *may not provide accreditations.* Hence statements such as "our laboratory is accredited by TÜV [German-based testing and certification organizations]" are incorrect, because the TÜVs are not accreditation bodies. A laboratory without an official accreditation may have some of its testing "recognized" by an accredited testing and certification body (such as the TÜVs) if the accredited body is satisfied, based on an evaluation, that the laboratory fulfills specific requirements. This kind of recognition based on a bilateral agreement, though, does not have the same level of validity as an official accreditation.

In an effort to promote national and international recognition national accreditation bodies have signed multilateral agreements or treaties with international accreditation organizations. A key objective of these international accreditation networks is the mutual recognition of the services and results of accredited bodies in order to prevent technical obstacles and multiple accreditations. Table 1.3 lists the main national accreditation bodies and international accreditation organizations.

The ISO/IEC 17000 international standard series, replacing older ISO guides and EN 45000 series standards, provide definitions and specify requirements for the operation of testing and certification schemes, as well as requirements for the accreditation of testing laboratories, certification bodies and CABs (see also Table 1.4).

The ISO/IEC 17000 standards represent a benchmark for best practices in running accreditation, testing and conformity assessment, and certification schemes. They are often referenced in Mutual Recognition Agreements (MRAs) or Multilateral Agreements (MLAs) between RAs in different countries as the basis for recognition and acceptance of each other's conformity assessments, largely eliminating the need for duplicative testing or re-certification [25].

A regulatory agency or certification body that is accredited in its country of origin for performing conformity assessments to specified requirements of another jurisdiction becomes a CAB recognized in the other jurisdiction.

Table 1.3 National accreditation bodies and international accreditation organizations

	Accreditation bodies	Jurisdiction
A2LA	American Association for Laboratory Accreditation	United States
ANAB	ANSI-ASQ National Accreditation Board	United States
NRTL	Nationally Recognized Testing Laboratory Program	United States
NVLAP	National Voluntary Laboratory Accreditation Program	United States
TPRB	FDA Third Party Recognition Board	United States
DakkS	Deutsche Akkreditierungsstelle	Germany
ZLG	Zentralstelle der Länder für Gesundheitsschutz bei Arzneimitteln und Medizinprodukten	Germany
UKAS	United Kingdom Accreditation Service	U.K.
COFRAC	Comité français d'accréditation	France
NATA	National Association of Testing Authorities, Australia	Australia
JAS-ANZ	Joint Accreditation Scheme Australia New Zealand	Australia, New Zealand
SCC	Standards Council of Canada/ Conseil canadien des normes	Canada
JAB	Japan Accreditation Board	Japan
CNAS	China National Accreditation Service	China
INMETRO	National Institute of Metrology, Quality and Technology	Brazil
EA	European co-operation for Accreditation	Europe
IAAC	Inter-American Accreditation Cooperation	Americas
IAF	International Accreditation Forum	International
ILAC	International Laboratory Accreditation Cooperation	International

The diagram in Fig. 1.6 illustrates the relationship between accreditation, certification and conformity assessment: accreditation bodies accredit CABs/certification bodies, which test, calibrate, inspect and certify products, quality systems and personnel.

The FDA in the United States, Health Canada, the Therapeutic Goods Administration (TGA) in Australia and the Pharmaceuticals and Medical Devices Agency (PMDA) in Japan are designated CABs for medical devices. The laws governing medical devices in their respective countries are the basis for their designation as CABs.

In Europe, CABs are accredited by their national accreditation bodies to perform conformity assessments for medical devices to the EU medical devices directives. Nationally accredited CABs are designated or notified to the EC and become EU Notified Bodies. They can issue certificates of conformity for medical devices,

Table 1.4 Main standards in the ISO/IEC 17000 standard series for conformity assessment

ISO/IEC 17000 standard series		Old ISO guides	Old EN standards
ISO/IEC 17000:2004	Conformity assessment - Vocabulary and general principles	ISO Guide 2 clauses 12-17	EN 45020 clauses 12–17
ISO/IEC 17011:2004	Conformity assessment - General requirements for accreditation bodies accrediting Conformity Assessment Bodies	ISO Guide 58 and 61	EN 45003, EN 45010
ISO/IEC 17020:2012	Conformity assessment -: Requirements for the operation of various types of bodies performing inspection	ISO Guide 39	EN 45004
ISO/IEC 17021:2011	Conformity assessment -: Requirements for bodies providing audit and certification of management systems	ISO Guide 62	EN 45012
ISO/IEC 17024:2012	Conformity assessment - General requirements for bodies operating certification of persons	-	EN 45013
ISO/IEC 17025:2005 + Corrigendum:2006	General requirements for the competence of testing and calibration laboratories (also referred to as Good Laboratory Practices, or GLPs)	ISO Guide 25	EN 45001
ISO/IEC 17065:2012	Product certification bodies	ISO Guide 65	EN 45011

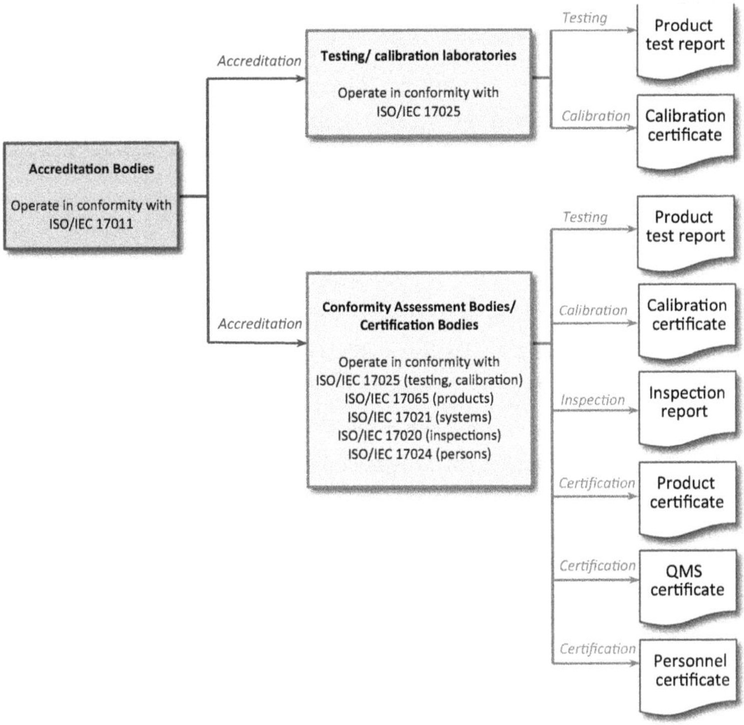

Figure 1.6 Diagram illustrating the concepts of accreditation, conformity assessment and certification and the relationship between them.

according to their scope of accreditation (and notification), which are recognized and accepted throughout the EU. Switzerland, Turkey and the European Economic Area (EEA) countries Norway, Iceland, and Liechtenstein have also Notified Bodies under the EU system, and they recognize the other EU Notified Bodies. Some EU Notified Bodies are recognized CABs in Australia [26], Canada [27] and the United States [28, 29] for certain categories of medical devices.

1.3 Medical Device Life Cycle

In established markets medical devices are, along with other therapeutic goods for human use such as medicines, vaccines,

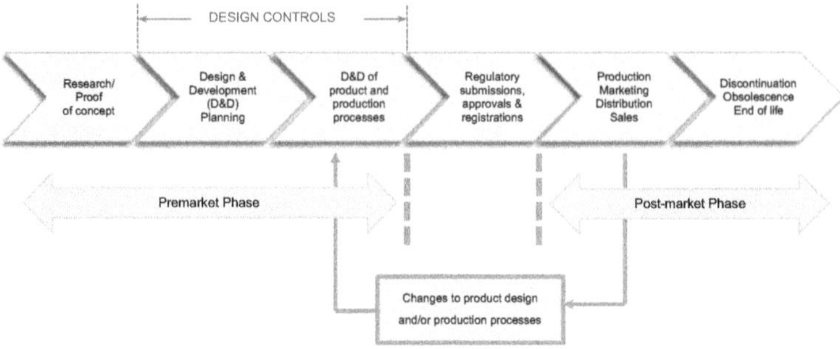

Figure 1.7 Typical medical device life cycle.

blood and biologics, among the highest-regulated products. Medical devices, like most other products, have a life cycle spanning from research and development, through production, marketing, sales and distribution, and then finally to obsolescence (Fig. 1.7).

Before making medical devices available for sale, manufacturers and sponsors must obtain marketing approvals and/or register their products with the RAs. After obtaining a marketing approval, manufacturers and sponsors are required to comply with any requirements that may apply to their products, including the obligation to notify the regulatory agency and get approvals for certain changes to the design or manufacturing process prior to implementation.

1.3.1 *Pre-Market Phase*

Novel medical devices evolve out of research or clinical activities using early prototypes. Many other devices are developed or modified by incremental innovation. Once the concept is proven to work, design and development (D&D) for a commercial product may commence. Design controls apply to all D&D activities – for novel or improved devices being developed in the pre-market phase, as well as for changes to existing, marketed devices. Design controls do not apply to research activities conducted during the proof of concept stage; however, these need to follow rigorous scientific practices, such as Design of Experiments (DoE) techniques, to ensure the quality and integrity of the research outcomes.

The D&D planning stage is not only a requirement in some jurisdictions but also good business practice to ensure that the D&D activities are clearly identified and responsibilities for implementation allocated. It is during the D&D planning stage that the regulatory strategy for the target markets is defined on the basis of the device risk classification and the intended purpose as declared by the manufacturer.

During the D&D process stage the medical device and the processes for its manufacturing are designed and tested until ready to be transferred to production and submitted to RAs for approval. In reality, the D&D process is iterative. As design issues are identified and fixed, the design is improved and optimized and tests may have to be repeated or specifications adjusted until all relevant requirements are met.

In a nutshell, D&D activities consist of:

- Defining of the design inputs and identifying the Essential Requirements (ERs) or Essential Principles (EPs) of safety and effectiveness applicable to the medical device.
- Designing of the product and production processes.
- Design verification and validation (V&V) and process validation; for higher-risk devices the evidence of safety and performance is usually required to include data generated from the actual use of the device, that is, from clinical trials also referred to as clinical investigations or studies.

D&D controls (or shortly, design controls) are covered in greater detail in Chapter 4 of this book.

1.3.2 *Regulatory Submissions, Approvals and Registrations*

The regulatory approvals and registrations stage involves the compilation and submission of documentation required for marketing applications to the relevant regulatory agencies and any administrative activities such as establishment registration and device listing. During this stage the regulatory professionals interface with the relevant authorities and coordinate efforts within their own organizations to address any questions or deficiencies raised during this process until the marketing approval is obtained.

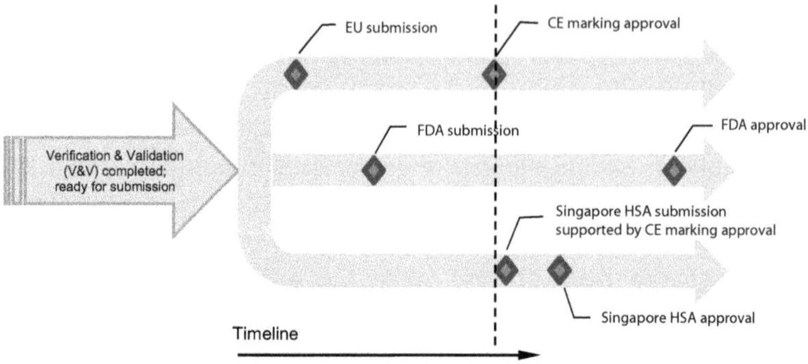

Figure 1.8 Example of a regulatory submissions and approvals process that branches into various regional and national streams.

The diagram in Fig. 1.7 representing a typical medical device life cycle looks linear, but in reality the process branches during the regulatory submissions, approvals and registrations stage, with applications and subsequent approvals and product launches running in parallel in various markets, for example, in Europe, the United States and Singapore (see Fig. 1.8).

The regulatory approvals and registration stage is covered in more detail in Chapter 5.

1.3.3 *Post-Market Phase*

Once a medical device receives regulatory approval in a country or region, it enters the post-market phase in that jurisdiction. Any promotion or advertising must be in line with the conditions of approval and for the indications for use and intended use that was originally approved.

Changes made to the device design or the production processes must be assessed, verified or validated, as applicable, to ensure that the modified design or production process maintains compliance with all applicable requirements for safety and effectiveness. If required by regulations, the changes must be submitted for approval to the relevant authorities. During this phase manufacturers are obliged to implement post-market surveillance controls and report adverse events involving their devices. Any claims made in the user instructions, promotion materials (brochures, websites) and advertising campaigns for a particular market must be within and according to the regulatory approval received in that market.

When a medical device reaches its end of life, the manufacturer needs to consider the implications of its discontinuation or obsolescence and plan accordingly before stopping production of the device.

The post-market stage is covered in more detail in Chapter 6.

1.4 Medical Devices

1.4.1 *Definitions of Medical Devices, Active Implantables and in vitro Diagnostics*

A medical device is defined in the European medical devices and active implantables directives as "any instrument, apparatus, appliance, software, material or other article, whether used alone or in combination, together with any accessories, including the software intended by its manufacturer to be used specifically for diagnostic and/or other purposes and necessary for its proper application intended by the manufacturer to be used for human beings for the purpose of:

- diagnosis, prevention, monitoring, treatment or alleviation of disease,
- diagnosis, monitoring, treatment, alleviation of or compensation for an injury or handicap,
- investigation, replacement or modification of the anatomy or of a physiological process,
- control of conception,

and which does not achieve its principal intended action in or on the human body by pharmacological, immunological or metabolic means, but which may be assisted in its function by such means".

An active implantable medical device is defined as "any active medical devices [i.e., relying for its function on a source of electrical energy or any source of power other than that directly generated by the human body or gravity] which is intended to be totally or partially introduced, surgically or medically, into the human body or by medical intervention into a natural orifice, and which is intended to remain after the procedure".

An IVD medical device is defined as "any medical device which is a reagent, reagent product, calibrator, control material, kit, instrument, apparatus, equipment or system, whether used alone or in combination, intended by the manufacturer to be used *in vitro* for the examination of specimens, including blood and tissue donations, derived from the human body, solely or principally for the purpose of providing information:

- concerning a physiological or pathological state, or
- concerning a congenital abnormality, or
- to determine the safety and compatibility with potential recipients, or
- to monitor therapeutic measures".

The FDA's definition of a medical device is "an instrument, apparatus, implement, machine, contrivance, implant, in vitro reagent, or other similar or related article, including a component part, or accessory which is:

- recognized in the official National Formulary, or the United States Pharmacopoeia, or any supplement to them,
- intended for use in the diagnosis of disease or other conditions, or in the cure, mitigation, treatment, or prevention of disease, in man or other animals, or
- intended to affect the structure or any function of the body of man or other animals, and which does not achieve its primary intended purposes through chemical action within or on the body of man or other animals and which is not dependent upon being metabolized for the achievement of any of its primary intended purposes".

IVD products are defined by the FDA as "reagents, instruments, and systems intended for use in the diagnosis of disease or other conditions, including a determination of the state of health, in order to cure, mitigate, treat, or prevent disease or its sequelae. Such products are intended for use in the collection, preparation, and examination of specimens taken from the human body. These products are devices as defined in section 201(h) of the federal Food, Drug, and Cosmetic Act (the act), and may also be biological products subject to section 351 of the Public Health Service Act".

The GHTF SG1/N071:2012 guidance, *Definition of the Terms "Medical Device" and "In Vitro Diagnostic (IVD) Medical Device"* includes IVD products in its definition of medical devices:

"Medical device" means any instrument, apparatus, implement, machine, appliance, implant, reagent for in vitro use, software, material or other similar or related article, intended by the manufacturer to be used, alone or in combination, for human beings, for one or more of the specific medical purpose(s) of:

- diagnosis, prevention, monitoring, treatment or alleviation of disease,
- diagnosis, monitoring, treatment, alleviation of or compensation for an injury,
- investigation, replacement, modification, or support of the anatomy or of a physiological process,
- supporting or sustaining life,
- control of conception,
- disinfection of medical devices,
- providing information by means of in vitro examination of specimens derived from the human body; and does not achieve its primary intended action by pharmacological, immunological or metabolic means, in or on the human body, but which may be assisted in its intended function by such means.

The term "medical devices", unless otherwise specified, will be used hereafter to mean medical devices other than IVDs as per the definitions in this section.

1.4.2 *Borderline Products*

It is important to check in every jurisdiction whether a particular product falls under medical device regulations, because certain products may be considered to be medical devices in some jurisdictions but not in others. Furthermore, the same product can be classified differently depending on the intended purpose declared by the manufacturer on the product labeling, instructions for use and promotional material.

To be classified as a medical device, a product must fulfill three conditions:

(1) It must be intended for human use.
(2) Its intended purpose, as stated in the manufacturer's labeling, instructions for use and promotional material, must include at least one of the *medical purposes* listed in the definition of medical devices (Section 1.4.1, "Definitions of Medical Devices, Active Implantables and in vitro Diagnostics").
(3) Its *primary mode of action* must not be metabolic, immunological or pharmacological.

Typically, the medical device function is achieved by physical means, including mechanical action, physical barrier, replacement of or support to organs or body functions. A medical device may be supported in its function by pharmacological, immunological or metabolic means (see definitions below), but if these become the primary mode of action, the product is no longer a medical device but instead it is regulated as a medicine [30].

- *Pharmacological means* is understood as an interaction between the molecules of the substance in question and a cellular constituent, usually referred to as a receptor, which either results in a direct response or which blocks the response to another agent. Although not a completely reliable criterion, the presence of a dose–response correlation is indicative of a pharmacological effect.
- *Immunological means* is understood as an action in or on the body by stimulation and/or mobilization of cells and/or products involved in a specific immune reaction.
- *Metabolic means* is understood as an action that involves an alteration, including stopping, starting or changing the speed of the normal chemical processes participating in, and available for, normal body function.

The following are a few examples of borderline products provided in published regulatory guidelines [31, 32] (33 p. 155).

Plain bone cement without antibiotics is a medical device since it achieves its principal intended action (the fixation of prosthesis) by physical means. Bone cements containing antibiotics, where the principal intended action remains fixation of prosthesis, are also medical devices. In this case the action of the antibiotic, which is to reduce the possibility of infection being introduced during surgery, is clearly ancillary. If, however, the principal intended action is to deliver the antibiotic, the product no longer fulfils the definition of a medical device and it is instead classified as a medicine.

Sterilants and disinfectants are not medical devices unless specifically intended to sterilize or disinfect other medical devices. Disinfectant products for use on humans (hand gels, washes and anti-microbial swabs and pre-injection wipes containing chlorhexidine, cetrimide or iodine) are regulated as medicines, but pre-injection alcohol-based wipes for use on humans are medical devices.

General-purpose products that can be used in a medical environment are usually not medical devices unless the manufacturer ascribes them a specific medical purpose. An exercise bike containing a heart rate measurement device is a fitness device; however, if the manufacturer declares that it is intended "for stroke patients in their rehabilitation therapy" it is a medical device.

Heat pads are general-purpose products as well, but if the manufacturer claims that they provide "pain relief" they are classified as medical devices. Foot massagers and footbaths (electrically operated devices with or without water that generate vibrations) are considered consumer products unless the manufacturer claims that they "improve circulation" or "relieve tension", in which case they are classified as medical devices.

Cosmetic and toiletry products without a specific primary medical purpose are not medical devices. For example, toothpaste is a cosmetic product unless the manufacturer claims to treat or prevent sensitive teeth or it contains an active ingredient known to have such an effect, in which case it is considered a medicinal product.

Other borderline products can be regulated either as medical devices or as personal protective equipment, depending on their main intended purpose. For example, latex, rubber, vinyl and neoprene gloves intended to be used for examination or during surgery are medical devices but if intended to be used in a medical laboratory they are personal protective devices.

Face masks intended for user protection against dust inhalation are classified as personal protective equipment, but if they are labelled as surgical masks intended for use in an operating theater, they are medical devices because they protect the *patient*, not the user, against infection and cross-contamination. Similarly, eye goggles, gowns and hats can be classified as either medical devices or personal protection equipment, depending on their primary intended use.

1.4.3 *Combination Products*

Combination products are therapeutic and diagnostic products that combine medicines (or drugs), devices and/or biological products. A combination product can be composed of two or more regulated components – a drug and a device; a biological product and a device; a drug and a biological product; or a drug, device and a biological product [34].

Combination products can be:

- Physically, chemically or otherwise combined or mixed and produced as a single entity (monoclonal antibody combined with a therapeutic drug, drug-eluting stent, orthopaedic implant with growth factors, pre-filled syringes)
- Packed together as separate entities in a single package or as a unit (drug or biological product packed together with a delivery device, surgical tray with surgical instruments, drapes, lidocaine or alcohol swabs)
- Provided separately but labelled for use together (photosensitizing drug and activating light source, iontophoretic drug delivery patch and controller) [35]

The main challenge with combination products is that their components (drug, device, biologic) are regulated by different types of RAs with different review procedures, and this complicates all aspects of product development and management, including pre-clinical testing, clinical investigation, marketing applications, manufacturing and quality control, adverse event reporting, promotion and advertising and post-approval modifications. The review process for combination products takes typically longer and is more expensive than the review for a device, drug or biologic on its own.

The pre-market review of a combination product is performed by the authority that has the primary jurisdiction for its regulation (drug, device or biologic); however, separate registration of the drug, device or biologic component with the relevant RA or agency department may be required in some markets.

Assignment of the primary jurisdiction is based on the determination of the primary mode of action of the combination product, that is, the single mode of action on the human body of a combination product that provides the most important therapeutic action of the combination product.

In general, drug device combination products where the device has merely a delivery function are classified as drugs, but combination products where the drug has only an ancillary function are classified as devices. Some typical examples are given in Table 1.5, but a manufacturer should always check with the relevant authorities what classification applies in a particular jurisdiction [30].

Table 1.5 Examples of drug device combination products classified as medical devices or medicinal products (drugs)

Medical devices	Medicinal products (drugs)
Kit containing reusable syringe and injectable drug	Pre-filled syringes
Reusable injector for use with insulin cartridge	Disposable pen injectors integral with insulin cartridge
Drug delivery pump	Nebulizers pre-charged with a specific medicinal product
Implantable infusion pump	Patches for transdermal drug delivery
Wound dressing with anti-microbial agent acting as physical barrier	Wound treatment product for delivery of anti-microbial agent
Drug-eluting coronary stents	Intrauterine contraceptives whose primary purpose is to release progestogens
Bone cements containing antibiotic	Implants containing medicinal products in a polymer matrix intended for the release of medicinal product

The regulatory framework for combination products is complex. The device component and the drug component have to comply with the applicable regulatory requirements of the medical devices and the medicines (drugs) regulations, respectively.

In some markets, the authority having primary jurisdiction over the combination product will coordinate with the other authorities to ensure that all components of the combination product (drug, device, biologic) are safe and effective. For example, a medical device that incorporates, as an integral part, an ancillary medicinal substance (drug) will be assessed under the medical device regulations by the relevant medical device RAs. The quality, safety and effectiveness of the drug will have to be determined under the drug regulations by the relevant drug RAs.

1.4.3.1 EU regulations for combination products

In Europe, combination products fall either under the medical devices directives (MDD, AIMDD and IVDD) or under Directive 2001/83/EC on medicinal products, depending on the primary mode of action. In addition to the evaluation by a Notified Body, medical devices incorporating medicinal substances must undergo a pharmaceutical dossier review by the European Medicines Agency (EMA) or by a national Competent Authority designated by an EU member state, a process that can take more than 210 days to complete.

The EC has recently updated its *Manual on Borderline and Classification in the Community: Regulatory Framework for Medical Devices*, which provides detailed guidance on interpreting the EU law on borderline and combination products [36]. Manufacturers should consult this manual when determining the classification and primary mode of action for combination products.

1.4.3.2 US regulations for combination products

In the United States, the FDA's Office of Combination Products (OCP) is responsible for the pre-market review of combination products, and it determines the appropriate regulatory process on the basis of a review of a product's primary mode of action. However, this determination alone can take up to two months before the actual pre-market review can commence [37].

The primary mode of action is defined in 21 CFR Part 3 as "the single mode of action of a combination product that provides the most important therapeutic action of the combination product. The most important therapeutic action is the mode of action expected to make the greatest contribution to the overall intended therapeutic effects of the combination product". The primary mode of action can be physical (medical devices); pharmacological, immunological or metabolic (drugs); or cellular (biologics).

Depending on the outcome of the primary mode of action analysis, the OCP will designate the lead review center – the Center of Devices and Radiological Health (CDRH), the Center for Drug Evaluation and Research (CDER) or the Center for Biologics Evaluation and Research (CBER). The lead review center will consult with the other centers, as necessary.

1.4.3.3 Australian regulations for combination products

In Australia, the primary intended purpose and the mode of action will determine whether a combination product is regulated as a device or a medicine. It is advisable to discuss with the TGA the characteristics and intended use of a combination product prior to submitting an application for conformity assessment and to ascertain the TGA's requirements for the medicinal component in relation to those characteristics [38].

If the combination product is considered to be a medical device, the assessment will be conducted by the Office of Devices Authorisation under the medical devices program, in consultation with other relevant departments for the medicine component.

If the combination product is considered to be a medicine, the assessment will be conducted by the relevant office for medicines regulation – the Office of Medicines Authorisation for prescription and over-the-counter (OTC) medicines or the Office of Complementary Medicines for "traditional" and "alternative" medicines – under the medicines program. For the assessment of the device component, the Office of Medicines Authorisation will consult with the Office of Devices Authorisation.

Blood, tissues and biologicals are assessed by the Office of Scientific Evaluation. Australian Regulations define biologicals as "a thing made from, or that contains, human cells or human tissues, and that is used to: treat or prevent disease, ailment, defect or injury; diagnose a condition of a person; alter the physiological processes of a person; test the susceptibility of a person to disease; replace or modify a person's body parts". Examples include human stem cells, tissue-based products (skin, bone, ocular, cardiovascular), cell-based products (genetically modified, in vitro cell expansion or depletion) and combined cell and tissue products (collagen matrices for localized cell delivery) [39].

Therapeutic products of human origin, such as vaccines and plasma derivatives, are not regulated as biologicals, they are (biological) prescription medicines and require assessment by the Office of Medicines Authorisation.

1.4.3.4 Canadian regulations for combination products

In Canada, the policy on drug device combination products effective May 13, 1999, states that "a combination product will be subject to either the Medical Devices Regulations or the Food and Drug Regulations according to the principal mechanism of action by which the claimed effect or purpose is achieved". The Therapeutic Products Classification Committee is responsible for assessing submissions for combination products referred to it and determining an appropriate classification and review mechanism for the submission [40].

The Therapeutic Products Directorate (TPD) and the Biologics Genetic Therapies Directorate (BGTD) have adopted the EU and US approach, whereby the risks associated with a combination product are managed under one set of regulations. Combination product classification decisions take into consideration the principal mechanism of action by which the claimed effect or purpose of the product is achieved, and then the entire product is regulated under either the Food and Drug Regulations or the Medical Devices Regulations. Both the principal and ancillary components must meet acceptable standards of safety, efficacy and quality.

Where the principal mechanism of action by which the claimed effect or purpose is achieved by pharmacological, immunological or metabolic means, the combination product is subject to the Food and Drug Regulations, unless that action occurs in vitro, without re-introducing a modified cellular substance to the patient, in which case the product is subject to the Medical Devices Regulations.

Where the principal mechanism of action by which the claimed effect or purpose is not achieved by pharmacological, immunological or metabolic means, but may be assisted in that effect or purpose by pharmacological, immunological or metabolic means, the combination product is subject to the Medical Devices Regulations.

1.4.3.5 Japanese regulations for combination products

Japanese regulations do not have a distinct definition for combination products, but it is generally accepted that a combination product is comprised of a drug and a medical device that are physically or chemically integrated [41].

Combination products are classified on a case-by-case basis, taking into consideration the primary mode of action, and then one set of regulations apply. It is recommendable to consult the PMDA prior to submitting an application for a combination product.

If a combination product is considered a device, the medical device regulatory scheme applies. If a combination product is considered a drug, the drug regulatory scheme applies. The PMDA department acting as lead reviewer will consult with other relevant PMDA departments, as necessary.

1.5 Risk-Based Classification

1.5.1 *Two Different Classification Philosophies*

The early medical device regulations established a nomenclature-based classification system whereby known, pre-determined categories of devices were assigned a risk classification – low, medium or high – and a level of regulatory scrutiny (or regulatory controls) directly proportionate with their risk class. The nomenclature-based medical device classification system is still used in the United States and Japan. The European IVDD also includes a nomenclature of high-risk IVDs in its Annex II.

The obvious difficulty with such a system is that it is not always easy to "fit" a particular medical device or medical device accessory in an existing category, so one is left with choosing the next closest generic type and use it even though it does not accurately describe the device. Things get even more difficult with new technologies for which there is no existing device type or even a category at all. Generating new regulatory guidelines for classification and assessment of novel devices can be a very lengthy process, making it difficult for regulations to keep up with the fast pace of scientific and technological advancements.

In 1993, the European Medical Devices Directives introduced a new philosophy for classifying medical devices. The European regulators recognized that while science and technology move at a faster pace than the regulations can keep up to, one thing remains unchanged and that is the human body. So instead of trying to fit all medical devices into pre-determined types and categories, they came up with a set of generic rules that can be applied to any medical device to determine its risk classification on the basis of the potential hazard posed to the human body. Article 9 of the MDD splits medical devices into four risk classes: low, low to medium, medium to high and high.

The classification philosophy using generic classification rules and four risk classes has since been adopted by the GHTF and the RAs in Australia and Canada, as well as by the AMDD.

1.5.2 *Nomenclature-Based Classification Systems*

1.5.2.1 US classification system for medical devices, including IVDs

Currently the FDA classification system has approximately 1700 generic categories of devices grouped into medical specialties overseen by expert panels [42]:

- Anesthesiology
- Cardiovascular
- Chemistry

- Dental
- Ear, Nose and Throat
- Gastroenterology and Urology
- General and Plastic Surgery
- General Hospital
- Hematology
- Immunology
- Microbiology
- Neurology
- Obstetrical and Gynecology
- Ophthalmic
- Orthopedic
- Pathology
- Physical Medicine
- Radiology
- Toxicology

The generic device categories are defined in the classification regulations in Parts 862 through 892 of the CFR. IVDs are listed in 21 CFR Parts 862, 864 and 866. Each classification regulation contains a general description and the applicable risk classification – Class I, II or III, with Class III being the highest risk classification – and information about marketing requirements. To correctly classify a medical device the manufacturer must ensure that the device meets the definition given in the particular section of the regulation.

The classification regulation is further defined through a product code nomenclature system. The Product Code Classification Database is available on the FDA's website. It contains device names and their associated product codes. The name and product code identify the generic category of a device for FDA. The product code assigned to a device is based upon the medical device product classification designated under 21 CFR Parts 862–892 [43].

For example, 21 CFR Part 870, *Cardiovascular Devices*, has 6 subparts containing approximately 140 generic device categories:

- Subpart A – General Provisions
- Subpart B – Cardiovascular Diagnostic Devices
- Subpart C – Cardiovascular Monitoring Devices
- Subpart D – Cardiovascular Prosthetic Devices

- Subpart E – Cardiovascular Surgical Devices
- Subpart F – Cardiovascular Therapeutic Devices

For instance, Section 870.3610 of Subpart D defines an *implantable pacemaker pulse generator* as "a device that has a power supply and electronic circuits that produce a periodic electrical pulse to stimulate the heart". There are two product codes covered by regulation 870.3610, both classified as Class III:

- Product Code DXY – Implantable Pacemaker Pulse Generator
- Product Code DSZ – Pacemaker Battery

Any changes in classification (proposed, implemented or withdrawn) are published in *Federal Register* [44].

1.5.2.2 Japanese classification system for medical devices, including IVDs

The Japanese medical device classification system, introduced by the Ministerial Notification or Yakushokuhatsu No. 0720022 in 2004, is based on nomenclature codes, which is similar to the US system of pre-defined medical device categories. The MHLW specifies Certification Standards, Approval Standards and Review Guidelines applicable to pre-determined types and categories of devices. Devices are classified as Class I, II, III and IV, with Class I being the lowest-risk class and Class IV being the highest-risk class.

Since April 2009, Japanese regulations also distinguish between generic ("me too"), improved (innovative) and new (novel) medical devices. This additional differentiation determines the kind of data required for regulatory submissions, for example, with or without clinical data; more details are provided in Chapter 5 of this book:

- Generic medical devices are devices substantially equivalent to one or more predicate devices marketed in Japan.
- New devices are devices that differ significantly from devices already approved in Japan, with regard to intended purpose, technology, principle of operation and performance.

- Improved devices are neither generic nor new, that is, they are not substantially equivalent to already approved devices but not novel enough to receive an instruction of reexamination.

The classification of IVDs in Japan is based on *Nomenclature of in vitro Diagnostics*, which was introduced by the Ministerial Notification or Yakushokuhatsu No. 0401031 in 2005 and which lists all IVD categories together with their risk classification. IVDs are classified as Class I, II and III; Class I and II are considered low risk, and Class III high risk.

1.5.3 *Classification Systems Using Generic Classification Rules*

1.5.3.1 Classification rules for medical devices other than IVDs

For medical devices other than IVDs, the generic classification rules are applied taking into consideration the intended purpose of a medical device as defined by the manufacturer, according to these four main criteria (refer also to Fig. 1.9):

- The duration of continuous contact with the patient
- The degree of invasiveness
- The part of the human body affected by the use of the device
- Whether it's an active device

The Canadian classification system differs in that only the "long term" duration, that is, 30 days or greater of continuous contact with the patient, is considered when classifying a medical device.

Article 9 of the European MDD identifies the four risk classes for medical devices: Class I (low risk), Class IIa, (low to moderate risk), Class IIb (moderate to high risk) and Class III (high risk). Active implantable medical devices covered by the EU AIMDD are automatically considered high risk. Annex IX of the MDD defines 12 general classification rules and 6 special classification rules for classifying medical devices into one of the four risk classes.

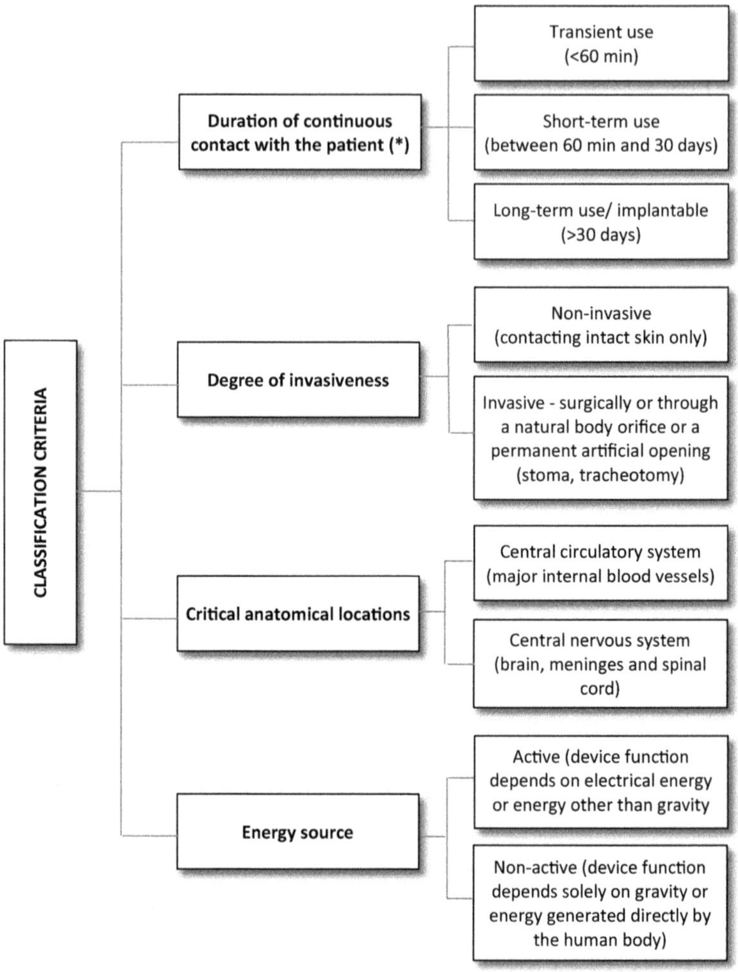

Figure 1.9 Classification criteria according to the "generic rules" philosophy used in the European MDD, the GHTF classification guidance and the ASEAN MDD.
*Except Canada, where only the "long term" duration, that is, 30 days or greater of continuous contact with the patient, is considered when classifying a medical device.

The 12 general rules cover:

- Non-invasive devices – rules 1, 2, 3 and 4;
- Invasive devices – rules 5, 6, 7 and 8; and
- Active devices – rules 9, 10, 11 and 12.

The 6 special rules cover:

- Devices incorporating medicines or drugs – rule 13;
- Devices used for contraception or prevention of sexually transmitted diseases (STDs) – rule 14;
- Equipment or substances used for disinfecting medical devices – rule 15;
- Devices intended for recording of X-ray diagnostic images – rule 16;
- Devices, other than contacting intact skin only, incorporating non-viable animal tissues or derivatives – rule 17; and
- Blood bags – rule 18.

The MEDDEV 2.4 guidance document, *Classification of medical devices*, contains details flowcharts and elaborates on each classification rule, including interpretations and examples that guide manufacturers in making the right risk class determination [45].

The GHTF guidance *Principles of Medical Devices Classification* defines 17 generic classification rules for classifying medical devices into one of the four risk classes – A, B, C or D, with A being the lowest-risk class and D the highest-risk class [46]. The GHTF classification has been adopted by the AMDD with only a minor difference, that is, GHTF rules 15 and 16 for medical device classification have been combined into rule 15 in the ASEAN MDD classification system [47].

Australian medical device regulations and guidelines define 22 classification rules grouped into 5 main rule categories and 4 risk classes that have the same designation as the European risk classes for medical devices: I, IIa, IIb, III and AIMD (48 pp. 74–104).

Canadian medical device regulations and guidelines define 16 classification rules and 4 risk classes: I, II, III and IV, with Class I being the lowest-risk class and Class IV the highest-risk class [49].

Although not identical, the classification rules are very similar and align quite well across various jurisdictions. A side-by-side comparison is provided in Table 1.6.

Table 1.6 Comparative table with generic classification rules for medical devices other than IVDs

Classification rules	GHTF AMDD	EU MDD	Australia	Canada
Duration of use	–	–	Rule 1	–
Non-invasive devices	Rules 1–4	Rules 1–4	Rules 2.1–2.4	Rules 4–7
Invasive devices	Rules 5–8	Rules 5–8	Rules 3.1–3.4	Rules 1–3
Active devices	Rules 9–12	Rules 9–12	Rules 4.1–4.4	Rules 8–12
Special rules	Rules 13–17 (GHTF) Rules 13–16 (AMDD)	Rules 13–18	Rules 5.1–5.9	Rules 13–16

When determining the risk class of a medical device it is important to walk through the classification rules of relevant regulations and guidelines in each jurisdiction, taking into consideration the manufacturer's intended use of the device. Classification guidelines have step-by-step decision flowcharts and examples to assist with this task.

The risk class will determine what regulatory controls and conformity assessment procedures apply in each market, and hence form the basis for defining the regulatory strategy. This assessment can be done early on in the development process as soon as the manufacturer has defined the intended purpose and principle of operation of the medical device.

1.5.3.2 Classification rules for IVDs

The European IVDD, published in 1998 and the first regulation dedicated to IVD medical devices, groups IVDs into four risk classes and specifies the categories of IVDs belonging to each class (listed below from the lowest to the highest risk):

- General IVDs that do not constitute a direct risk to patients, as they are used by competently trained professionals, and the results obtained can often be confirmed by other means;
- IVDs for self-testing, such as test kits that can be used by laypersons in a home environment, excluding self-test IVDs covered in Annex II of the IVDD;
- IVDs in Annex II List B, such as test kits for detecting rubella, chlamydia and cytomegalovirus (CMV); for determining prostate-specific antigen (PSA) tumor marker, human leuko-

cyte antigen (HLA) tissue typing groups – DR, A, B; or for measuring blood sugar; and
- IVDs in Annex II List A, such as test kits for detecting human immunodeficiency virus (HIV) – HIV 1 and 2; human T-lymphotropic virus (HTLV) – HTLV I and II; and hepatitis B, C or D; and for determining the major blood groups – ABO system, rhesus (C, c, D, E, e) anti-Kell.

The general IVDs represent the large majority of IVDs for which the conformity assessment procedures can be carried out, as a general rule, under the sole responsibility of the manufacturer. The IVDs for self-testing and those listed in Annex II of the IVDD (List A and List B) require an optimum level of safety and reliability; hence the conformity assessment procedures must involve EU Notified Bodies.

In 2012 the EC published a proposal for a revised regulation for IVDs. According to this proposal, IVDs will be subject to generic classification rules for IVDs that allocate products to one of the four risk classes, similar to the classification structure that already exists for the other medical devices in the EU [50].

Since the publishing of the European IVDD, Australia [51] and Canada [52] have released their own IVD regulations and guidelines defining generic classification rules and four risk classifications for IVDs: I, II, III and IV, with Class I being the lowest-risk and Class IV the highest-risk class. The classification rules in Australia and Canada are not identical, though, so a manufacturer will need to apply them separately when classifying a device. Also, in Australia, Regulations define in-house IVDs as those developed within a laboratory or laboratory network that are not supplied commercially outside the laboratory or laboratory network.

The GHTF classification rules for IVDs, documented in the *Principles of IVD Medical Devices Classification* guideline [53], have been adopted by the AMDD [54].

IVD classification rules are applied taking into consideration the intended purpose of the IVD medical device as defined by the manufacturer, as well as the level of risk to the individual patient and to the public health, according to these four main criteria (see also Table 1.7):

- The use with respect to transmissible agents;
- Uses other than for transmissible agents (self-testing);

Table 1.7 Comparative table with generic classification rules for IVDs

Classification rules	GHTF AMDD	Australia	Canada
IVDs for use with respect to transmissible agents	Rules 1, 3	Rules 1.1, 1.3	Rules 1–3
IVDs for immunological typing	Rule 2	Rule 1.2	Rule 5
IVDs for uses other than for transmissible agents (self-test)	Rule 4	Rule 1.4	Rule 4
Special rules	Rules 5–7	Rules 1.5–1.8	Rules 6–9

- For immunological typing; and
- Other uses covered by special rules.

1.5.4 *Medical Devices Risk Classes: Comparison between Main Jurisdictions*

A side-by-side comparison between the risk classifications of medical devices other than IVDs across various jurisdictions is shown in Table 1.8. Note that there are differences between the various classification systems, so the comparison is indicative only.

Although classification principles and most risk classes seem to align relatively well, it does not mean that same medical devices are classified in the same way or that they are assigned the same level of risk across these jurisdictions.

For instance, hip, knee and shoulder joint replacements (see Fig. 1.10) are classified as Class III in Europe (EU Directive 2005/50/EC) and as Class IIb in Australia (Schedule 2, Part 3.4(2) of the Regulations).

Another example: all devices intended to come in direct contact with the central nervous system, like neuroendoscopes (see example in Fig. 1.11), are classified as Class III in Europe (Annex IX, rules 6, 7 and 8 of the MDD amended by 2007/47/EC), whereas in Australia, such devices are classified as Class I, IIa or IIb if duration of contact is transient (Schedule 2, Part 3.2 of the Regulations) and as Class III or Class AIMD if duration of contact is short term, long term or implantable (Schedule 2, Parts 3.3 and 3.4 of the Regulations).

Furthermore, there are products that, depending on their intended use, can take on different classifications as medical devices

Table 1.8 Comparative table with medical devices risk classes

Hazard level	GHTF AMDD	EU MDD, AIMDD	Australia	Canada	Japan	United States
Low	Class A	Class I	Class I	Class I	Class I	Class I
Low to moderate	Class B	Class $I^{s/m}$ (see Note); Class IIa	Class I $^{s/m}$ (see Note); Class IIa	Class II	Class II	Class II
Moderate to high	Class C	Class IIb	Class IIb	Class III	Class III	
High	Class D	Class III, AIMD	Class III, AIMD	Class IV	Class IV	Class III

Note: Under EU and Australian medical device regulations Class $I^{s/m}$ devices are Class I devices supplied sterile or incorporating a measuring function; these require additional controls compared to non-sterile, non-measuring Class I devices.

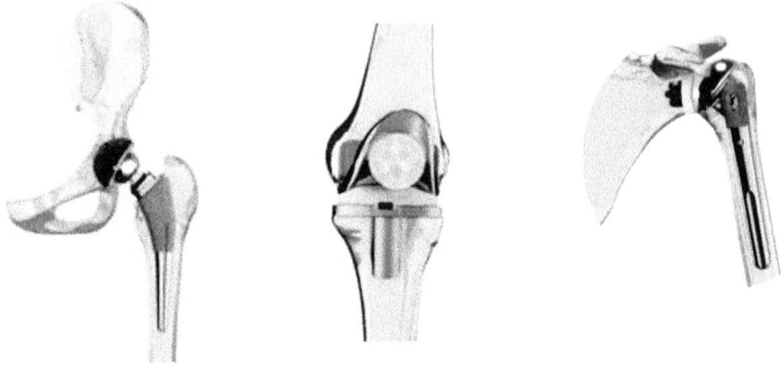

Figure 1.10 Examples of hip, knee and shoulder joint replacements. *Source*: Zimmer.

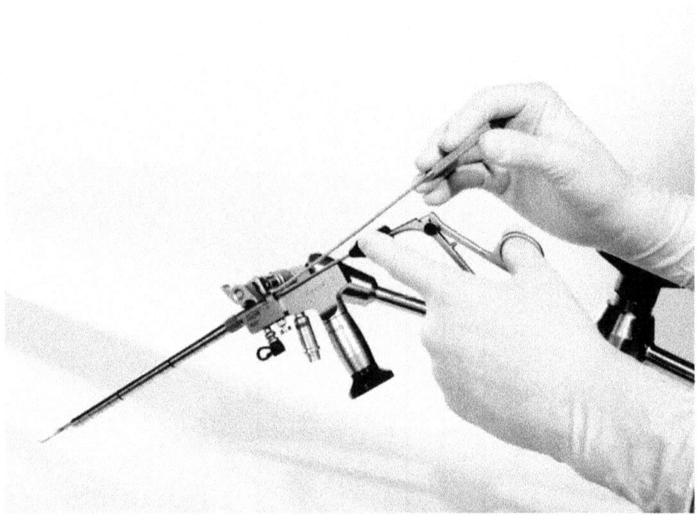

Figure 1.11 Neuroendoscope used in neurosurgery. *Source*: Aesculap.

or are not classified as medical devices at all. Disinfectants and sterilants are medical devices if intended to be used for disinfecting or sterilizing other medical devices. In Europe, they are classified as Class IIb if specifically intended for invasive devices and as Class IIa if specifically intended for non-invasive devices. In Australia, they are classified as Class IIb irrespective of whether they are intended for invasive or non-invasive devices. Disinfectants intended to be used by healthcare professionals to disinfect the skin of patients are regulated as medicinal products, not medical devices.

1.5.5 *IVD Risk Classes: Comparison between Main Jurisdictions*

A side-by-side comparison between the IVD medical device risk classifications across various jurisdictions is shown in Table 1.9. Note that the classification rules are different in the various classification systems, so the comparison is indicative only.

1.6 Components, Spare Parts, Accessories, Device Families, Kits, Systems and Procedure Packs

1.6.1 *Components and Spare Parts*

Medical devices and IVDs are products with a *medical purpose*. The medical purpose is defined by the manufacturer and it relates to finished devices. A *finished device* means any device or accessory to any device that is suitable for use or capable of functioning, whether it is packaged, labeled or sterilized [55].

A *component* means any raw material, substance, piece, part, software, firmware, labeling or assembly that is intended to be included as part of the finished, packaged and labeled device [55]. Raw materials, components or intermediate products, although they may need to poses properties or characteristics that are determinant for the safety and quality of finished products, are not considered medical devices themselves.

Spare parts supplied for replacement of existing components of a device, the conformity of which has already been established, are not medical devices. If spare parts, however, change significantly the characteristics or performances of a device with regard to its already established conformity, such spare parts are considered medical devices in their own right [56].

Table 1.9 Comparative table with IVD medical device risk classes

Level of risk	GHTF AMDD	EU IVDD	Australia	Canada	Japan	United States
Low or no public health risk and/or low individual risk	Class A	General IVDs	Class 1 IVD	Class I	Class I (low risk)	Class I (low)
Low public health risk and/or moderate individual risk	Class B	Self-test IVDs not covered in Annex II	Class 2 IVD	Class II	Class II (low risk)	Class II (moderate)
Moderate public health risk and/or high individual risk	Class C	Annex II List B	Class 3 IVD	Class III	Class III (high risk)	
High public health risk and/or high individual risk	Class D	Annex II List A	Class 4 IVD	Class IV		Class III (high)

1.6.2 *Accessories*

Accessories are devices specifically intended by the manufacturer to be used together with a medical device in order to enable the medical device to be used in accordance with its intended use. The intended use of the accessory must be such as to enable a device to be used in accordance with its intended use. Therefore a product can only become an accessory to a medical device if the manufacturer of such a product establishes an intended use in conjunction with one or several medical devices [56].

Some regulations and guidelines specify how accessories are to be treated. Some key points are listed hereafter.

In the United States:

- Accessories to classified devices take on the same classification as the "parent" device. An accessory such as software that accepts input from multiple devices usually takes on the classification of the parent device with the highest risk, that is, class [57].

In Europe:

- Accessories to active implantable medical devices are by definition medical devices according to the EU AIMDD; all AIMDs and AIMD accessories are regulated under the AIMDD and are treated in an equivalent manner to Class III medical devices in the EU MDD.
- A distinction is made between *devices* and *accessories* according to the EU MDD; although being treated as devices, accessories are considered as medical devices in their own right and are classified separately from the devices they are used with [56].

In Australia:

- Accessories including software are classified separately from the devices they are used with; software is considered an accessory when it is not essential to the operation of the device.

- Accessories to AIMDs are classified in their own right and may be classified as Class I, Class I sterile, Class I measuring, Class IIa, Class IIb or Class III, depending on the intended purpose.
- Implantable accessories to AIMDs are Class III; this means implantable pacing leads (Class III) are classified differently than the implantable pulse generator (Class AIMD).
- Active medical devices intended for controlling, monitoring or directly influencing the performance of active implantable medical devices are also classified as Class III; this means devices that are not implanted, such as pacemaker programmers and external cochlea implant speech processors, are Class III and are classified differently to the implantable pulse generator, which is Class AIMD.

1.6.3 *Device Families*

Often manufacturers produce more than one variant of the same device. Similar devices can be grouped into a product family and there are significant advantages of doing so. Conformity assessment for the whole product family can be performed by testing a representative model – usually the most complex variant – and assessing only the differences for the other models in the family, instead of fully testing each variant individually. Also, regulatory applications can be submitted for a whole product family, saving time and money. Variants can be subsequently added to an approved product family, leveraging on already submitted and accepted technical documentation.

In general, medical devices can be grouped into a product family if they have the same:

- Manufacturer or sponsor;
- Indications for use and intended use;
- Risk classification;
- Technology and principle of operation;
- Basic design and performance characteristics; and
- GMDN code – GMDN codes are available from the Global Medical Device Nomenclature Database, a system of inter-

nationally agreed generic descriptors used to identify all medical device products [58].

Definitions from regulations and guidelines for device families are provided in Section 4.5.3, "Product Grouping".

1.6.4 *Kits, Systems and Procedure Packs*

The terms "kit", "system" and "procedure pack" are often used interchangeably, but they are regulated differently across jurisdictions.

In the United States, the FDA defines *convenience kits* as being comprised of legally marketed devices that are simply being assembled in kit form strictly for the "convenience" of the user. According to the FDA's terminology, the terms "kit", "set", and "tray" are considered synonymous. They are classified according to the FDA's nomenclature-based classification system [59].

In Europe, *systems and procedure packs* are covered in Article 12 of the MDD. Procedure packs are treated as medical devices in their own right and classified according to the MDD classification rules. In those cases where the intended use of the procedure pack is not specific enough to determine the classification, the classification of the pack is at the level of the highest-classified device included in the pack, where applicable, taking into account the new intended use of the device [45].

In Australia, *systems or procedure packs* are products that are packaged together and used as a unit, either in combination as a system or in a medical or surgical procedure. Such a package must include at least one medical device, but it can also contain medicines, other therapeutic goods and non-therapeutic goods. A group of products packaged together that meets the definition of *system or procedure pack* is considered to be a medical device under Australian legislation. The medical device component with the highest classification determines the overall classification for the system or procedure pack [60].

Also, according to Australian Regulations, *composite packs* and *therapeutic kits* are regulated as medicines. Composite packs are therapeutic goods containing only medicines and their containers and are used for a single treatment or for a single course of treatment. Therapeutic kits contain medicines, other therapeutic goods and non-therapeutic goods [60].

In Canada, a *system* is a medical device or an IVD that is sold under a single name and contains components or parts intended to be used together to fulfill some or all the device's intended functions. In other words, a system consists of a device and accessories that are intended to be used together with the device and that enable the device to be used in accordance with its intended use. IVD systems are referred to as *test kits.* A *procedure pack* is a collection of medical devices that is sold under a single name, also referred to as a *medical device group.* Systems, test kits and procedure packs are classified according to the rules outlined in the classification guidance documents for medical devices and IVDs, as applicable [49, 52].

Definitions from regulations and guidelines for kits, systems and procedure packs are provided in Section 4.5.3, "Product Grouping".

1.7 Risk-Based Approach for Regulatory Controls and Conformity Assessment

Generally, to ensure regulatory compliance for medical devices and IVDs, three main sets of requirements must be met:

(1) The device design and manufacturing process must comply with applicable state-of-the-art requirements for safety and effectiveness, also known as Essential Requirements or Essential Principles of safety and effectiveness (referred to shortly as ERs or EPs).
(2) The quality management system (QMS) under which the device is made must comply with requirements defined in EN/ISO 13485, *Medical devices - Quality management systems - Requirements for regulatory purposes,* as well as any additional regulatory requirements for post-market surveillance and adverse event reporting.
(3) Manufacturers must register their place of business and the devices they place on the market according to the administrative provisions in each jurisdiction.

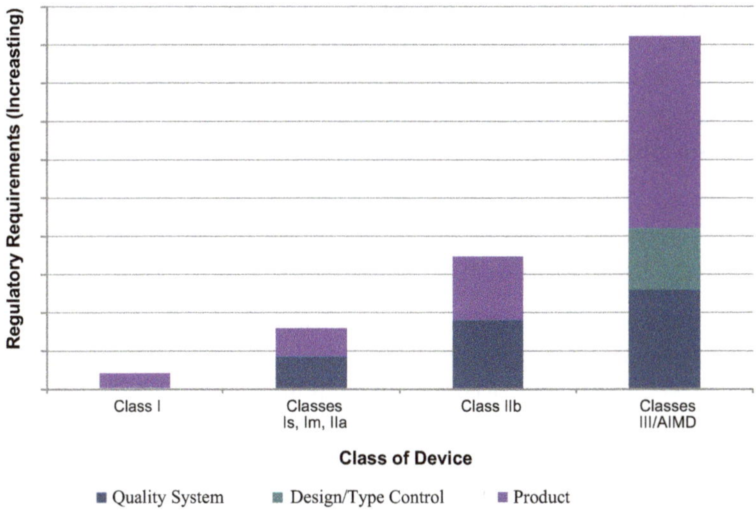

Figure 1.12 Regulatory requirements increase with the risk classification of medical devices. *Source*: TGA ARGMD, p. 21 of 337.

Although the methods of applying regulatory controls differ across jurisdictions, authorities in countries with established medical device regulations are guided by the same principle, namely to impose a degree of regulation that is proportional to the potential hazard inherent in the device. In other words, the involvement of the regulatory agency and the stringency of its scrutiny increase with the increased risk classification of a medical device (see Fig. 1.12). This approach is known as risk management.

1.7.1 *Regulatory Controls in the United States*

Medical devices marketed in the United States are subject to the regulatory controls in the federal Food, Drug, and Cosmetic Act (FD&C Act) and the regulations in 21 CFR Parts 1–58 and 800–1299. Medical devices that emit radiation are, in addition, subject to regulations for radiation-emitting electronic products in 21 CFR Parts 1000–1050.

The level of regulatory controls applied depends on the risk classification of the medical device:

- Class I (low risk) subject to general controls;
- Class II (moderate risk) subject to general controls and special controls (performance standards, post-market surveillance, specific guidelines); and
- Class III (high risk) subject to general controls and Premarket Approval (PMA) [61].

1.7.1.1 General controls

General controls are basic statutory provisions of the US FD&C Act that provide the regulatory framework for medical devices [62]. They include regulatory controls pertaining to:

- Adulteration: A device is adulterated if it includes any filthy, putrid or decomposed substance; if it is prepared, packed or held under unsanitary conditions; if it contains any poisonous or deleterious substance or an unsafe color additive; or if its strength differs from, or its purity or quality falls below, that which it claims to represent.
- Misbranding: Examples of misbranding include false and misleading labeling; missing of important information on device packaging such as name and place of business of manufacturer, packer or distributor; a lack of adequate directions for use; and failure to comply with the color additive provisions listed under Section 706 of the FD&C Act.
- Establishment registration and device listing: Manufacturers and other specified processors of devices (re-packers, relabelers and importers) must register their establishments with the FDA and provide to the FDA a list of all devices processed in any establishment that they operate, and medical device manufacturers must submit to the FDA a list of all devices they produce or process.
- Banned devices: The FDA is authorized to ban devices that present substantial deception or unreasonable and substantial risk of illness or injury.
- Notification of risk and of repair, replacement and refund: Manufacturers have an obligation to notify device prescribers, users, importers, distributors and retailers, as

appropriate, of health risks resulting from the use of a device in violation of applicable requirements; hazardous products in the hands of consumers and other users must be repaired, replaced or refunded.

- Records and reports: Manufacturers, importers and distributors of devices must maintain records and reports to ensure that devices are not adulterated or misbranded.
- Restricted devices: The FDA is authorized to restrict the sale, distribution or use of a device if there is no reasonable assurance of its safety and effectiveness; a restricted device can only be sold on oral or written authorization by a licensed practitioner or under conditions specified by the relevant regulation.
- *Quality System Regulation* (QSR) defined in 21 CFR Part 820, *Good Manufacturing Practices* (GMPs): The FDA has the authority to promulgate regulations covering manufacturing, packing, storage and installation of a device.

Section 702 of the FD&C Act confers the FDA the authority to conduct examinations and investigations (inspections) at facilities or other locations falling under the scope of the regulations [63].

In a nutshell, the general controls are about ensuring that medical devices are designed and manufactured under a quality assurance (QA) program, are fit for the intended use, are adequately packaged and labeled and have establishment registration and device listing forms on file with the FDA.

The general controls apply to all medical devices with some exemptions. A few Class I devices, other than devices labelled or otherwise represented as sterile, are exempt from general controls but not from requirements concerning record keeping (820.180) and complaint files (820.198). These exemptions are marked with an asterisk (*) in the lists of exempt devices defined in Parts 862 to 892 of the CFR [64]. For example, CFR Part 862, *Clinical Chemistry and Clinical Toxicology Devices,* lists exempt device categories, defined in regulations Sections 862.1030 through 862.2920. Section 862.2050, "General Purpose Laboratory Equipment Labeled or Promoted for a Specific Medical Use", is marked with an asterisk (*), indicating that all product codes in this category, which include centrifuges, freezers, blenders and mixers, are exempt from general controls [65].

1.7.1.2 Special controls

Special controls apply to Class II devices and are usually device specific. They include:

- Performance standards and guidelines;
- Pre-market data requirements;
- Special labelling requirements;
- Post-market surveillance requirements; and
- Patient registries.

For example, resuscitators (powered emergency ventilators; see Fig. 1.13) defined by Regulation 868.5925 are Class II. The performance standards and guidance documents applicable to powered resuscitators are:

- ISO 5356-1, Anaesthetic and respiratory equipment – Conical connectors; Part 1: cones and sockets;
- ISO 10651-2, Lung ventilators for medical use – Particular requirements for basic safety and essential performance – Part 5: Gas-powered emergency resuscitators;
- CGA V-5, Diameter-Index Safety System (Non-interchangeable Low-pressure Connections for Medical Gas Applications);
- FDA *Emergency Resuscitator Guidance* (draft); and
- FDA *Reviewer Guidance for Ventilators* (draft) [66].

Class I and Class II devices, unless exempt, require a Premarket Notification, as mandated by Section 510(k) of the FD&C Act [67] and must obtain clearance from the FDA before being placed on the market. The 510(k) Premarket Notification, referred to simply as "510(k)", involves a comparison of the manufacturer's new device to one or more legally marketed (predicate) devices and must include evidence that the new device is substantially equivalent with, in other words it is as safe and effective as, the predicate device.

Most Class I devices (over 800 generic types) and 60 Class II devices are exempt from a 510(k) submission. These are:

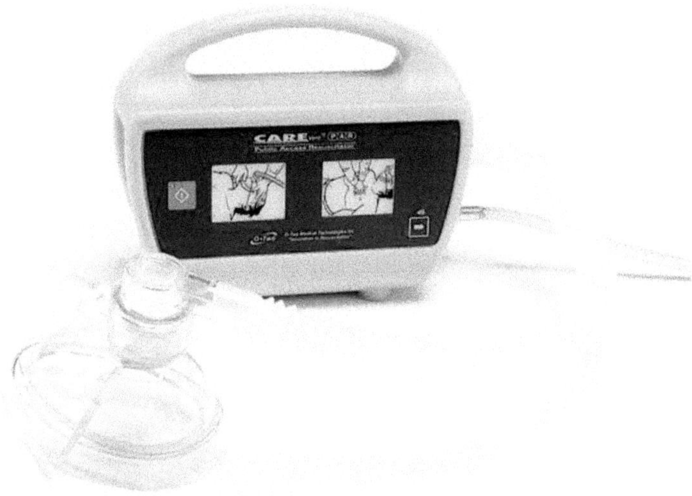

Figure 1.13 Example of a powered resuscitator. *Source*: O-Two Medical Technologies, Inc.

- Grandfathered (also known as pre-amendment) devices that have been in commercial distribution on the US market prior to the 1976 Amendment to the FD&C Act that introduced the 510(k) section and that have not been significantly changed or modified since then and for which there is no regulation requiring a PMA application.
- Class I/II devices specifically exempted by regulations; a consolidated list of devices exempt from 510(k) is available from the FDA's website [68]. This list is compiled from Parts 862–892 of the CFR that define the generic medical device categories and is updated by the FDA as new Class I/II exemptions are added to the list (see Table 1.10). Any limitations to an exemption from 510(k) are covered in Section XXX.9 of each part, where XXX refers to Parts 862–892.

For example, the list containing Part 888, "Orthopedic Devices", exempted from 510(k) – third row from the bottom in Table 1.10 – includes Class I and Class II devices. Class II devices are indicated by "(II)"; Class I devices marked with an asterisk (*) are also

Table 1.10 FDA-compiled list containing Class I and Class II exempt devices grouped according to 21 CFR Parts 862–892 (status as of September 1, 2014)

Part 862	Clinical Chemistry and Clinical Toxicology Devices
Part 864	Hematology and Pathology Devices
Part 866	Immunology and Microbiology Devices
Part 868	Anesthesiology Devices
Part 870	Cardiovascular Devices
Part 872	Dental Devices
Part 874	Ear, Nose, and Throat Devices
Part 876	Gastroenterology-Urology Devices
Part 878	General and Plastic Surgery Devices
Part 880	General Hospital and Personal Use Devices
Part 882	Neurological Devices
Part 884	Obstetrical and Gynecological Devices
Part 886	Ophthalmic Devices
Part 888	Orthopedic Devices
Part 890	Physical Medicine Devices
Part 892	Radiology Devices

exempted from the GMP regulation 21 CFR Part 820, except for general requirements concerning records (820.180) and complaint files (820.198), as long as the device is not labeled or otherwise represented as sterile (see Table 1.11).

Section 888.9 lists the limitations to exempting orthopaedic devices from 510(k), such as using "a different fundamental scientific technology than a legally marketed device in that generic type of device" [69].

1.7.1.3 Pre-market approval

The highest level of regulatory controls in the United States is the PMA and it applies to Class III devices. Devices other than pre-amendment devices are classified automatically as Class III under US federal law.

In addition, the FDA classifies into Class III devices intended to be used in supporting or sustaining human life or preventing impairment of human health, those that may present a potential unreasonable risk of illness or injury for which general controls

Table 1.11 FDA-compiled list of orthopaedic devices covered by Part 888 – third row from the bottom in Table 1.10 (status as of September 1, 2014)

888.1100	Arthroscope: Only the following manual arthroscopic instruments: cannulas, currettes, drill guides, forceps, gouges, graspers, knives, obturators, osteotomes, probes, punches, rasps, retractors, rongeurs, suture passers, suture knotpushers, suture punches, switching rods and trocars, are 510(k) exempt.
888.1250	Nonpowered dynamometer
888.1500	Goniometer (II)
888.1500	Goniometer
888.1520	Nonpowered goniometer
888.3000	Bone cap
888.4150	Calipers for clinical use
888.4200	Cement dispenser
888.4210	Cement mixer for clinical use
888.4220	Cement monomer vapor evacuator
888.4230	Cement ventilation tube
888.4300	Depth gauge for clinical use
888.4540	Orthopedic manual surgical instrument
888.4600	Protractor for clinical use
888.4800	Template for clinical use
888.5850	Nonpowered orthopedic traction apparatus and accessories*
888.5890	Noninvasive traction component*
888.5940	Cast component*
888.5960	Cast removal instrument
888.5980	Manual cast application and removal instrument*

and special controls are insufficient to provide reasonable assurance of the safety and effectiveness of a device, or for which there is insufficient information to make such a determination. Pacemakers, ventricular bypass (assist) devices, joint replacement prostheses, intravascular catheters, intraocular lenses and IVD devices for STD testing are only a few examples of devices classified as Class III by the FDA.

1.7.2 *Regulatory Controls in Japan*

The Japanese Medical Device Nomenclature (JMDN) code determines the regulatory controls applicable to medical devices, depending on their risk classification. It is therefore important that a manufacturer apply the correct JMDN code for its device before starting the application process. There are four risk classifications for medical devices other than IVDs and three risk classifications for IVDs.

The regulatory controls applicable to medical devices other than IVDs are summarized in Table 1.12 [70].

Class I devices, classified as extremely low risk (equivalent to low risk in other jurisdictions) and categorized as *general medical devices*, can be placed on the Japanese market after notifying the Pharmaceuticals and Medical Devices Agency (PMDA), with no pre-market approval required.

Class II devices, classified as low risk (equivalent to low to moderate risk in other jurisdictions) and categorized as *controlled medical devices*, require either certification or premarket approval, depending on whether they comply with Certification Standards designated by the MHLW or not:

- Controlled medical devices that comply with Certification Standards are also known as *specified controlled medical devices*. Assessment and certification to applicable Japanese Industrial Standards (JIS) can be performed by a third-party Registered Certification Body, or RCB, accredited by the MHLW (71 p. 24).
- Controlled medical devices that do not meet or for which there are no designated Certification Standards, require approval by the PMDA, which reviews conformance with the Essential Requirements of safety and efficacy (ERs).

Class III and IV devices, classified as moderate and high risk, respectively (equivalent to moderate to high and high risk in other jurisdictions), are categorized as *specially controlled medical devices* and require pre-market approval by the PMDA. Evaluation is performed according to Approval Standards (JIS, ISO/IEC) or Review Guidelines specified by the MHLW, if available.

Since the enactment of the new Pharmaceutical and Medical Devices (PMD) Act in November 2014 certain generic (me-too) Class III devices can also use the certification by the RCB option. As the PMDA moves gradually toward allowing more Class III devices to

Table 1.12 Regulatory controls for medical devices in Japan

Risk-based classification of medical devices		Regulatory controls	GHTF classification
Class I	General medical devices Extremely low risk to the human body, for example, stainless steel surgical instruments, X-ray film	Notification to the PMDA is required.	Class A
Class II	Controlled medical devices designated by the MHLW for which applicable Certification Standards are specified by the MHLW Low risk to the human body, for example, MRI, diagnostic X-ray machines, EtO sterilizers, intravascular guiding catheters, digestive catheters	Certification by a registered third-party Registered Certification Body (RCB) is required according to Certification Standards.	Class B
	Other controlled medical devices for which there are no specified product standards Low risk to the human body	Approval by the PMDA is required; evaluation is performed using Approval Standards and Review Guidelines. Some generic (me-too) Class III devices can use third-party certification option.	
Class III	Specially controlled medical devices Moderate risk to the human body, for example, artificial bones, dialyzer		Class C
Class IV	Specially controlled medical devices Highly invasive to patients High risk to the human body, for example, pacemaker, artificial heart valves		Class D

Source: PMDA official website

Table 1.13 Regulatory controls for IVDs in Japan

	Risk-based classification of IVDs	Regulatory controls
Class I	IVDs for which diagnostic accuracy represents a relatively low risk Applicable Standard Reference Materials for Calibration specified by the MHLW	Notification to the PMDA is required; the manufacturer ensures self-compliance with Standard Reference Materials for Calibration.
Class II	IVDs for which diagnostic accuracy represents a relatively low risk IVDs for over-the-counter (OTC) use Applicable Certification Standards specified by the MHLW	Certification by a Registered Certification Body (RCB) is required according to Certification Standards.
Class III	IVDs for which diagnostic accuracy represents a relatively high risk	Approval by the PMDA is required; evaluation is performed using Approval Standards.

Source: *Fundamentals of Japanese Regulatory Affairs*, First Edition, RAPS

be assessed via third-party review, (foreign) manufacturers should check with their in-country representatives to confirm whether their products can use the RCB certification process.

The regulatory controls applicable to IVDs are summarized in Table 1.13. The type of submission depends on the risk classification and the compliance with specified standards. However, regardless of classification, all radioactive IVDs require PMDA approval. Novel IVDs require review by the PMDA to determine their classification, and the approval process is used until a Ministerial Announcement specifies applicable standards for the new IVDs [72].

Class I IVDs can be placed on the Japanese market after notification to the PMDA. Manufacturers must ensure compliance with specified Standard Reference Materials for Calibration. In case a Class I IVD is not compliant with the applicable standard, the manufacturer must lodge an application for approval with the PMDA.

Class II IVDs must demonstrate compliance with applicable Certification Standards specified by the MHLW. Assessment and certification can be performed by an accredited third-party RCB. If a Class II IVD is not compliant with the relevant Certification Standard, the manufacturer must apply for approval from the PMDA.

Class III IVDs require PMDA approval prior to marketing in Japan. The assessment is done using specified Approval Standards.

MHLW Ordinance No. 169, *Standard of Manufacturing Control and Quality Control for Medical Devices and In-vitro Diagnostic Reagents*, of 2004 is the main regulation specifically listing QMS requirements. It applies to:

- Specially controlled medical devices – Class III and IV
- Controlled medical devices – Class II
- Some General medical devices – Class I, specified in MHLW Ordinance No. 440 from 2004
- IVDs

Japanese QMS requirements defined in Ordinance 169 align with the international standard ISO 13485, *Medical devices - Quality* Management *Systems - Requirements for regulatory purposes*, but some key differences exist:

- Specific requirements for documents defining the product specifications (*Seihin Hyojun Sho*);
- Specific retention periods defined for documents and records;
- Additional requirements for facilities and infrastructure, including for the manufacturing of sterile devices;
- Manufacturing control and quality controls for labelers;
- Manufacturing control and quality control for manufacturing of biological-origin medical devices; and
- Manufacturing control and quality control for manufacturing of IVDs.

The requirements for design controls apply to specially controlled medical devices (Class III and IV) and to designated medical devices (Class II) (73 pp. 5–6).

1.7.3 *Regulatory Controls in Australia and the EU*

1.7.3.1 Regulatory controls in Australia and the EU for medical devices other than IVDs

EU regulations have a modular, relatively flexible approach to applying regulatory controls and defining the processes for conformity assessment of medical devices. Depending on the device risk classification, the paths to demonstrating conformity can range from the manufacturer's self-declaration of conformity (no involvement of RAs other than for administrative establishment registration and device listing) to examination of device design and a full QMS audit.

Although the terminology and statutory references are different, the regulatory controls in the EU and Australia have one important thing in common, namely a set of conformity assessment elements or modules that can be combined into distinct conformity assessment procedures. Each conformity assessment procedure has a well-defined level of regulatory oversight that is directly proportionate with the device class it applies to. Where there are alternative conformity assessment procedures with an equivalent or higher level of regulatory scrutiny, the manufacturer may choose the one that it wants to use.

Irrespective of their risk classification, all medical devices must have technical documentation with information demonstrating compliance with the ERs/EPs, must have a Declaration of Conformity (DoC) and must be manufactured under a QA program. Establishment registration and device listing also apply according to specific requirements in each jurisdiction.

Manufacturers of Class I non-sterile, non-measuring devices (low risk) can self-declare conformity with regulations and after completing the administrative obligations can legally market their products.

For all other risk classes of medical devices, including for Class I devices supplied sterile or with a measuring function, manufacturers must involve a Conformity Assessment Body (CAB) – an EU Notified Body in the EU and the TGA in Australia, respectively.

Manufacturers of Class I devices supplied sterile must ensure that sterility is consistently maintained. They may choose one the following conformity assessment procedures:

- Self-declaration of conformity with ERs/EPs combined with the production QA audit; or
- Full QMS certification not including design examination.

Manufacturers of Class I devices with a measuring function must ensure that the measurement function is provided with the required accuracy and stability. They may choose one of the following conformity assessment procedures:

- Self-declaration combined with either: a production QA audit or a final inspection process also known as product QA or product verification – either 100% or based on statistical sampling; or
- Full QMS certification not including design examination.

Manufacturers of Class IIa devices (low to moderate risk) may apply one of the following conformity assessment procedures:

- Self-declaration of conformity with ERs/EPs combined with either: production QA certification or product QA (not appropriate for Class B sterile devices) or product verification – either 100% or based on a statistical sampling (not appropriate for Class B sterile devices); or
- Full QMS certification not including design examination.

Manufacturers of Class IIb devices (moderate to high risk) may apply one of the following conformity assessment procedures:

- Type examination, whereby the CAB undertakes testing of a device type in order to determine compliance of its design with the ERs/EPs, combined with either: production QA; or product QA (not appropriate for Class C sterile devices); or product verification – either 100% or based on a statistical sampling (not appropriate for Class C sterile devices); or
- Full QMS certification not including design examination.

Manufacturers of Class III devices and AIMDs (high risk) must undergo an assessment of the device design. Either this can be based on manufacturer's data ("Design Examination" module), or the CAB can undertake or arrange for type testing ("Type Examination/Type Testing" module). Manufacturers may apply one of the following conformity assessment procedures:

- Design examination combined with a full QMS audit and certification; or
- Type examination combined with one of the following modules: full QMS certification; or production QA; or

product verification – 100% or statistical sampling (not appropriate for Class D sterile devices).

1.7.3.2 Regulatory controls in Australia and the EU for IVDs

The EU and Australian conformity assessment procedures for IVDs are applied taking into consideration the risk classification of the IVDs.

The conformity assessment procedures in the two jurisdictions are similar for higher-risk IVDs but differ for the lower-risk IVDs, mainly due to the differences in classification of IVDs. It is expected that after the implementation of the revised EU IVDD [74] the EU and Australian IVD classification and conformity assessment procedures will be much closely aligned with each other.

Irrespective of their risk classification, all IVDs must have technical documentation with information demonstrating compliance with the ERs/EPs, must have a DoC and must be manufactured under a QA program. Establishment registration and device listing also apply according to specific requirements in each jurisdiction.

Manufacturers of IVDs posing low individual risk and low or no public health risk can self-declare conformity with regulations and after completing the administrative obligations can legally market their products. In the EU general IVDs (other than self-testing and those listed in Annex II of the IVDD) and in Australia Class 1 IVDs such as reagents and instruments fall under this category.

For all other risk classes of IVDs, manufacturers must involve a CAB – an EU Notified Body in the EU and the TGA in Australia, respectively.

Self-test IVDs not covered in Annex II of the IVDD in Europe and Class 2 IVDs in Australia have a risk profile similar to the IVDs posing moderate individual risk and/or low public health risk. Manufacturers can choose one of the following conformity assessment procedures:

- Design examination and certification by a Notified Body (in the EU only);
- Type examination combined with either product verification – 100% or statistical sampling or with production QA (in the EU only);

- Self-declaration combined with production QA (Australia only); and
- Full QMS certification except design examination (the EU and Australia).

IVDs listed in Annex II List B of the EU IVDD and Class 3 IVDs in Australia fall have a risk profile similar to IVDs posing high individual risk and/or moderate public health risk. Manufacturers can apply one of the following conformity assessment procedures:

- Type examination of the device design combined with either product verification - 100% or statistical sampling (the EU only) - or production QA (the EU and Australia); or
- Full QMS certification except design examination (the EU and Australia).

IVDs listed in Annex II List A of the EU IVDD and Class 4 IVDs in Australia have a risk profile similar to IVDs posing high individual risk and high public risk. Manufacturers can apply one of the following conformity assessment procedures:

- Type examination of the device design combined with production QA (the EU and Australia); or
- Full QMS certification, including design examination (the EU and Australia).

1.7.4 *Regulatory Controls in Canada*

The conformity assessment procedures defined in the Canadian regulations are arguably more straightforward but less flexible than the previous model.

Health Canada requires that all devices comply with the safety and effectiveness requirements defined in the regulations (also referred to as ERs) and manufacturers must keep that information on record.

Manufacturers of Class I devices must fulfill the administrative provisions for establishment registration. They must either hold a Medical Device Establishment License (MDEL) themselves or import or distribute solely through an importer or distributor that holds a MDEL.

Manufacturers of Class II, III and IV devices are required to have a valid Medical Device License (MDL) and a QMS certified to ISO 13485, *Medical devices - Quality* management systems - *Requirements for regulatory purposes*, issued by a Canadian Medical Devices Conformity Assessment System (CMDCAS)-recognized registrar. For Class II devices at least the manufacturing (or production QA) must be certified. For Class III and IV devices the full QMS (D&D and production QA) must be certified.

1.7.5 *GHTF Model for Conformity Assessment Procedures*

The GHTF has published the following guidelines for a modular approach to conformity assessment of medical devices and IVDs inspired by the European MDD conformity assessment procedures:

- *Principles of Conformity Assessment for Medical Devices* [75]; and
- *Principles of Conformity Assessment for In Vitro Diagnostic (IVD) Medical Devices* [76].

These GHTF guidelines emphasize the three main elements required for ensuring regulatory compliance for medical devices, which are also mentioned at the beginning of Section 1.7, "Risk-Based Approach for Regulatory Controls and Conformity Assessment", in this chapter:

- Conformity assessment of device safety and performance – to ensure compliance with applicable state-of-the-art requirements for safety and effectiveness (EPs);
- Conformity assessment of the QMS – to ensure consistency and continued compliance with regulatory requirements, including post-market surveillance and adverse event reporting; and
- Registration – an administrative measure whereby manufacturers inform local RAs of their place of business and the devices they place on the market.

The GHTF terminology also defines RAs that may be involved in applying the conformity assessment procedures (see also Table 1.14):

Table 1.14 Regulatory Authorities (RAs) and Conformity Assessment Bodies (CABs) in the established markets

Jurisdiction	Regulatory Authorities (RAs)	Conformity Assessment Bodies (CABs)
Australia	Therapeutic Goods Administration (TGA)	TGA CABs recognized via Mutual Recognition Agreements (MRAs) [77]
Canada	Health Canada (HC)	HC Canadian Medical Devices Conformity Assessment System (CMDCAS)-recognized registrars [27]
EU	EU National Competent Authorities (CAs)	EU Notified Bodies Non-EU CABs recognized via Mutual Recognition Agreements (MRAs), such as TGA [78]
Japan	Pharmaceuticals and Medical Devices Agency (PMDA)	PMDA Registered Certification Bodies (RCBs) [79]
United States	Food and Drug Administration (FDA)	FDA FDA Accredited Persons under Third-Party Review program [80] FDA Accredited Persons for (post-market) Inspection [28]

- Regulatory Authority (RA): A government body or other entity that exercises a legal right to control the use or sale of medical devices within its jurisdiction and that may take enforcement action to ensure that medical products marketed within its jurisdiction comply with legal requirements.
- Conformity Assessment Body (CAB): A body, other than an RA, engaged in determining whether the relevant requirements in technical regulations or standards are fulfilled. A CAB is authorized to undertake specified conformity assessment activities by an RA that will ensure performance of the CAB is monitored and, if necessary, withdraw designation.

The appointment or designation of CABs is undertaken by the government regulatory agency in each jurisdiction. In some jurisdictions, such as Australia, Canada, Japan and the United States, the agency performing the designation task can also be responsible for assessments. In others, such as the EU, the agency performing the assessments is a commercial organization appointed by the regulatory agency. RAs may also appoint CABs to perform

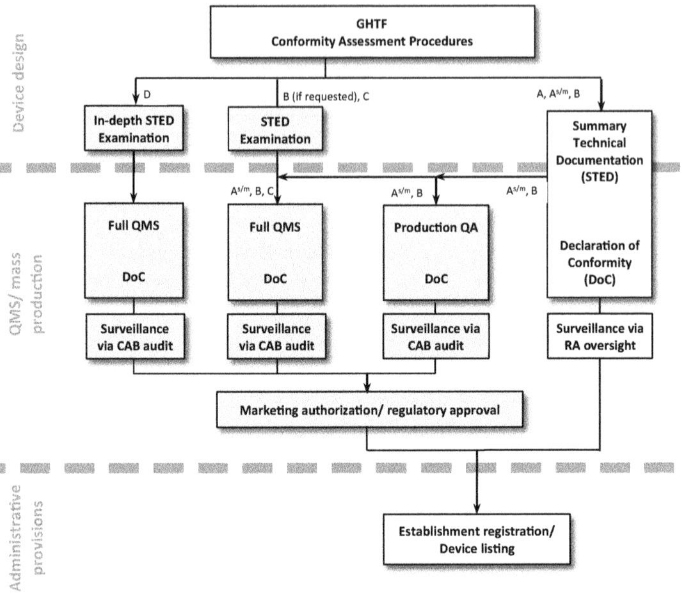

Figure 1.14 GHTF model for medical device conformity assessment procedures. Letters "s" and "m" in superscript indicate Class A devices (low risk) supplied sterile or with a measuring function, respectively. Shaded boxes represent modules for which a CAB must be involved.

conformity assessment to regulations in other countries with which they have a Mutual Recognition Agreement (MRA).

The regulatory controls and conformity assessment procedures proposed by the GHTF model for medical devices and IVDs are described in the next sections. The GHTF proposal strikes a balance between the level of regulatory scrutiny and the product risk classification and it may well be the model adopted in emerging markets sometime in the future.

1.7.5.1 GHTF model for medical devices

The diagram in Fig. 1.14 and the following tables (Tables 1.15–1.18) summarize the conformity assessment procedures for medical devices of all risk classes – A, B, C and D – according to GHTF guideline *Principles of Conformity Assessment for Medical Devices* [75].

Table 1.15 Regulatory compliance elements for Class A medical devices (low risk)

Regulatory compliance elements	Conformity assessment element	Manufacturer responsibility	RA/CAB responsibility
Conformity assessment of the quality management system (QMS)	QMS	Establish and maintain a full QMS or a QMS without design controls.	Regulatory audit normally not required except where assurance of sterility or of a measuring function is required
	Post-market surveillance	Establish and maintain an adverse event–reporting procedure.	May audit post-market to investigate specific safety or regulatory concerns
Conformity assessment of device safety and performance	Technical documentation	Establish and keep up-to-date technical documentation and prepare and submit a Summary Technical Documentation (STED) only at the request of an RA/CAB.	Pre-market submission of STED normally not requested
	Declaration of Conformity (DoC)	Prepare, sign and maintain.	Submission normally not requested
Registration	Registration of manufacturers and their devices	Perform according to regulatory requirements.	To maintain and verify, as appropriate

Table 1.16 Regulatory compliance elements for Class B medical devices (low to moderate risk)

Regulatory compliance elements	Conformity assessment element	Manufacturer responsibility	RA/CAB responsibility
Conformity assessment of the quality management system (QMS)	QMS	Establish and maintain a full QMS or a QMS without design controls.	Be satisfied that a current and appropriate QMS is in place or otherwise conduct a QMS audit prior to marketing authorization.
	Post-market surveillance	Establish and maintain an adverse event–reporting procedure.	Be satisfied that a current and appropriate adverse event–reporting procedure is in place as part of the QMS.
Conformity assessment of device safety and performance	Technical documentation	Establish and keep up-to-date technical documentation and prepare and submit a Summary Technical Documentation (STED) only at the request of an RA/CAB.	Do not normally review pre-market. If submission is requested, receive and conduct a pre-market review of the STED sufficient to determine conformity to EPs.
	Declaration of Conformity (DoC)	Prepare, sign and make available for review.	Review and verify compliance with requirements.
Registration	Registration of manufacturers and their devices	Perform according to regulatory requirements.	Maintain and verify, as appropriate.

Table 1.17 Regulatory compliance elements for Class C medical devices (moderate to high risk)

Regulatory compliance elements	Conformity assessment element	Manufacturer responsibility	RA/CAB responsibility
Conformity assessment of the quality management system (QMS)	QMS	Establish and maintain a full QMS.	Be satisfied that a current and appropriate QMS is in place or otherwise conduct a QMS audit prior to marketing authorization.
	Post-market durveillance	Establish and maintain an adverse event–reporting procedure.	Be satisfied that a current and appropriate adverse event–reporting procedure is in place as part of the QMS.
Conformity assessment of device safety and performance	Technical documentation	Establish and keep up-to-date technical documentation and prepare and submit a Summary Technical Documentation (STED) for review.	Undertake a pre-market review of the STED to determine conformity to Essential Principles (EPs).
	Declaration of Conformity (DoC)	Prepare, sign and submit.	Review and verify compliance with requirements.
Registration	Registration of manufacturers and their devices	Perform according to regulatory requirements.	Maintain and verify, as appropriate.

Table 1.18 Regulatory compliance elements for Class D medical devices (high risk)

Regulatory compliance elements	Conformity assessment element	Manufacturer responsibility	RA/CAB responsibility
Conformity assessment of the quality management system (QMS)	QMS	Establish and maintain a full QMS.	Be satisfied that a current and appropriate QMS is in place or otherwise conduct a QMS audit prior to marketing authorization.
	Post-market surveillance	Establish and maintain an adverse event–reporting procedure.	Be satisfied that a current and appropriate adverse event–reporting procedure is in place as part of the QMS.
Conformity assessment of device safety and performance	Technical documentation	Establish and keep up-to-date technical documentation and prepare and submit a Summary Technical Documentation (STED) for review.	Undertake an in-depth pre-market review of the STED to determine conformity to Essential Principles (EPs).
	Declaration of Conformity (DoC)	Prepare, sign and submit.	Review and verify compliance with requirements.
Registration	Registration of manufacturers and their devices	Perform according to regulatory requirements.	Maintain and verify, as appropriate.

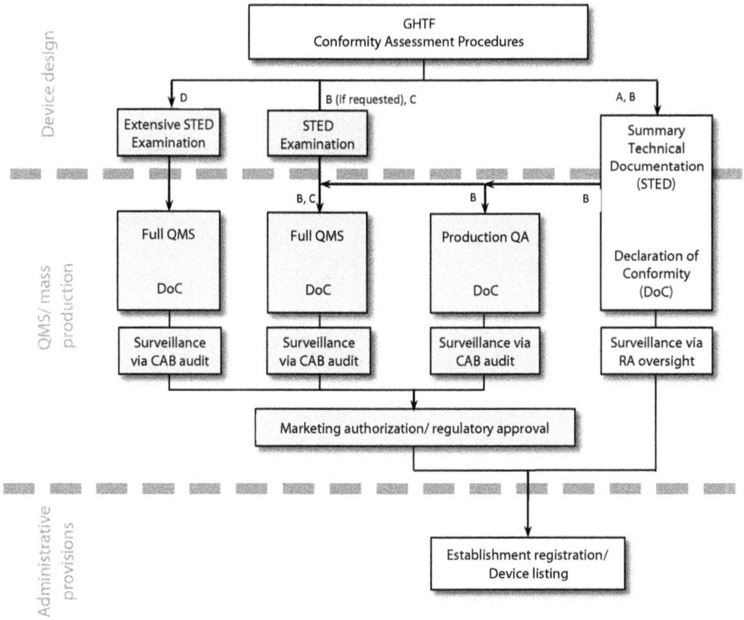

Figure 1.15 GHTF model for IVDs conformity assessment procedures. Shaded boxes represent modules for which a CAB must be involved.

1.7.5.2 GHTF model for IVD

The diagram in Fig. 1.15 and the following tables (Tables 1.19–1.22) summarize the conformity assessment procedures for IVDs of all risk classes – A, B, C and D – according to GHTF guideline *Principles of Conformity Assessment for In Vitro Diagnostic (IVD) Medical Devices* [76]. Shaded boxes represent modules for which a CAB must be involved.

Table 1.19 Regulatory compliance elements for Class A IVDs (low individual risk and low or no public health risk)

Regulatory compliance elements	Conformity assessment element	Manufacturer responsibility	RA/CAB responsibility
Conformity assessment of the quality management system (QMS)	QMS	Establish and maintain a full QMS or a QMS without design and development controls.	Pre-market regulatory audit not required.
	Post-market surveillance	Establish and maintain an adverse event–reporting procedure.	May audit post-market to investigate specific safety or regulatory concerns.
Conformity assessment of device safety and performance	Technical documentation	Establish and keep up-to-date technical documentation and prepare and submit a Summary Technical Documentation (STED) only at the request of an RA/CAB.	Pre-market submission of STED not required May be requested to investigate specific safety or regulatory concerns.
	Declaration of Conformity (DoC)	Prepare, sign and maintain.	On file with the manufacturer; available upon request.
Registration	Registration of manufacturers and their devices	Perform according to regulatory requirements.	To maintain and verify, as appropriate.

Table 1.20 Regulatory compliance elements for Class B IVDs (moderate individual risk and/or low public health risk)

Regulatory compliance elements	Conformity assessment element	Manufacturer responsibility	RA/CAB responsibility
Conformity assessment of the quality management system (QMS)	QMS	Establish and maintain a full QMS or a QMS without design and development controls.	Be satisfied that a current and appropriate QMS is in place or otherwise conduct a QMS audit prior to marketing authorization.
	Post-market surveillance	Establish and maintain an adverse event–reporting procedure.	Be satisfied that a current and appropriate adverse event–reporting procedure is in place as part of the QMS.
Conformity assessment of device safety and performance	Technical documentation	Establish and keep up-to-date technical documentation and prepare and submit a Summary Technical Documentation (STED) only at the request of an RA/CAB.	Pre-market submission is normally not required. If requested, receive and conduct a review of the STED to determine conformity to Essential Principles (EPs).
	Declaration of Conformity (DoC)	Prepare, sign and make available for review.	Review and verify compliance with requirements.
Registration	Registration of manufacturers and their devices	Perform according to regulatory requirements.	Maintain and verify, as appropriate.

Table 1.21 Regulatory compliance elements for Class C IVDs (high individual risk and/or moderate public health risk)

Regulatory compliance elements	Conformity assessment element	Manufacturer responsibility	RA/CAB responsibility
Conformity assessment of the quality management system (QMS)	QMS	Establish and maintain a full QMS.	Be satisfied that a current and appropriate QMS is in place or otherwise conduct a QMS audit prior to marketing authorization.
	Post-market surveillance	Establish and maintain an adverse event–reporting procedure.	Be satisfied that a current and appropriate adverse event–reporting procedure is in place as part of the QMS.
Conformity assessment of device safety and performance	Technical documentation	Establish and keep up-to-date technical documentation and prepare and submit a Summary Technical Documentation (STED) for review.	Receive and conduct a pre-market review of the STED to determine conformity to Essential Principles (EPs).
	Declaration of Conformity (DoC)	Prepare, sign and submit.	Review and verify compliance with requirements.
Registration	Registration of manufacturers and their devices	Perform according to regulatory requirements.	Maintain and verify, as appropriate.

Table 1.22 Regulatory compliance elements for Class D IVDs (high individual risk and high public risk)

Regulatory compliance elements	Conformity assessment element	Manufacturer responsibility	RA/CAB responsibility
Conformity assessment of the quality management system (QMS)	QMS	Establish and maintain a full QMS.	Be satisfied that a current and appropriate QMS is in place or otherwise conduct a QMS audit prior to marketing authorization.
	Post-market surveillance	Establish and maintain an adverse event–reporting procedure.	Be satisfied that a current and appropriate adverse event–reporting procedure is in place as part of the QMS.
Conformity assessment of device safety and performance	Technical documentation	Establish and keep up-to-date technical documentation, including a full performance evaluation report. Prepare and submit a Summary Technical Documentation (STED) for review.	Receive and conduct a pre-market review of the STED sufficient to determine conformity to Essential Principles (EPs).
	Declaration of Conformity (DoC)	Prepare, sign and submit.	Review and verify compliance with requirements.
Registration	Registration of manufacturers and their devices	Perform according to regulatory requirements.	Maintain and verify, as appropriate.

1.8 Concluding Summary

Chapter 1 introduces some fundamentals of medical device regulations. It covers:

- An overview on how medical devices are regulated worldwide, in both established and emerging markets, and the regulatory agencies in the main markets
- Terminology related to and bodies issuing accreditations and certifications conferring credibility and authority of approvals
- Medical device definitions – medical devices, active implantables, IVDs – including examples of borderline and combination products
- Phases of a typical medical devices life cycle – pre-market; regulatory submissions, approvals and registrations; and post-market
- Risk-based medical device classification systems in established markets and the two different classification philosophies – nomenclature based and generic rule based – and what the risk classes in the major markets are
- Regulatory controls in established jurisdictions and the underlying philosophy in applying them, namely the higher the risk class of a medical device, the more stringent the regulatory oversight and involvement of regulatory agencies.

References

1. Bartels, H.G., et al. Promoting access to medical technologies and innovation – Intersections between public health, intellectual property and trade. *www.wto.org.* [Online] 2013. [Cited: April 28, 2014.] http://www.wto.org/english/res_e/booksp_e/pamtiwhowipowtoweb13_e.pdf.
2. IMDRF. About IMDRF. *www.imdrf.org.* [Online] [Cited: April 28, 2014.] http://www.imdrf.org/about/about.asp.

3. Food and Drug Administration. Device Regulation and Guidance – Overview. *www.fda.gov.* [Online] [Cited: April 28, 2014.] http://www.fda.gov/MedicalDevices/DeviceRegulationandGuidance/Overview/ucm134499.htm.
4. Food and Drug Administration. Device Regulation and Guidance – Guidance Documents. *www.fda.gov.* [Online] [Cited: April 28, 2014.] http://www.fda.gov/MedicalDevices/DeviceRegulationandGuidance/GuidanceDocuments/default.htm.
5. Food and Drug Administration. Device Regulation and Guidance – Standards. *www.fda.gov.* [Online] [Cited: April 28, 2014.] http://www.fda.gov/MedicalDevices/DeviceRegulationandGuidance/Standards/default.htm.
6. Therapeutic Goods Administration. Legislation & legislative instruments. *www.tga.gov.au.* [Online] [Cited: April 28, 2014.] http://www.tga.gov.au/industry/legislation.htm#.U12gx_mSx8E.
7. Therapeutic Goods Administration. www.tga.gov.au. *Australian regulatory guidelines for medical devices (ARGMD).* [Online] [Cited: April 28, 2014.] http://www.tga.gov.au/industry/devices-argmd.htm#.U12iA_mSx8G.
8. Therapeutic Goods Administration. Standards, guidelines & publications (medical devices & IVDs). *www.tga.gov.au.* [Online] [Cited: April 28, 2014.] http://www.tga.gov.au/industry/ devices-sgp.htm#.U12idfmSx8E.
9. Health Canada. Legislation and Guidelines. *www.hc-sc.gc.ca.* [Online] [Cited: April 28, 2014.] http://www.hc-sc.gc.ca/dhp-mps/md-im/legislation/index-eng.php.
10. Health Canada. Guidance Documents. *www.hc-sc.gc.ca.* [Online] [Cited: April 14, 2014.] http://www.hc-sc.gc.ca/dhp-mps/md-im/applic-demande/guide-ld/index-eng.php.
11. Health Canada. Standards. *www.hc-sc.gc.ca.* [Online] September 26, 2014. [Cited: October 3, 2014.] http://www.hc-sc.gc.ca/dhp-mps/md-im/standards-normes/index-eng.php.
12. Ministry of Health, Labour and Welfare. New Direction of Japanese Regulations on MD/IVD. *www.pmda.go.jp.* [Online] March 31, 2014. [Cited: October 3, 2014.] http://www.imdrf.org/docs/imdrf/final/meetings/imdrf-meet-140829-washington-japan-update.pdf.
13. Pharmaceuticals and Medical Devices Agency. Regulations and Procedures. *www.pmda.go.jp.* [Online] 2014. [Cited: November 1, 2014.] http://www.pmda.go.jp/english/service/regulation.html.

14. Pharmaceuticals and Medical Devices Agency. Standards for Medical Devices. *www.std.pmda.go.jp.* [Online] [Cited: April 28, 2014.] http://www.std.pmda.go.jp/stdDB/index_e.html.
15. European Commission. Application of EU law – What is EU law? *ec.europa.eu.* [Online] [Cited: April 28, 2014.] http://ec.europa.eu/eu_law/introduction/treaty_en.htm.
16. European Commission. Application of EU law; Directives – definitions. *ec.europa.eu.* [Online] [Cited: April 28, 2014.] http://ec.europa.eu/eu_law/directives/directives_en.htm.
17. European Commission. Reference documents. *ec.europa.eu.* [Online] [Cited: April 28, 2014.] http://ec.europa.eu/health/medical-devices/documents/index_en.htm.
18. European Commission. Revision of the medical devices directives. [Online] [Cited: April 28, 2014.] http://ec.europa.eu/health/medical-devices/documents/index_en.htm.
19. European Commission. Application of EU law – What are EU regulations? *ec.europa.eu.* [Online] [Cited: April 28, 2014.] http://ec.europa.eu/ eu_law/introduction/what_regulation_en.htm.
20. European Commission. Application of EU law – What are EU decisions? *ec.europa.eu.* [Online] [Cited: April 28, 2014.] http://ec.europa.eu/eu_law/introduction/what_decision_en.htm.
21. European Commission. Guidance MEDDEVs. *ec.europa.eu.* [Online] [Cited: April 28, 2014.] http://ec.europa.eu/health/medical-devices/documents/guidelines/index_en.htm.
22. European Commission. European standardisation policy. *ec.europa.eu.* [Online] [Cited: April 28, 2014.] http://ec.europa.eu/enterprise/policies/european-standards/standardisation-policy/index_en.htm.
23. ASEAN. ASEAN Agreement on Medical Device Directive. *www.hsa.gov.sg.* [Online] May 8, 2012. [Cited: April 28, 2014.] http://ec.europa.eu/enterprise/policies/european-standards/standardisation-policy/index_en.htm.
24. Opening Address by Dr Amy Khor, Minister of State, at the Town Hall Session with Medical Device Industry. *www.hsa.gov.sg.* [Online] April 20, 2012. [Cited: April 28, 2014.] http://webcache.googleusercontent.com/search?q=cache:http://www.hsa.gov.sg/publish/hsaportal/en/news_events/speeches/2012/opening_address_by.html.
25. Therapeutic Goods Administration. Medical device amendments to the EU-Australia MRA on conformity assessment to come into effect 1 January 2013. *www.tga.gov.au.* [Online] January 1, 1999. [Cited: July 1, 2014.] http://www.austlii.edu.au/au/other/dfat/treaties/1999/2.html.

26. Therapeutic Goods Administration. Approved 'Conformity Assessment Bodies' for the purposes of the EC-MRA. *www.tga.gov.au.* [Online] June 23, 2009. [Cited: August 10, 2014.] http://www.tga.gov.au/industry/devices-ecmra-cab.htm#.U-MMTPmSx8E.
27. Health Canada. List of Registrars Recognized by Health Canada under section 32.1 of the Medical Devices Regulations (MDR). *www.hc-sc.gc.ca.* [Online] December 4, 2013. [Cited: August 10, 2014.] http://www.hc-sc.gc.ca/dhp-mps/md-im/qualsys/list_liste_regist-eng.php.
28. Food and Drug Administration. List of Accredited Persons for Inspection. *www.fda.gov.* [Online] March 12, 2014. [Cited: August 10, 2014.] http://www.fda.gov/medicaldevices/deviceregulationandguidance/postmarketrequirements/thirdpartyinspection/ucm125410.htm#list.
29. Food and Drug Administration. Current List of Accredited Persons for 510(k) Review under the FDA Modernization Act of 1997. *www.accessdata.fda.gov.* [Online] August 4, 2014. [Cited: August 10, 2014.] http://www.accessdata.fda.gov/scripts/cdrh/cfdocs/cfthirdparty/accredit.cfm.
30. European Commission. MEDDEV 2.3/1 Rev. 3 Borderline products, drug delivery products and medical devices incorporating, as an integral part, an ancillary medicinal substance or an ancillary human blood derivative. *ec.europa.eu.* [Online] March 21, 2010. [Cited: May 10, 2014.] http:// ec.europa.eu/health/medical-devices/files/meddev/2_1_3_rev_3-12_2009_en.pdf.
31. European Commission. Borderline and classification issues. *ec.europa.eu.* [Online] June 2013. [Cited: July 1, 2014.] http://ec.europa.eu/health/medical-devices/documents/borderline/index_en.htm.
32. MHRA. Borderlines. *www.mhra.gov.uk.* [Online] March 19, 2014. [Cited: July 1, 2014.] http://www.mhra.gov.uk/Howweregulate/Devices/ Borderlines/index.htm.
33. Therapeutic Goods Administration. Australian regulatory guidelines for medical devices (ARGMD) – Part 1 Introduction. *www.tga.gov.au.* [Online] May 2011. [Cited: July 1, 2014.] http://www.tga.gov.au/pdf/devices-argmd-p1-01.pdf.
34. Food and Drug Administration. 21 CFR Part 3 Product jurisdiction, Sec. 3.2 Definitions. *www.accessdata.fda.gov.* [Online] June 1, 2013. [Cited: July 1, 2014.]
35. Food and Drug Administration. About combination products. *www.fda.gov.* [Online] October 20, 2009. [Cited: July 1, 2014.] http://www.fda.gov/CombinationProducts/AboutCombinationProducts/default.htm.

36. European Commission. Manual on Borderline and Classification in the Community – Regulatory Framework for Medical Devices. *ec.europa.eu.* [Online] July 2014. [Cited: October 3, 2014.] http://ec. europa.eu/health/medical-devices/files/wg_minutes_member_lists/borderline_manual_ol_en.pdf.
37. Food and Drug Administration. Combination Products. *www.fda.gov.* [Online] August 22, 2013. [Cited: October 3, 2014.] http://www.fda.gov/CombinationProducts/default.htm.
38. *Australian Regulatory Guidance for Medical Devices* (ARGMD) – Part 2 Section 14 Medical devices incorporating a medicine. *www.tga.gov.au.* [Online] May 2011. [Cited: October 3, 2014.] https://www.tga.gov.au/sites/default/files/devices-argmd-p2.pdf.
39. Therapeutic Goods Administration. Products regulated as biologicals. *www.tga.gov.au.* [Online] January 8, 2013. [Cited: October 3, 2014.] https://www.tga.gov.au/products-regulated-biologicals.
40. Health Canada. Drug/Medical Device Combination Products. *www.hc-sc.gc.ca.* [Online] May 13, 1999. [Cited: October 3, 2014.] http://www.hc-sc.gc.ca/dhp-mps/prodpharma/applic-demande/pol/combo_mixte_pol_2006-eng.php.
41. Onodera, Y., Pharmaceuticals and Medical Devices Agency. Regulation on Combination Products in Japan. *www.fda.gov.tw.* [Online] January 11, 2013. [Cited: October 3, 2014.] http://www.fda.gov.tw/upload/189/Content/2013011111572280721.pdf.
42. Food and Drug Administration. Classify Your Medical Device. *www.fda.gov.* [Online] [Cited: April 28, 2014.] http://www.fda.gov/MedicalDevices/DeviceRegulationandGuidance/Overview/ClassifyYourDevice/default.htm.
43. Food and Drug Administration. Product Code Classification Database. *www.fda.gov.* [Online] June 6, 2014. [Cited: September 1, 2014.] http://www.fda.gov/MedicalDevices/DeviceRegulationandGuidance/Overview/ClassifyYourDevice/ucm051637.htm.
44. Food and Drug Administration. Federal Register Volume 79, Number 178. *www.gpo.gov.* [Online] September 15, 2014. [Cited: September 4, 2014.] http://www.gpo.gov/fdsys/pkg/FR-2014-09-15/html/2014-21816.htm?source=govdelivery&utm_medium=email&utm_source=govdelivery.
45. European Commission. MEDDEV 2.4/1 Rev 9 June 2012 – Classification of medical devices. *ec.europa.eu.* [Online] June 2012. [Cited: April 28, 2014.] http://ec.europa. eu/health/medical-devices/files/meddev/2_4_1_rev_9_classification_en.pdf.

46. Global Harmonization Taskforce. GHTF SG1/N77:2012 Principles of Medical Devices Classification. *www.imdrf.org.* [Online] November 2, 2012. [Cited: May 10, 2014.] http://www.imdrf.org/docs/ghtf/final/sg1/technical-docs/ghtf-sg1-n77-2012-principles-medical-devices-classification-121102.pdf.
47. ASEAN Medical Device Product Working Group (MDPWG). ASEAN Medical Devices Directive (Version 11) – Annex 2 Risk Classification Rules for medical devices other than IVDs. *www.hsa.gov.sg.* [Online] May 8, 2012. [Cited: July 1, 2014.] http://www.hsa.gov.sg/publish/etc/medialib/hsa_library/health_products_regulation/medical_devices/files_2.Par.69318.File.tmp/AMDD%20-%20Draft%20for%20consultation%20-%2002%20Aug%202012.pdf.
48. Therapeutic Goods Administration. Australian regulatory guidelines for medical devices (ARGMD) – Part 1 Introduction, Section 4 Classification of medical devices. *www.tga.gov.* [Online] May 2011. [Cited: April 28, 2014.] http://www.tga.gov.au/pdf/devices-argmd-p1-01.pdf.
49. Health Canada. Guidance for the risk based classification system (Draft). *www.hc-sc.gc.ca.* [Online] May 4, 1998. [Cited: April 28, 2014.] http://www.hc-sc.gc.ca/dhp-mps/md-im/applic-demande/guide-ld/risk5_risque5-eng.php.
50. European Commission. Proposal for a Regulation of the European Parliament and of the Council on in vitro diagnostic medical devices – Annex VII Classification criteria. *ec.europa.eu.* [Online] September 26, 2012. [Cited: August 10, 2014.] http://ec.europa.eu/health/medical-devices/files/revision_docs/proposal_2012_541_en.pdf.
51. Therapeutic Goods Administration. Classification of IVD medical devices. *www.tga.gov.au.* [Online] November 2011. [Cited: May 10, 2014.] http://www.tga.gov.au/pdf/ivd-classification.pdf.
52. Health Canada. Guidance for the risk based classification system of in vitro diagnostic devices (Draft). *www.hc-sc.gc.ca.* [Online] April 24, 1998. [Cited: May 10, 2014.] http://www.hc-sc.gc.ca/dhp-mps/alt_formats/hpfb-dgpsa/pdf/md-im/ivd-rsk_idiv-rsq-eng.pdf.
53. Global Harmonization Taskforce. GHTF/SG1/N045:2008 Principles of IVD Medical Devices Classification. *www.imdrf.org.* [Online] February 19, 2008. [Cited: May 10, 2014.] http://www.imdrf.org/docs/ghtf/final/sg1/procedural-docs/ghtf-sg1-n045-2008-principles-ivd-medical-devices-classification-080219.pdf.
54. ASEAN Medical Device Product Working Group (MDPWG). ASEAN Medical Devices Directive (Version 11) – Annex 3 Risk Classification rules

for IVDs. *www.hsa.gov.sg.* [Online] May 8, 2012. [Cited: July 1, 2014.] http://www.hsa.gov.sg/publish/etc/medialib/hsa_library/health_products_regulation/medical_devices/files_2.Par.69318.File.tmp/AMDD%20-%20Draft%20for%20consultation%20-%2002%20Aug%202012.pdf.

55. Food and Drug Administration. 21 CFR Part 820 Quality System Regulation, Section 820.3 Definitions. *www.accessdata.fda.gov.* [Online] June 1, 2013. [Cited: August 30, 2014.] http://www.accessdata.fda.gov/scripts/cdrh/cfdocs/cfcfr/CFRSearch.cfm?fr=820.3.
56. European Commission. MEDDEV 2.1/1 Definitions of "medical devices", "accessory" and "manufacturer". *ec.europa.eu.* [Online] April 1994. [Cited: August 30, 2014.] http://ec.europa.eu/health/medical-devices/files/meddev/2_1-1___04-1994_en.pdf.
57. Food and Drug Administration. Content of a 510(k) – General Information. *www.fda.gov.* [Online] August 11, 2014. [Cited: September 1, 2014.] http://www.fda.gov/MedicalDevices/DeviceRegulationandGuidance/HowtoMarketYourDevice/PremarketSubmissions/PremarketNotification510k/ucm142651.htm.
58. GMDN. GMDN Database. *www.gmdnagency.com.* [Online] [Cited: August 30, 2014.] https://www.gmdnagency.com/Info.aspx?pageid=1091.
59. Food and Drug Administration. Convenience Kits Interim Regulatory Guidance. *www.fda.gov.* [Online] May 7, 2014. [Cited: August 30, 2014.] http://www.fda.gov/medicaldevices/deviceregulationandguidance/guidancedocuments/ucm080216.htm.
60. Therapeutic Goods Administration. Australian regulatory guidelines for medical devices (ARGMD), Section 16. Systems and procedure packs. *www.tga.gov.au.* [Online] May 2011. [Cited: August 30, 2014.] http://www.tga.gov.au/pdf/devices-argmd-01.pdf.
61. Food and Drug Administration. Regulatory Controls – Introduction. *www.fda.gov.* [Online] June 26, 2014. [Cited: August 30, 2014.] http://www.fda.gov/MedicalDevices/DeviceRegulationandGuidance/Overview/GeneralandSpecialControls/.
62. Food and Drug Administration. General Controls for Medical Devices. *www.fda.gov.* [Online] June 26, 2014. [Cited: August 30, 2014.] http://www.fda.gov/MedicalDevices/DeviceRegulationandGuidance/Over-view/GeneralandSpecialControls/ucm055910.htm#records_and_reports.
63. Food and Drug Administration. FD&C Act Chapter VII, Section 702 (Title 21, §372) Examinations and investigations. *www.gpo.gov.* [Online]

[Cited: April 28, 2014.] http://www.gpo.gov/fdsys/pkg/USCODE-2010-title21/pdf/USCODE-2010-title21-chap9-subchapVII-partA-sec372.pdf.

64. Food and Drug Administration. Medical Device Exemptions 510(k) and GMP Requirements – Class I and Class II Exempt Devices. *www.accessdata.fda.gov.* [Online] [Cited: April 28, 2014.] http://www.accessdata.fda.gov/scripts/cdrh/cfdocs/cfpcd/315.cfm.
65. Food and Drug Administration. Medical Device Exemptions 510(k) and GMP Requirements – Part 862 Clinical Chemistry and Clinical Toxicology Devices. *www.accessdata.fda.gov.* [Online] [Cited: April 28, 2014.] http://www.accessdata.fda.gov/scripts/cdrh/cfdocs/cfpcd/315.cfm?GMPPart=862#start.
66. Food and Drug Administration. Product Classification – Ventilator, Emergency, Powered (Resuscitator). *www.accessdata.fda.gov.* [Online] August 4, 2014. [Cited: August 10, 2014.] http://www.accessdata.fda.gov/scripts/cdrh/cfdocs/cfPCD/classification.cfm?ID=19.
67. Food and Drug Administration. FD&C Act Chapter V, Section 510(k) (Title 21, §360) Report preceding introduction of devices into interstate commerce. *www.gpo.gov.* [Online] [Cited: April 28, 2014.] http://www.gpo.gov/fdsys/pkg/USCODE-2010-title21/pdf/USCODE-2010-title21-chap9-subchapV-partA-sec360.pdf.
68. Food and Drug Administration. Medical Device Exemptions 510(k) and GMP Requirements. *www.accessdata.fda.gov.* [Online] September 1, 2014. [Cited: September 1, 2014.] http://www.accessdata.fda.gov/scripts/cdrh/cfdocs/cfpcd/315.cfm.
69. Food and Drug Administration. 21 CFR Part 888 – Orthopaedic Devices, Section 888.9 Limitations of Exemptions from Section 510(k) of the FD&C Act. *www.accessdata.fda.gov.* [Online] June 1, 2013. [Cited: August 30, 2014.] http://www.accessdata.fda.gov/scripts/cdrh/cfdocs/cfcfr/CFRSearch.cfm?fr=888.9.
70. Pharmaceuticals and Medical Devices Agency. Regulatory system for Medical Devices in Japan. *www.std.pmda.go.jp.* [Online] [Cited: April 28, 2014.] http://www.std.pmda.go.jp/scripts/stdDB/pubeng/stdDB_pubeng_regulation.cgi.
71. Ministry of Health, Labor and Welfare. Medical Device Registration in Japan. *www.emergogroup.com.* [Online] April 2012. [Cited: August 10, 2014.] http://www.emergogroup.com/files/japan-webinar-presentation-slides-april-2012.pdf.

72. Regulatory Affairs Professionals Society. *Fundamentals of Japanese Regulatory Affairs, First Edition.* Rockville, MD 20852 : Regulatory Affairs Professionals Society, 2010.
73. Pharmaceuticals and Medical Devices Agency. MHLW Ministerial Ordinance No. 169. *www.pmda.go.jp.* [Online] December 17, 2004. [Cited: April 28, 2014.] http://www.pmda.go.jp/english/service/pdf/ministerial/050909betsu3.pdf.
74. European Commission. Directive 98/79/EC of the European Parliament and of the Council of 27 October 1998 on in vitro diagnostic medical devices. *eur-lex.europa.eu.* [Online] [Cited: April 28, 2014.] http://eur-lex.europa.eu/legal-content/en/ALL/?uri=CELEX:31998L0079.
75. Global Harmonization Taskforce. GHTF SG1/N78:2012 Principles of Conformity Assessment for Medical Devices. *www.imdrf.org.* [Online] November 2, 2012. [Cited: April 28, 2014.] http://www.imdrf.org/docs/ghtf/final/sg1/technical-docs/ghtf-sg1-n78-2012-conformity-assessment-medical-devices-121102.pdf.
76. Global Harmonization Taskforce. GHTF SG1/N046:2008 Principles of Conformity Assessment for In Vitro Diagnostic (IVD) Medical Devices. *www.imdrf.org.* [Online] July 31, 2008. [Cited: August 10, 2014.] http://www.imdrf.org/docs/ghtf/final/sg1/procedural-docs/ghtf-sg1-n046-2008-principles-of-ca-for-ivd-medical-devices-080731.pdf.
77. Therapeutic Goods Administration. International cooperation. *www.tga.gov.au.* [Online] October 28, 2014. [Cited: October 30, 2014.] https://www.tga.gov.au/international-cooperation.
78. European Commission. Mutual recognition agreements. *ec.europa.eu.* [Online] October 16, 2014. [Cited: October 30, 2014.] http://ec.europa.eu/enterprise/policies/single-market-goods/international-aspects/mutual-recognition-agreement/index_en.htm.
79. Pharmaceuticals and Medical Devices Agency. PMDA List of Registered certification Bodies (RCBs). *www.pmda.go.jp.com.* [Online] [Cited: October 3, 2014.] http://www.pmda.go.jp/operations/shonin/info/attestation/ninsyokikan.html.
80. Food and Drug Administration. Third Party Review. *www.fda.gov.* [Online] June 25, 2014. [Cited: October 3, 2014.] http://www.fda.gov/medicaldevices/deviceregulationandguidance/howtomarketyourdevice/premarketsubmissions/thirdparyreview/default.htm.

Chapter 2

Safety and Effectiveness

This chapter explains what safety and effectiveness mean in the context of Medical Devices Regulations and what is required to demonstrate that a medical device is safe and effective. There are two main areas a manufacturer needs to address, product compliance with Essential Requirements/Principles of safety and effectiveness and quality management system compliance with relevant standards and regulations. The reader is introduced to standards and their use, the risk management process and clinical evaluation.

2.1 What are Safety and Effectiveness?

Intuitively, we know that a safe and effective medical technology is one that works as intended and causes no undue harm. The main purpose of regulations concerning healthcare products such as drugs, biologics and medical devices is to ensure that only safe and effective products are placed on the market or put into service, in the interest of public health and the welfare of patients, healthcare

Medical Device Regulatory Practices: An International Perspective
Val Theisz

ISBN 978-981-4669-10-8 (Hardcover), 978-981-4669-11-5 (eBook)
www.panstanford.com

professionals and the wider community. But what do *safety* and *effectiveness* actually mean?

2.1.1 *Safety*

Safety is a relative concept defined in terms of a risk. A definition of safety can be found in the International Organization for Standardization/International Electrotechnical Commission (ISO/IEC) Guide 51, which states that safety is "freedom from risk which is not tolerable", risk being the combination of the probability of occurrence of harm and the severity of that harm. Tolerable risk is the "level of risk that is accepted in a given context based on the current values of society" [1]. Obviously, as science and technology advance and society expectations grow, risk that was considered tolerable at one point in time may subsequently become unacceptable.

According to the Food and Drug Administration (FDA) regulations:

> There is reasonable assurance that a device is safe when it can be determined, based upon valid scientific evidence, that the probable benefits to health from use of the device for its intended uses and conditions of use, when accompanied by adequate directions and warnings against unsafe use, outweigh any probable risks. The valid scientific evidence used to determine the safety of a device shall adequately demonstrate the absence of unreasonable risk of illness or injury associated with the use of the device for its intended uses and conditions of use [2].

No healthcare product, be it a medical device, drug or biologic, is 100% safe. They inherently carry a certain degree of risk, and often a problem cannot be detected until sufficient experience is gained from their use. The current approach is to manage the risk, that is, to identify and mitigate hazards as much as possible, and accept residual risks if, on the whole, the benefits outweigh the risks. For medical devices this approach is illustrated in the Essential Requirements or Essential Principles of safety and effectiveness (also referred to as ERs or EPs), defined in various medical device regulations and the Global Harmonization Taskforce (GHTF) SG1/N68:2012 guidance *Essential Principles of Safety and Performance of Medical Devices.* The first Essential Principle states the following:

> Medical devices should be designed and manufactured in such a way that, when used under the conditions and for the purposes intended and, where applicable, by virtue of the technical knowledge, experience, education or training of intended users, they will not compromise the clinical condition or the safety of patients, or the safety and health of users or, where applicable, other persons, provided that any risks which may be associated with their use constitute acceptable risks when weighed against the benefits to the patient and are compatible with a high level of protection of health and safety [3].

Product safety standards, including safety standards for medical devices, require that safety be maintained, not just during normal operation when the device is used as intended by the manufacturer, but also in single-fault conditions, for instance, due to a component failure. In other words, the device must not cause harm even when a single abnormal condition is present or when a single means for reducing a risk is defective. Although the device is not expected to continue to function normally under single-fault conditions, it must fail safely, that is, it must remain free of unacceptable risk.

The IEC 60601-1 safety standard for medical electrical equipment distinguishes between basic safety and essential performance. Basic safety is defined as "freedom from unacceptable risk directly caused by physical hazards when medical electrical equipment is used under normal condition and single fault condition", whereas essential performance is defined as "performance of a clinical function, other than that related to basic safety, where loss or degradation beyond the limits specified by the manufacturer results in an unacceptable risk" [4]. Essential performance is closely related to effectiveness.

2.1.2 *Effectiveness*

Effectiveness is a relative concept defined in terms of a benefit. Every medical device is designed for a purpose that must be declared by the manufacturer in the medical device labelling (user manual, instructions for use, advertising and promotional material). A device is effective when it delivers the outcome for which it was designed. For example, a ventricular assist device (VAD) is expected to provide circulatory support in patients with heart failure, and the manufacturer must provide objective, scientific evidence that the device does in fact work as intended. Providing circulatory support represents essential performance for a VAD, because loss or degradation beyond the limits specified by the manufacturer would result in an unacceptable risk.

Effectiveness is expressed as a statistically significant effect on a clinically meaningful endpoint. The FDA frames effectiveness as follows:

> There is reasonable assurance that a device is effective when it can be determined, based upon valid scientific evidence, that in a significant portion of the target population, the use of the device for its intended uses and conditions of use, when accompanied by adequate directions for use and warnings against unsafe use, will provide clinically significant results [2].

The terms "effectiveness" and "efficacy" are often used interchangeably, but there is a subtle difference between them. In its guidance *Providing Clinical Evidence of Effectiveness for Human Drug and Biological Products* the FDA states that *effectiveness* refers to the regulatory determination that is made on the basis of clinical efficacy and other data (i.e., reality), whereas *efficacy* refers to the findings in an adequate and well-controlled clinical trial or the intent of conducting such a trial (i.e., expectation). Efficacy is a narrower definition that means how well something works in an ideal or controlled setting, such as a clinical trial, whereas effectiveness describes how well it works under real-world conditions [5]. In other words, efficacy is effectiveness under an ideal controlled setting.

2.1.3 *Related Terminology*

Safety and effectiveness are minimum requirements for a medical device to be acceptable and receive regulatory approval. They are good indicators of a device's overall *performance*. Performance, however, encompasses technical functionalities in addition to the clinical effectiveness. For example, the performance of medical devices with measuring functions and in vitro diagnostics (IVD) would typically include characteristics and measures such as:

- Sensitivity – estimation of the proportion of subjects with the target condition in whom a test is positive;
- Specificity – estimation of the proportion of subjects without the target condition in whom the test is negative;
- Accuracy – trueness and precision when compared to a reference standard;
- Repeatability and reproducibility; and
- Control of known relevant interference and limits of detection.

Effectiveness is always expressed in relation to the intended purpose of a medical device. The terms "indications for use" and "intended use" are often used interchangeably, but regulators make a distinction between the two.

Indications for use are defined by FDA regulations as "a general description of the disease or condition the device will diagnose, treat, prevent, cure, or mitigate, including a description of the patient population for which the device is intended" [6].

Intended use means the general purpose of the medical device, as declared by the manufacturer in the device labelling and it includes the indications for use. ISO 14971 standard *Medical devices — Application of risk management to medical devices* defines *intended use* as the "intended purpose use for which a product, process or service is intended according to the specifications, instructions and information provided by the manufacturer" [7].

Differences in the indications for use, such as the population for which a device is intended or the disease a device is intended to treat, may result in a new intended use if they affect (or may affect) the safety and/or effectiveness of the device. For example, changing from an adult to a paediatric population represents a change in indications for use that raises new questions of safety and effectiveness hence results in a new intended use (8 pp. 15–18).

2.2 Essential Requirements/Principles of Safety and Effectiveness

The European Union (EU) pioneered the New Approach concept in 1985, which confined the content of legislation to *essential requirements* leaving the technical details to European Harmonised Standards. This represented a significant departure from the old approach, in which national authorities drew up technical legislation, going into great detail – usually motivated by a lack of confidence in the rigour of economic operators on issues of public health and safety.

The aim of the New Approach has been to eliminate barriers to trade and facilitate the free movement of goods within the EU, while ensuring that only safe and otherwise compliant products find their way on to the market, in such a way that honest economic operators can benefit from a level playing field, thus promoting at the same time an effective protection of EU consumers and professional users and a competitive single EU market (9 p. 6).

European medical devices directives were the first medical device regulations to define a generic set of high-level Essential Requirements of safety and effectiveness for medical devices (ERs), initially in 1990 as part of the Active Implantable Medical Device (AIMD) Directive (AIMDD), then in 1993 as part of the MDD and in 1998 in the IVD Directive (IVDD).

- The AIMDD defines 16 ERs – 5 general requirements and 11 requirements regarding design and construction [10].
- The MDD defines 13 ERs – 6 general requirements and 7 requirements regarding design and construction [11].
- The IVDD defines 13 ERs – 5 general requirements and 8 design and manufacturing requirements [12].

In 1995 GHTF Study Group 1 published the first version of its guidance document *Essential Principles of Safety and Performance of Medical Devices*, which formed the basis for similar generic safety and effectiveness requirements in regulations in Australia, Canada and Japan, as well as the Association of Southeast Asian Nations (ASEAN) MDD, or shortly AMDD.

- The GHTF guidance lists 6 EPs applicable to all medical devices, including IVDs, and 14 EPs applicable to medical devices other than IVDs [3].
- Australian regulations define 6 general EPs and 9 EPs about design and constructions covering medical devices and IVDs [13]
- Canadian regulations define 11 safety and effectiveness requirements and 3 labelling requirements [14]
- Japanese regulations define 6 general ERs and 10 ERs for design and manufacturing (15 pp. 170–171)
- The AMDD has 19 EPs - 7 general requirements and 12 design and manufacturing requirements [16].

The FDA regulations pre-date the EU medical devices directives and the GHTF; hence they do not define a similar list of generic ERs or EPs. Instead, the FDA publishes guidance documents for specific categories of medical devices such as hearing aid devices, apnea monitors and pacemakers. A closer look at the FDA guidance documents for the content of a Premarket Notification 510(k) [17] and a Premarket Approval (PMA) [18] reveals that the elements required in an FDA submission align quite well with the ERs or EPs, as shown in Table 1.1.

Depending on what the target markets are, the Australian, Canadian and Japanese ERs/EPs can be added to Table 1.1 to provide the consolidated regulatory input into the design and development process (see Fig. 2.1).

Identifying applicable ERs/EPs upfront helps development project teams to plan the verification and validation activities and build the required traceability to demonstrate that the ERs/EPs for a particular jurisdiction have been met. This approach will avoid re-work caused by situations where not enough or too much testing is done during development [19].

Table 2.1 Comparative table with ERs for medical devices from the EU MDD, AIMDD and IVDD; GHTF N68 guidance; draft AMDD; and FDA requirements for submission contents

EU AIMDD ERs 90/385/EEC (2007 status)	EU MDD ERs 93/42/EEC (2007 status)	EU IVD ERs 98/79/EC (2009 status)	GHTF EPs SG1/N68:2012	AMDD EPs (2012 draft)	FDA 510(k) substantial equivalence information	FDA PMA content: checklist for acceptance review
I. General requirements						
1. Risk management	1. Risk management and usability	A1 Risk management	A1 Risk management and usability B12 Usability for laypersons	1 Risk management and usability	Human factors	Risk–benefit analysis
6. Safety principles and state of the art	2. Safety principles for risk reduction and state of the art	A2 Safety principles for risk reduction and state of the art	A2 Safety principles and state of the art	2 Safety principles and state of the art	Standards met	-
2. Performance according to indications for use and intended use	3. Performance according to indications for use and intended use	A3 Performance according to indicated purpose and state of the art (sensitivity, specificity, repeatability, reproducibility)	A3 Performance according to indications for use and intended use	3 Performance according to indications for use and intended use	Intended use; where used (hospital, home, ambulance) Indications for use; target population; anatomical sites Performance	Indications for use Principle of operation
3. Reliability	4. Reliability	A4 Reliability	A4 Reliability	4 Reliability	Performance	Engineering studies (stress, wear)

4. Transport and storage	5. Transport and storage	A5 Transport and storage	A5 Transport and storage	5 Transport and storage	Performance	Engineering studies (stress, wear) Shelf life studies
5. Undesirable side effects and clinical evaluation	6. Undesirable side effects and clinical evaluation	–	A6 Undesirable side effects	6 Undesirable side effects 7 Clinical evaluation	Performance	Contraindications, Warnings and pre-cautions Potential adverse effects
II. Requirements regarding design and construction/manufacturing					Standards met	Laboratory studies, animal studies, additional studies
9. Material toxicity; biocompatibility; compatibility with other substances; ingress and egress protection; combination with medicinal substances, blood derivatives	7. Chemical, physical and biological properties	B1 Chemical and physical properties – leakage, contaminants and residues	B1 Chemical, physical and biological properties B3 Combination with medicinal product/drug	8 Chemical, physical and biological properties	Materials Biocompatibility Chemical safety	Biological/ microbiological studies Immunological studies Toxicological/ biocompatibility studies Chemistry/analytical studies
7. Non-reusable sterile packs	8. Infection and microbial contamination: non-reusable sterile packs	B2 Infection and microbial contamination – biological substances; sterile packs	B2 Infection and microbial contamination B4 Materials of biological origin	9 Infection and microbial contamination	Sterility	Sterilization

(*Contd.*)

Table 2.1 *(Contd.)*

EU AIMDD ERs 90/385/EEC (2007 status)	EU MDD ERs 93/42/EEC (2007 status)	EU IVD ERs 98/79/EC (2009 status)	GHTF EPs SG1/N68:2012	AMDD EPs (2012 draft)	FDA 510(k) substantial equivalence information	FDA PMA content: checklist for acceptance review
8. Physical features; interference with other equipment 9. Connections	9. Construction and environmental properties – physical and ergonomic features, flammability, interferences	B3 Manufacturing and environmental properties – physical and ergonomic features, flammability, safe waste disposal	B5 Environmental properties B9 Active implantable medical devices and devices connected to them	10 Manufacturing and environmental properties 16 Active implantable medical devices	Design Compatibility with the environment and other devices Mechanical safety	Safety and effectiveness studies
8. Accuracy of measuring and control mechanisms	10.Devices with a measuring function	B4 Instruments or apparatus with a measuring function	B6 Devices with a diagnostic or measuring function	11 Devices with a diagnostic or measuring function	Performance	Safety and effectiveness studies
8. Ionizing radiation	11. Protection against radiation	B5 Protection against radiation	B7 Protection against radiation	12 Protection against radiation	Radiation safety	Safety and effectiveness studies

8. Electrical safety; thermal risks; electromagnetic compatibility (EMC) 9. Reliability of energy source; software	12. Requirements for medical devices connected to or equipped with an energy source – programmable systems	B6 Requirements for medical devices connected to or equipped with an energy source – programmable systems	B8 Software B9 AIMDs and devices connected to them B10 Mechanical safety B11 Supplied energy or substances	13 Requirements for medical devices connected to or equipped with an energy source 14 Mechanical safety 15 Supplied energy or substances	Electrical safety Mechanical safety Thermal safety	Safety and effectiveness studies
–	–	B7 Requirements for devices for self-testing	–	17 Devices for self-testing or self-administration	Performance	Safety and effectiveness studies
11. Identification of device and component parts 12. Unique code readable without surgical operation 13. Visual indicators 14. Markings on the device and its packaging 15. Instructions for use (IFUs)	13. Information supplied by the manufacturer	B8 Information supplied by the manufacturer	B13 Label and instructions for use (IFUs)	18 Information supplied by the product owner	Device labeling	Physician labelling Patient labelling Technical/operators manual
16. Clinical evaluation	6. Clinical evaluation	–	–	19 Clinical investigation	–	Clinical studies

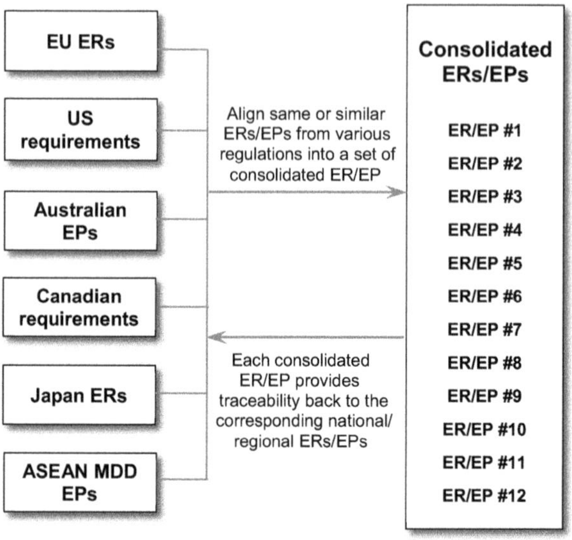

Figure 2.1 Diagram representing the concept of aligning ERs/EPs defined by various regulations into a consolidated set of ERs/EPs to be used as input into the product development process.

2.3 Quality Management System

Ensuring that the design and manufacturing of a medical device comply with the safety and effectiveness requirements is essential but in itself not enough. A manufacturer must also ensure that these requirements are met *consistently*, and this is achieved by establishing and maintaining a quality management system (QMS) according to relevant regulations, standards and guidelines.

The main processes in a medical device manufacturer that typically require regulatory controls are:

- Design controls
- Device identification and tracking controls
- Document controls
- Change controls
- Manufacturing process controls, including sterilization process controls, if applicable
- Equipment and facilities environmental controls

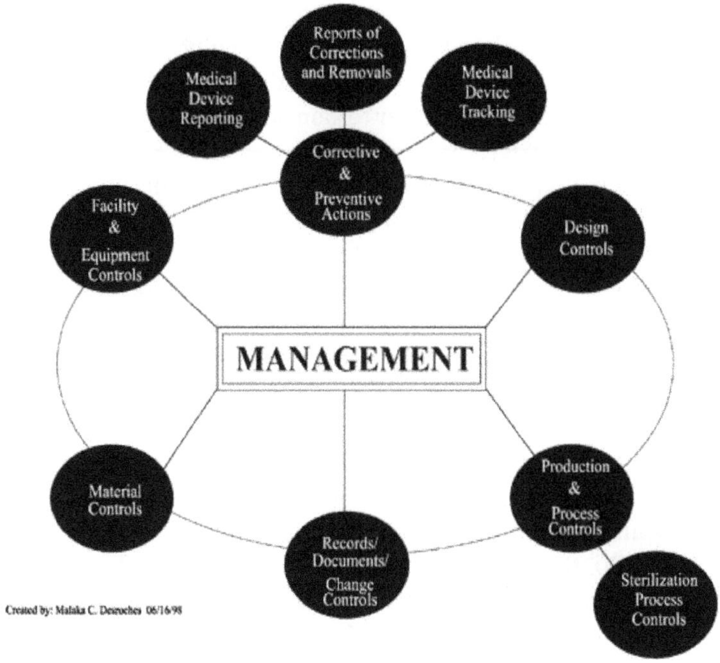

Figure 2.2 A representation of QMS sub-systems. *Source*: FDA *Quality System Inspection Technique (QSIT) Manual.*

- Suppliers and material controls
- Corrective actions and preventive actions (CAPAs), including reporting of corrections, product removals and adverse events

The management of an organization is responsible for putting in place an adequate organizational structure with well-defined roles and responsibilities, for making available adequate resources and for appointing a management representative who is independent from all other functions and who reports regularly on the suitability and effectiveness of the quality system. The diagram in Fig. 2.2 represents the typical QMS sub-systems and processes with management at its centre.

In the United States, the regulatory requirements for quality systems are stipulated in *Code of Federal Regulations* (CFR): 21

CFR Part 820, *Quality System Regulation* (QSR). The QSR, effective since June 1997, replaced the 1978 Good Manufacturing Practice (GMP) regulation. The FDA emphasizes the importance of reading the preamble to the QSR in order to gain an insight into the meaning and intent of the QSR [20].

In other regions and countries compliance with the international standard ISO 13485:2003, *Medical devices – Quality management systems – Requirements for regulatory purposes*, is the best way to demonstrate quality system compliance with regulatory requirements. ISO 13485:2003 is the second edition that has been technically revised by a corrigendum in 2009; therefore the revised version of the second edition will be referred to as ISO 13485:2009.

The ISO/TR 14969:2004 technical report provides guidance on the application of the ISO 13485:2003 standard. It has useful interpretations and examples that guide medical device manufacturers in establishing a quality management system (QMS).

In the EU, the European version of ISO 13485 is a harmonized European Norms (EN) standard published in *Official Journal of the European Union* (*OJ*) (EN ISO 13485:2012) and as such it provides a presumption of conformity with most, but not all, quality systems requirements of the medical devices directives. Annexes ZA, ZB and ZC in EN ISO 13485 include comparative tables showing the relationship between the clauses in the standard and the regulatory requirements for quality systems in the AIMD, the MD and the IVD directive, respectively. For example, the following requirements in Annex II of the MDD are not covered in EN ISO 13485:2012:

> 3. Quality system
>
> 3.1 The manufacturer must lodge an application for assessment of his quality system with a notified body.
>
> The application must include:
>
> - the name and address of the manufacturer and any additional manufacturing site covered by the quality system,
> - all the relevant information on the product or product category covered by the procedure,
> - a written declaration that no application has been lodged with any other notified body for the same product-related quality system, [...]

- an undertaking by the manufacturer to institute and keep up to date a systematic procedure to review experience gained from devices in the post-production phase, including the provisions referred to in Annex X [Clinical Evaluation], and to implement appropriate means to apply any necessary corrective action. This undertaking must include an obligation for the manufacturer to notify the competent authorities of the following incidents immediately on learning of them:
  (i) any malfunction or deterioration in the characteristics and/or performance of a device, as well as any inadequacy in the instructions for use which might lead or might have led to the death of a patient or user or to a serious deterioration in his state of health;
  (ii) any technical or medical reason connected with the characteristics or performance of a device leading for the reasons referred to in subparagraph (i) to systematic recall of devices of the same type by the manufacturer.

Although there are some differences between the FDA QSR and the ISO 13485:2009 standard, there are no conflicting requirements. For instance, the QSR includes specific requirements on device labelling and packaging, which do not need to be included in the ISO 13485 because they are covered in the ERs/EPs of various regulations. Also, the ISO 13485 standard has sections on customer focus that the FDA QSR does not, and that's because ISO 13485 is based on the ISO 9001 standard for generic quality systems, which includes requirements on customer satisfaction [21].

Table 2.2 provides a side-by-side comparison between the main requirements of the FDA QSR and the ISO 13485 standard. Obviously, the most efficient and effective way is to put in place one set of coherent QMS procedures describing the processes and controls that meet both the FDA QSR and the ISO 13485 requirements.

The new revision of ISO 13485, still in draft at the time this book went to print but expected to be released sometime in the near future will, once published, replace the existing version of the standard. The new revision of ISO 13485 puts even more emphasis on compliance with regulatory requirements, such as:

Table 2.2 Comparison between FDA QSR and ISO 13485:2009

FDA QSR: 1997	ISO 13485:2009
Subpart A General Provisions	-
§820.1 Scope	**Section 1 Scope**
-	**Section 2 Normative References**
§820.3 Definitions	**Section 3 Terms and Definitions**
§820.5 Quality system	Sub-section 4.1 General requirements
Subpart B Quality System Requirements	Sub-section 4.1 General requirements
§820.20 Management responsibility	**Section 5 Management Responsibility**
-	Sub-section 5.2 Customer focus
§820.22 Quality audit	Sub-section 8.2.2 Internal audit
§820.25 Personnel	Sub-section 6.2 Human resources
Subpart C Design Controls	**Section 7 Product Realization**
§820.30 Design controls	Sub-section 7.3 Design and development
Subpart D Document Controls	**Section 4 Quality Management System**
§820.40 Document controls	Sub-section 4.2.3 Control of documents
Subpart E Purchasing Controls	**Section 7 Product Realization**
§820.50 Purchasing controls	Sub-section 7.4 Purchasing
Subpart F Identification and Traceability	**Section 7 Product Realization**
§820.60 Identification	Sub-section 7.5.3 Identification and traceability
§820.65 Traceability	Sub-section 7.5.3 Identification and traceability
Subpart G Production and Process Controls	**Section 7 Product Realization**
§820.70 Production and process controls	Sub-section 6.3 Infrastructure Sub-section 6.4 Work environment
§820.72 Inspection, measuring and test equipment	Sub-section 7.6 Control of monitoring and measuring devices
§820.75 Process validation	Sub-section 7.5.2 Validation of processes for production and service provision
Subpart H Acceptance Activities	**Section 8 Measurement, Analysis and Improvement**
§820.80 Receiving, in-process, and finished device acceptance	Sub-section 8.2.4 Monitoring and measurement of product
§820.86 Acceptance status	Sub-section 8.2.4 Monitoring and measurement of product
Subpart I Nonconforming product	**Section 8 Measurement, Analysis and Improvement**
§820.90 Nonconforming product	Sub-section 8.3 Control of nonconforming product
Subpart J Corrective and Preventive Action	**Section 8 Measurement, Analysis and Improvement**

(Contd.)

Table 2.2 *(Contd.)*

FDA QSR: 1997	ISO 13485:2009
§820.100 Corrective and preventive action	Sub-section 8.5 Improvement
Subpart K Labeling and Packaging Controls	-
§820.120 Device labeling	Covered in the ERs/EPs
§820.130 Device packaging	Covered in the ERs/EPs
Subpart L Handling, Storage, Distribution and Installation	**Section 8 Measurement, Analysis and Improvement**
§820.140 Handling	Sub-section 6.4 Work environment Sub-section 7.5.1.2.1 Cleanliness of product and contamination control
§820.150 Storage	Sub-section 6.4 Work environment Sub-section 7.5.1.2.1 Cleanliness of product and contamination control
§820.160 Distribution	Sub-section 7.5.1.1 General requirements (Control of production and service provision) Sub-section 7.5.3.2.2 Particular requirements for implants
§820.170 Installation	Sub-section 7.5.1.2.2 Installation activities
Subpart M Records	**Section 4 Quality Management System**
§820.180 General requirements	Sub-section 4.2.4 Control of records
§820.181 Device master record	-
§820.184 Device history record	-
§820.186 Quality system record	Sub-section 4.2.2 Quality manual
§820.198 Complaint files	Sub-section 7.2.3 Customer communication
Subpart N Servicing	**Section 7 Product Realization**
§820.200 Servicing	Sub-section 7.5.1.2.3 Servicing activities
Subpart O Statistical Techniques	**Section 8 Measurement, Analysis and Improvement**
§820.250 Statistical techniques	Sub-section 8.1 General (Measurement, analysis and improvement)

- Risk-based approach and risk management;
- Clinical data;
- Post-market surveillance;
- Validation of the application of computer software used in the QMS;
- Particular requirements for sterile medical devices;
- Communication with regulatory authorities;
- Design and development transfer; and
- Design and development records.

2.4 Standards

2.4.1 *General Principles and the Use of Standards*

Standards are technical specifications that provide solutions for compliance with a legal provision at a level of detail that cannot be included in regulations. They reflect the opinion of experts in a particular area, such as sterilization, biocompatibility, electrical safety and electromagnetic compatibility, or for a particular category of devices. Unless specified otherwise in regulations, compliance with standards is voluntary.

International standards represent a tool for harmonizing requirements for safety, quality and performance of medical devices. By encouraging convergence at the international level standards facilitate trade and promote the use of state-of-the-art best practices for the benefit of patients, healthcare professionals and the larger community. The voluntary nature of standards allows individual countries to regulate the protection of public health by means they consider the most appropriate.

In Europe, compliance with Harmonised Standards published in the *OJ* confers a presumption of conformity with mandatory ERs. The relationship between clauses of an EN standard and ERs of a European directive is tabled in annexes of the EN standard. The list of standards applicable to each European directive is available from the official website of the European Commission [22].

In the United States, conformance with Recognized Consensus Standards can support a reasonable assurance of safety and effectiveness for many applicable aspects of medical devices and may help establish the substantial equivalence of a new device to a legally marketed predicate device. A searchable database with consensus standards recognized by the FDA is available on the agency's website [23].

Medical device regulators in Australia, Canada and Japan also publish lists of standards that can be used to demonstrate compliance with the requirements for safety and effectiveness in their respective jurisdictions [24–27].

However, conformance with standards may not always be a sufficient basis for obtaining regulatory approvals if, for instance, a specific device may raise a safety or effectiveness issue not addressed by any published standard or a specific regulation may require additional information beyond what conformity to standards provides [28].

The ISO ISO/TR 16142:2006 technical report, *Medical devices – Guidance on the selection of standards in support of recognized essential principles of safety and performance of medical devices*, defines three categories of standards:

- **Basic or horizontal standards** – include fundamental concepts, principles and requirements with regard to general aspects applicable to a wide range of products, processes or services (e.g., risk management, clinical investigation, symbols and the QMSs for medical devices);
- **Group or semi-horizontal standards** – cover safety and essential performance aspects applicable to several or a family of similar products, processes or services dealt with by two or more technical committees or subcommittees, making reference, as far as possible, to basic standards (e.g., EMC, software and programmable electrical medical systems, stability of IVD reagents, sterility); and
- **Product or vertical standards** – cover all necessary safety and essential performance aspects of a specific or a family of products, processes or services within the scope of a single technical committee or subcommittee, making reference, as far as possible, to basic standards and group standards (e.g., standards for infusion pumps, for anaesthetic machines or for blood glucose meters for self-testing).

The following are examples of basic, group and product standards applicable to electrically powered medical devices:

- IEC 60601-1, *Medical electrical equipment – Part 1: General requirements for basic safety and essential performance*, is a basic/horizontal standard. Its structure is hazard specific in that it provides requirements for evaluating the common hazards associated with electrical medical devices.
- IEC 60601-1-2, *Medical electrical equipment – Part 1-2: General requirements for basic safety and essential perfor-*

mance – Collateral standard: Electromagnetic disturbances – Requirements and tests, is a group/semi-horizontal standard covering EMC requirements for all electrical medical equipment.

- IEC 60601-1-6, *Medical electrical equipment – Part 1-6: General requirements for basic safety and essential performance – Collateral standard: Usability*, is a group/semi-horizontal standard covering usability requirements for all electrical medical equipment.
- IEC 60601-2-4, *Medical electrical equipment – Part 2-4: Particular requirements for the basic safety and essential performance of cardiac defibrillators*, is a product-specific/vertical standard for cardiac defibrillators.

Collateral (group) and product standards refer to certain basic standards they are related to for compliance with common hazards. When basic standards are revised, the related collateral and product standards may have to be revised as well to bring them in line with the basic standards.

Manufacturers need to manage carefully claims of compliance to standards in their technical documentation, as compliance with a particular version of a collateral standard is always linked to the version of the basic standard that is referenced in the collateral standard (see also example in Fig. 2.3).

Collateral standards IEC 60601-1-2 Ed. 3.0 and IEC 60601-1-6 Ed. 2.0 were the versions related to basic standard IEC 60601-1:2005 Ed. 3.0.

2.4.2 *Standards Organizations*

International and European standards organizations are independent, not-for-profit, non-governmental bodies, whose members are national standardization bodies (see also Table 2.3). Standards are developed on a consensus-based approach by a panel of experts, within a technical committee. The technical committees are made up of experts from the relevant industry and other stakeholders such as regulators, consumer associations, science and academia.

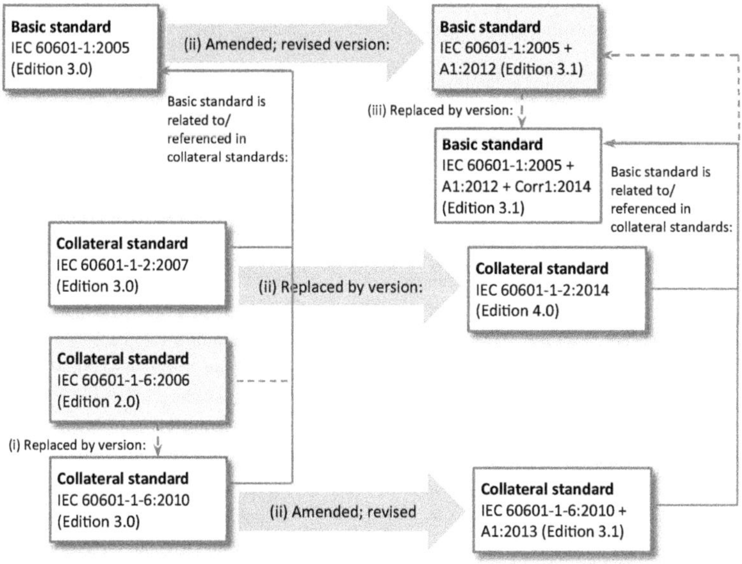

Figure 2.3 Referencing versions of related basic and collateral standards correctly; example of IEC 60601-1 basic standard and two of its collateral standards - IEC 60601-1-2 and IEC 60601-1-6.

(i) In 2010 IEC 60601-1-6 Ed. 2.0 was revised to Ed. 3.0, which became related to IEC 60601-1:2005 Ed. 3.0.

(ii) In 2012 the basic standard IEC 60601-1 was revised from Ed. 3.0 to Ed. 3.1. Collateral standards IEC 60601-1-2 and IEC 60601-1-6 had to be revised to Ed. 4.0 and 3.1, respectively, to align with IEC 60601-1:2012 Ed. 3.1.

(iii) In 2014 a corrigendum was added to the basic standard IEC 60601-1:2012 Ed. 3.1, so the latest version of the basic standard became IEC 60601-1:2014 Ed. 3.1. Since the corrigendum did not affect the collateral standards, the same versions of IEC 60601-1-2 and IEC 60601-1-6 remain related to IEC 60601-1:2014 Ed. 3.1.

Typically, international standards (ISO, IEC) are published first and then adopted with or without modifications (deviations) by European and national standardization bodies.

Manufacturers need to manage carefully situations where they need to comply both with state-of-the-art requirements defined in the latest version of an international standard (refer also to

Table 2.3 International and European standards organizations developing standards relevant to medical devices including IVDs

International and European standards organizations		Membership (as of October 2014)
ISO	International Organization for Standardization	165 member countries
IEC	International Electrotechnical Commission	83 member countries: 60 full members and 23 associate members
CISPR	International Special Committee on Radio Interference	40 full members: 27 participating countries and 13 observer countries
CEN	European Committee for Standardization	28 EU countries, Republic of Macedonia, Turkey plus three EFTAS countries: Iceland, Norway and Switzerland
CENELEC	European Committee for Electrotechnical Standardization	33 full members: 28 EU countries, Iceland, Norway, Switzerland, Republic of Macedonia, Turkey plus 13 affiliates from Eastern Europe, the Middle East and Africa
ETSI	European Telecommunications Standards Institute	Over 750 member organizations from 63 countries across 5 continents worldwide

Table 1.1, second row after I. General requirements) and the version of a standard listed as providing a presumption of conformity with ERs/EPs, for instance, an EN Harmonised Standard that may be equivalent to a previous version of the same international standard. Especially when relevant to existing or potential safety adverse events the new scientific knowledge contained in the latest international standards should be taken into consideration as part of the risk management process [29].

2.4.3 *Example of List of Standards Applicable to Medical Devices*

Manufacturers need to determine which standards apply to their products (see example in Table 2.4) and whether there are any national deviations applicable to their target markets.

Table 2.4 Example of a list of standards that may apply to a company's medical devices (shown standards versions may not be the most current at the time of going to print)

Standard category	Title	International standards	EN Harmonised Standards	FDA Recognized Consensus Standards
Risk management (basic)	Medical devices – Application of risk management to medical devices; Guidance on the application of ISO 14791	ISO 14971:2007 Ed. 2.0 ISO TR 24971:2013	EN ISO 14971:2012	ISO 14971:2007 ANSI/AAMI/ISO 14971:2007/(R)2010
General safety – medical electrical equipment (basic)	Medical electrical equipment – Part 1. General requirements for basic safety and essential performance	IEC 60601-1:2014 Ed. 3.1	EN 60601-1:2006 +A1:2013 Ed. 3.0	ANSI/AAMI ES60601-1:2005/(R)2012 +C1:2009/(R)2012
General safety – medical electrical systems (collateral)	Medical electrical equipment – Part 1-1: General requirements for safety – Collateral standard: Safety requirements for medical electrical systems	Withdrawn, incorporated in clause 16 of IEC 60601-1:2014	Withdrawn, incorporated in clause 16 of EN 60601-1:2013	–
General safety – programmable electrical medical electrical systems (collateral)	Medical electrical equipment – Part 1-4: General requirements for safety – Collateral standard: Safety requirements for programmable electrical medical systems	Withdrawn, incorporated in clause 14 of IEC 60601-1:2014	Withdrawn, incorporated in clause 14 of EN 60601-1:2013	–
Ingress protection (IP code)	Degrees of protection provided by enclosures (IP code)	IEC 60529:2013 Ed. 2.2	–	–

(*Contd.*)

Table 2.4 *(Contd.)*

Standard category	Title	International standards	EN Harmonised Standards	FDA Recognized Consensus Standards
Electromagnetic compatibility (EMC) (collateral)	Medical electrical equipment – Part 1-2: General requirements for safety – Collateral standard: Electromagnetic disturbances – Requirements and tests	IEC 60601-1-2:2014 Ed. 4.0	EN 60601-1-2:2007 + Corr:2010	IEC 60601-1-2:2014 Ed. 4.0 ANSI/AAMI/IEC 60601-1-2:2007 Ed. 3.0/(R)2012
Exposure to electromagnetic fields	Assessment of electronic and electrical equipment related to human exposure restrictions for electromagnetic fields (0 Hz – 300 GHz)	IEC 62311: 2007 Ed. 1.0	EN 62311:2008	–
	International Commission on Non-Ionizing Radiation Protection (ICNIRP) – Guidelines for limiting exposure to time-varying electric, magnetic and electromagnetic fields up to 300 GHz	ICNIRP Guidelines 1998	–	–
	Safety Levels with Respect to Human Exposure to Radio Frequency Electromagnetic Fields, 3 kHz to 300 GHz	IEEE C95.1:2005 + C95.1a:2010	–	–

	Other regulations and standards for protection against exposure to RF fields:	**Australia**: Radiation Protection Standard:2002 – Maximum Exposure Levels to Radiofrequency Fields; 3 kHz to 300 GHz (Australian Radiation Protection and Nuclear Safety Agency [ARPANSA]) **Canada**: Safety Code 6:2009 Radiofrequency Exposure Guidelines – Limits of Human Exposure to Radiofrequency Electromagnetic Energy in the Frequency Range from 3 kHz to 300 GHz; Technical Guide for Interpretation and Compliance Assessment of Health Canada's Radiofrequency Exposure Guidelines **EU**: Directive 2013/35/EU of the European Parliament and of the Council of June 26, 2013, on the minimum health and safety requirements regarding the exposure of workers to the risks arising from physical agents (electromagnetic fields up to 300 GHz) (20th individual directive within the meaning of Article 16(1) of Directive 89/391/EEC) and repealing Directive 2004/40/EC **Japan**: Exposure limits identical to those of US FCC **United States**: FCC 47 CFR Part 1 §1.1307(b), §1.1310; Part 2 §2.1091, §2.1093; Office of Engineering and Technology – OET Bulletin No. 65 (August 1997)		
Usability (collateral)	Medical electrical equipment – Part 1-6: General requirements for basic safety and essential performance - Collateral standard: Usability;	IEC 60601-1-6:2010 Ed. 3.1	EN 60601-1-6:2010	IEC 60601-1-6:2010 Ed. 3.1
	Application of usability engineering to medical devices	IEC 62366:2014 Ed. 1.1	EN 62366:2008	IEC 62366:2014 Ed. 1.1 AAMI/ANSI/IEC 62366:2007/(R)2013

(*Contd.*)

Table 2.4 *(Contd.)*

Standard category	Title	International standards	EN Harmonised Standards	FDA Recognized Consensus Standards
Alarm signals (collateral)	Medical electrical equipment – Part 1-8: General requirements for basic safety and essential performance – Collateral standard: General requirements, tests and guidance for alarm systems in medical electrical equipment and medical electrical systems	IEC 60601-1-8:2012 Ed. 2.1	EN 60601-1-8:2013 + Corr:2010 + Corr:2014	IEC 60601-1-8:2012 Ed. 2.1 AAMI/ANSI/IEC 60601-1-8 :2006 + A1:2012
Home use (collateral)	Medical electrical equipment – Part 1-11: General requirements for basic safety and essential performance – Collateral Standard: Requirements for medical electrical equipment and medical electrical systems used in the home healthcare environment	IEC 60601-1-11:2010 Ed. 1.0	EN 60601-1-11:2010	IEC 60601-1-11:2010 Ed. 1.0 ANSI/AAMI HA60601-1-11:2011
Medical device software (collateral)	Medical Device Software – Software Life Cycle Processes	IEC 62304:2006 Ed. 1.0	EN 62304:2006 +Corr:2008	IEC 62304:2006 Ed. 1.0 AAMI/ANSI/IEC 62304:2006
	Medical device software – Part 1: Guidance on the application of ISO 14971 to medical device software Part 3: Medical device software – Part 3: Process reference model of medical device software life cycle processes (IEC 62304)	IEC TR 80002-1:2009 Ed 1.0 IEC TR 80002-3:2014 Ed. 1.0	–	–

Off-the-Shelf (OTS) Software (group)	Software engineering - Systems and software product Quality Requirement and Evaluation (SQuaRE)-Requirements for quality of Ready to Use Software Product (RUSP) and instructions for testing	ISO IEC 25051: 2014	–	–
AIMDs (product)	Implants for surgery – Active implantable medical devices – Part 1: General requirements for safety, marking and for information to be provided by the manufacturer	ISO 14708-1:2014 Ed. 2.0	EN 45502-1:1997	–
Implantable neurostimulators (product)	Implants for surgery - Active implantable medical devices - Part 3: Implantable neurostimulators	ISO 14708-3:2008 Ed. 1.0	–	ISO 14708-3:2008 AAMI/ANSI/ISO 14708-3:2008/(R)2011
Magnetic resonance imaging (MRI) for patients with an AIMD (group)	Assessment of the safety of magnetic resonance imaging for patients with an active implantable medical device	ISO/TR 10974:2012	–	–
Packaging, sterile (group)	Packaging for terminally sterilized medical devices — Part 1: Requirements for materials, sterile barrier systems and packaging systems	ISO 11607-1:2006 + A1:2014 Ed. 1.0	EN ISO 11607-1:2009	ISO 11607-1:2006 Ed. 1.0 AAMI/ANSI/ISO 11607:2006/(R)2010
	Packaging for terminally sterilized medical devices — Part 2: Validation requirements for forming, sealing and assembly processes	ISO 11607-2:2006 + A1:2014 Ed. 1.0	EN ISO 11607-2:2006	ISO 11607-2:2006 Ed. 1.0 ANSI/AAMI/ISO 11607-1:2006/(R)2010

(*Contd.*)

Table 2.4 (*Contd.*)

Standard category	Title	International standards	EN Harmonised Standards	FDA Recognized Consensus Standards
Conditioning containers (group)	Standard Practice for Conditioning Containers, Packages, or Packaging Components for Testing	–	–	ASTM D4332:2013
Internal pressurization test methods (group)	Standard Test Methods for Internal Pressurization Failure Resistance of Unrestrained Packages	–	–	ASTM F1140/F1140M 2013
	Standard Test Method for Burst Testing of Flexible Package Seals Using Internal Air Pressurization Within Restraining Plates	–	–	ASTM F2054/F2054M 2013
	Standard Test Method for Detecting Gross Leaks in Packaging by Internal Pressurization (Bubble Test)	–	–	ASTM F2096: 2011
Integrity of seals (group)	Standard Test Method for Measuring Package and Seal Integrity Using Helium as the Tracer Gas	–	–	ASTM F2391: 2005/(R)2011
Detecting seal leaks (group)	Standard Test Method for Detecting Seal Leaks in Porous Medical Packaging by Dye Penetration	–	–	ASTM F1929: 2012
Accelerated ageing (group)	Standard Guide for Accelerated Aging of Sterile Barrier Systems for Medical Devices	–	–	ASTM F1980: 2007/(R)2011
Bubble test (group)	Standard Test Method for Detecting Gross Leaks in Packaging by Internal Pressurization (Bubble Test)	–	–	ASTM F2096: 2011

Evaluation flexible packaging (group)	Standard Guide for Design and Evaluation of Primary Flexible Packaging for Medical Products	–	–	ASTM F2097: 2010
Printed inks and coatings (group)	Standard Practice for Evaluation of Chemical Resistance of Printed Inks and Coatings on Flexible Packaging Materials	–	–	ASTM F2250: 2013
Seal strength – flexible barrier (group)	Standard Test Method for Seal Strength of Flexible Barrier Materials	–	–	ASTM F88/F88M: 2009
Cold	Environmental testing – Part 2-1: Tests – Test A: Cold	IEC 60068-2-1: 2007 Ed. 6.0	–	–
Dry heat	Environmental testing - Part 2-2: Tests - Test B: Dry heat	IEC 60068-2-2: 2007	–	–
Temperature change	Environmental testing. Tests. Test N. Change of temperature	IEC 60068-2-14: 2009 Ed. 6.0	–	–
Test Ea – Shock	Environmental testing - Part 2-27: Tests - Test Ea and guidance: Shock	IEC 60068-2-27: 2008 Ed. 4.0	–	–
Test Fh – Vibration, digital control	Environmental testing - Part 2-64: Tests - Test Fh: Vibration, broadband random and guidance	IEC 60068-2-64: 2008 Ed. 2.0	–	–
Test Eh – Hammer tests	Environmental testing - Part 2-75: Tests - Test Eh: Hammer tests	IEC 60068-2-75: 2014 Ed. 2.0	–	–

(*Contd.*)

Table 2.4 *(Contd.)*

Standard category	Title	International standards	EN Harmonised Standards	FDA Recognized Consensus Standards
Storage and transportation (basic)	International Safe Transit Association (ISTA) tests for: • Handling drop and impact • Transportation vibration • Stacking load • Atmospheric conditions	ISTA 2A for packaged products $\leq$ 68 kg ISTA 2B for packaged products $>$68 kg	-	-
Graphical symbols and labelling (basic)	Medical devices - Symbols to be used with medical device labels, labelling and information to be supplied - Part 1: General requirements	ISO 15223-1:2012 Ed. 2.0	EN 980:2008	ISO 15223-1:2012 Ed. 1.0 ANSI/AAMI/ISO 15223-1:2012
	Symbol for use in the labelling of medical devices - Requirements for labelling of medical devices containing phthalates	-	EN 15986:2011	-
	Information supplied by the manufacturer of medical devices	-	EN 1041:2008	-
	Sterilization of medical devices – Information to be provided by the manufacturer for the processing of resterilizable medical devices	ISO 17664:2004 Ed. 1.0	EN ISO 17664:2004	-
Biocompatibility (basic)	Biological evaluation of medical devices - Part 1: Evaluation and testing within a risk management process	ISO 10993-1:2009 +Corr1:2010 Ed. 4.0	EN ISO 10993-1:2009 +Corr:2010	ISO 10993-1:2009 Ed. 4.0 ANSI AAMI ISO 10993-1:2009/(R)2013

Genotoxicity, carcinogenicity and reproductive toxicity	Biological evaluation of medical devices – Part 3: Tests for genotoxicity, carcinogenicity and reproductive toxicity	ISO 10993-3:2013 Ed. 2.0 ISO FDIS 10993-3: 2014	EN ISO 10993-3:2009	ISO 10993-3:2003 Ed. 2.0 ANSI AAMI ISO 10993-3:2003/(R)2013
Haemocompatibility	Biological evaluation of medical devices - Part 4: Selection of tests for interaction with blood	ISO 10993-4:2002 + A1:2006 Ed. 2.0	EN ISO 10993-4:2009	-
In vitro cytotoxicity	Biological evaluation of medical devices – Part 5: Tests for in vitro cytotoxicity	ISO 10993-5:2009 Ed. 3.0	EN ISO 10993-5:2009	ANSI AAMI ISO 10993-5:2009/(R)2014
Implantation	Biological evaluation of medical devices – Part 6: Tests for local effects after implantation	ISO 10993-6:2007 Ed. 2.0	EN 10993-6:2009	ANSI AAMI ISO 10993-6:2007/(R)2010
Ethylene oxide (EtO) sterilization residuals	Biological evaluation of medical devices - Part 7: Ehtylene oxide sterilization residuals	ISO 10993-7:2008 +Corr1:2009 Ed. 2.0	EN ISO 10993-7:2008 +Corr:2009	ISO 10993-7:2008 Ed. 2.0 ANSI AAMI ISO 10993-7:2008/(R)2012
Potential degradation products	Biological evaluation of medical devices - Part 9: Framework for identification and quantification of potential degradation products	ISO 10993-9:2009 Ed. 2.0	EN ISO 10993-9:2009	ISO 10993-9:2009 Ed. 2.0 AAMI ANSI ISO 10993-9:2009

(*Contd.*)

Table 2.4 (*Contd.*)

Standard category	Title	International standards	EN Harmonised Standards	FDA Recognized Consensus Standards
Irritation and delayed-type hyper-sensitivity	Biological evaluation of medical devices - Part 10: Tests for irritation and skin sensitization	ISO 10993-10:2010 Ed. 3.0	EN ISO 10993-10: 2013 (not published in the *OJ* as of October 2014)	ISO 10993-10:2010 Ed. 3.0 AAMI ANSI ISO 10993-10: 2010
Systemic toxicity	Biological evaluation of medical devices - Part 11: Tests for systemic toxicity	ISO 10993-11:2006 Ed. 2.0	EN ISO 10993-11: 2009	ISO 10993-11:2006 Ed. 2.0 ANSI/AAMI 10993-11: 2006/(R)2010
Sample preparation and reference materials	Biological evaluation of medical devices - Part 12: Sample preparation and reference materials	ISO 10993-12:2007 Ed. 4.0	EN ISO 10993-12: 2012	ISO 10993-12:2012 Ed. 4.0 AAMI ANSI ISO 10993-12:2012
Degradation products from polymeric devices	Biological evaluation of medical devices - Part 13: Identification and quantification of degradation products from polymeric medical devices	ISO 10993-13:2010 Ed. 2.0	EN ISO 10993-13: 2010	ISO 10993-13:2010 Ed. 2.0 AAMI ANSI ISO 10993-13:2010
Degradation products from ceramics	Biological evaluation of medical devices - Part 14: Identification and quantification of degradation products from ceramics	ISO 10993-14:2001 Ed. 1.0	EN ISO 10993-14: 2009	ISO 10993-14:2001 Ed. 1.0 AAMI ANSI ISO 10993-14:2001/(R)2011

Degradation products from metals and alloys	Biological evaluation of medical devices - Part 15: Identification and quantification of degradation products from metals and alloys	ISO 10993-15:2000 Ed. 1.0	EN ISO 10993-15: 2009	-
Toxicogenetic study design for degradation products and leachables	Biological evaluation of medical devices - Part 16: Toxicokinetic study design for degradation products and leachables	ISO 10993-16:2010 Ed. 2.0	EN ISO 10993-16: 2010	ISO 10993-16:2010 Ed. 2.0 AAMI ANSI ISO 10993-16: 2010
Leachable substances	Biological evaluation of medical devices - Part 17: Establishment of allowable limits for leachable substances	ISO 10993-17:2002 Ed. 1.0	EN ISO 10993-17: 2009	-
Chemical characterization of materials	Biological evaluation of medical devices - Part 18: Chemical characterization of materials	ISO 10993-18:2005 Ed. 1.0	EN ISO 10993-18: 2009	-
Physico-chemical, morphological and topographical	Biological evaluation of medical devices – Part 19: Physico-chemical, morphological and topographical characterization of materials	ISO TS 10993-19: 2006 Ed. 1.0	-	ISO TS 10993-19:2006 Ed. 1.0 ANSI AAMI ISO TIR 10993-19: 2006

(*Contd.*)

Table 2.4 *(Contd.)*

Standard category	Title	International standards	EN Harmonised Standards	FDA Recognized Consensus Standards
Immunotoxicity	Biological evaluation of medical devices – Part 20: Principles and methods for immunotoxicology testing of medical devices	ISO TS 10993-20: 2006 Ed. 1.0	–	–
Sterilization (group)	Sterilization of medical devices - Requirements for medical devices to be designated 'STERILE' Part 1: Requirements for terminally sterilized medical devices Part 2: Requirements for aseptically processed medical devices	–	EN 556-1:2001 +Corr:2006; EN 556-2:2003	–
	Sterilization of health care products - Ethylene oxide - Part 1: Requirements for development, validation and routine control of a sterilization process for medical devices	ISO 11135-1:2007 (withdrawn)	EN ISO 11135-1:2007	ISO 11135: 2014 Ed. 2.0
	Product adoption and process equivalence for ethylene oxide sterilization	–	–	AAMI TIR28:2009/(R)2013 (not an FDA Recognized Consensus Standard as of October 2014)
	Sterilization of health care products - Radiation Part 1: Requirements for development, validation and routine control of a sterilization process for medical devices Part 2: Establishing the sterilization dose Part 3: Guidance on dosimetric aspects	ISO 11137-1:2006 +A1:2013 Ed. 1.0 ISO 11137-2: 2013 Ed. 3.0 ISO 11137-3: 2006 Ed. 1.0	EN ISO 11137-1:2006 EN ISO 11137-2:2012	ISO 11137-1:2006 Ed. 1.0 AAMI ANSI ISO 11137-1:2006/(R)2010 ISO 11137-2: 2013 Ed. 3.0 AAMI ANSI ISO 1137-2:2013 ISO 11137-3: 2006 Ed. 1.0 AAMI ANSI ISO 11137-3:2006/(R)2010

	Sterilization of health care products Biological indicators Part 1: General requirements Part 2: Biological indicators for ethylene oxide sterilization processes Part 3: Biological indicators for moist heat sterilization processes	ISO 11138-1: 2006 Ed. 2.0 ISO 11138-2: 2006 Ed. 2.0 ISO 11138-3: 2006 Ed. 2.0	EN ISO 11138-2:2009 EN ISO 11138-3:2009	ISO 11138-1: 2006 Ed. 2.0 AAMI ANSI ISO 11138-1: 2006/(R)2010
	Sterilization of health care products. Chemical indicators. Part 1. General requirements	ISO 11140-1: 2005 Ed. 2.0	EN ISO 11140-1:2009	ISO 1140-1: 2005 Ed. 2.0 AAMI ANSI ISO 11140-1:2005/(R)2010
	Sterilization of medical devices Microbiological methods Part 1: Determination of a population of microorganisms on products Part 2: Tests of sterility performed in the definition, validation and maintenance of a sterilization process	ISO 11737-1: 2006 Ed. 2.0 ISO 11737-2: 2009 Ed. 2.0	EN ISO 11737-1:2006 EN ISO 11737-2:2009	ISO 11737-1: 2006 Ed. 2.0 AAMI ANSI ISO 11737-1:2006/(R)2011 ISO 11737-2: 2009 Ed. 2.0 AAMI ANSI ISO 11737-2:2009

(Contd.)

Table 2.4 *(Contd.)*

Standard category	Title	International standards	EN Harmonised Standards	FDA Recognized Consensus Standards
	Aseptic processing of health care products Part 5: Sterilization in place	ISO 13408-5: 2006 Ed. 1.0	EN ISO 13408-5:2011	ISO 13408-5: 2006 Ed. 1.0 AAMI ANSI ISO 13408-5:2006/(R)2012
	Sterilization of health care products — General requirements for characterization of a sterilizing agent and the development, validation and routine control of a sterilization process for medical devices	ISO 14937: 2009 Ed. 2.0	EN ISO 14937:2009	ISO 14937: 2009 Ed. 2.0 AAMI ANSI ISO 14937:2009/(R)2013
	Sterilization of health care products Moist heat Part 1: Requirements for the development, validation and routine control of a sterilization process for medical devices	ISO 17665-1: 2006 Ed. 1.0	EN ISO 17665-1:2006	ISO 17665-1: 2006 Ed. 1.0 AAMI ANSI ISO 17665-1:2006/(R)2013
Devices operating in the radio frequency (RF) spectrum	EMC and RF spectrum Matters (ERM); Wideband transmission systems; Data transmission equipment operating in the 2,4 GHz ISM band and using wide band modulation techniques; Harmonized EN covering the essential requirements of article 3.2 of the R&TTE Directive	-	ETSI EN 300 328 v1.8.2: 2014 (Wireless LAN Bluetooth)	-

EMC and RF spectrum Matters (ERM); Short range devices; Radio equipment to be used in the 1 GHz to 40 GHz frequency range; Part 2: Harmonized EN covering the essential requirements of article 3.2 of the R&TTE Directive	–	ETSI EN 300 440-2 v1.4.1: 2010 (RF remote short range)	–
EMC and RF spectrum Matters (ERM); EMC standard for radio equipment and services; Part 3: Specific conditions for Short-Range Devices (SRD) operating on frequencies between 9 kHz and 40 GHz	–	ETSI EN 301 489-3 v1.6.1: 2013	–
Other national regulations and standards applicable to RF devices	**Australia**: Radio Communications (short-range devices) Standards 2014 – refers to AS/NZS 4268: 2003 Radio equipment and systems - Short range devices - Limits and methods of measurement; **Canada**: RSS-210 Issue 8:2010 Licence-Exempt Radio Apparatus (All Frequency Bands): Category I Equipment **EU**: Directive 2014/53/EU of the European Parliament and of the Council of 16 April 2014 on harmonization of the laws of the member states to the making available on the market of radio equipment and repealing Directive 1999/5/EC **Japan**: ARIB STD-T66 v3.6:2012 Second Generation Low Power Data Communication System/Wireless LAN System **United States**: FCC – 47 CFR Part 15, Subpart C – Intentional Radiators		

(*Contd.*)

Table 2.4 (*Contd.*)

Standard category	Title	International standards	EN Harmonised Standards	FDA Recognized Consensus Standards
Airborne equipment	Aircraft – Environmental conditions and test procedures for airborne equipment	ISO 7137:1995 Ed. 4.0	–	–
Clinical trials (basic)	Clinical investigation of medical devices for human subjects – Good clinical practice	ISO 14155-1:2011 +Corr1:2011 Ed. 2.0	EN ISO 14155:2011	ISO 14155:2011 Ed. 2.0 AAMI ANSI ISO 14155: 2011
Quality assurance (basic)	Medical devices - Quality management systems - Requirements for regulatory purposes Medical devices Quality management systems Guidance on the application of ISO 13485:2003	ISO 13485:2003 + Corr1:2009 ed. 2.0 ISO DIS 13485: 2014 ISO TR 14969:2004 Ed. 1.0	EN ISO 13485:2012 +Corr:2012 EN ISO TR 14969: 2005 (not published in the *OJ*)	–

2.5 Risk Management

Risk management is a methodology for the systematic assessment and mitigation of risks associated with the use of medical devices. The manufacturer is responsible for implementing risk management processes, taking into account the generally accepted state of the art, and for maintaining risk management files for its devices. Risk management must be an integral part of a manufacturer's QMS.

The international standard ISO 14971:2007, *Medical devices - Application of risk management to medical devices,* defines the ongoing life cycle process for managing risks associated with medical devices and IVDs. The ISO 14971 standard has been adopted as an EN Harmonised Standard as well as an FDA Recognized Consensus Standard.

In a nutshell, the risk management process for medical devices and IVDs is comprised of the following steps:

(1) Risk analysis: Identify known or foreseeable hazards (potential sources of harm) and then estimate risks by combining the severity of each harm and the probability of occurrence of that harm for each hazardous situation (see Fig. 2.4).
(2) Risk evaluation: Determine if risk reduction is required according to risk acceptability criteria identified in the risk management plan.
(3) Risk control: Analyze mitigation options, implement risk control measures, evaluate residual risks, perform risk–benefit analysis, determine any risks arising from risk control measures, complete risk control and evaluate overall acceptability of residual risks.
(4) Monitoring: Monitor the effectiveness of the controls; any new hazards are added to the risk analysis (back to step 1).

In this example, the risk evaluation matrix has five levels for the severity of harm - from negligible to catastrophic - and five levels for the frequency of occurrence - from improbable to frequent.

For each identified hazard the severity of harm is combined with the probability of occurrence of that harm. The resulting risk $R(i)$ is placed in the corresponding box in the risk evaluation matrix.

Severity of harm

Frequency of occurrence	Negligible	Minor	Serious	Critical	Catastrophic
Frequent					
Probable	R1	R3			
Occasional		R4, R5			
Remote	R2			R9, R10	
Improbable		R6, R7	R8	R11	R12

Figure 2.4 Example of a risk evaluation matrix (based on Figure D.7 in ISO 14971:2012).

The risk acceptance levels should be established using information from scientific literature, regulatory agencies databases for adverse events, alerts and recalls and in accordance with the generally accepted state of the art for that type of devices. The red area represents an unacceptable risk level, the yellow area represents a risk level requiring further investigation and reduction, and the green area represents an acceptable risk level.

Risk control measures need to bring all risks from the red area down into the yellow and green areas. The effectiveness of control measures must be monitored on an ongoing basis. Any new hazards identified from the actual use of the device in the field must be added to the risk evaluation matrix and controlled, as necessary.

The ERs/EPs cover known generic hazards such as toxicity, infection, microbial contamination, electric shock, flammability, mechanical and thermal hazards, electromagnetic interference and radiation, and most of them can be mitigated by complying with standards that define requirements and technical specifications that reflect industry best practice. Standards, however, cannot always fully replicate real-life situations; hence compliance with their requirements will only ensure a minimum level of safety. For a particular device, the risk analysis needs to identify the specific clinical hazards related to its intended use – for example, bleeding, arterial embolism and cardiac tamponade, among others, in a ventricular assist device (VAD) [30].

Risk assessment draws on the knowledge of experienced healthcare professionals, scientists and engineers. Regulatory guidelines utilize this expertise in defining risk classification rules and assigning risk classes to medical devices and IVDs. While risk control measures may lower the risk to the patient and thus improve the safety of a device, they do not change the device risk classification. For instance, a poorly designed pacemaker prone to malfunction and failure has the same risk classification as a well-designed, safe and reliable pacemaker. Both are classified as Class III in the United States, AIMDs in Australia and the EU and Class IV in Canada and Japan. Both are subject to the same level of regulatory controls. The difference between them is that the poorly designed pacemaker poses an unacceptable risk.

Depending on a medical device's intended use, composition- and technology-specific hazards may have to be addressed, for example, in relation to:

- Software and firmware;
- Wireless technology and the use of the radio frequency (RF) spectrum;
- Cybersecurity;
- Hazardous substances contained in electronic devices;
- Medicinal substances and biologics;
- Tissues of animal origin susceptible to transmissible spongiform encephalopathy (TSE);
- Phthalates; and
- Latex and other allergens.

2.5.1 *Software and Firmware*

Many electrically powered medical devices nowadays contain software components, parts or accessories. Others, such as medical apps, are comprised solely of software. Software is very different from hardware; it is intangible with many different internal states, which makes it highly complex. Failures in software are systematic in nature, that is, if a software failure can happen, it will happen with 100% probability. This requires systematic management of software life cycle processes. The international standard IEC

62304:2006, *Medical device software – Software life cycle processes*, defines the following stages in the software life cycle: development, maintenance, risk management, configuration management and software problem resolution.

In general, to be considered a medical device, software must have a *medical purpose*. If software does not meet the definition of a medical device or an IVD (see Section 1.4.1, "Definitions of Medical Devices, Active Implantables and in vitro Diagnostics") but is intended by the manufacturer to be an accessory to a medical device or an IVD, it still falls under the scope of medical device or IVD regulations. On the other hand, software for general purposes, even if used in a healthcare setting, is not a medical device.

Examples of software that fall under the definition of medical devices/IVDs include:

- Software embedded in, incorporated as a component or part of accessory of a medical device and supplied with the medical device, also known as firmware – for example, pacemaker firmware, embedded patient monitor software or software that controls insulin pump delivery rate.
- Software as an accessory to a medical device that can be supplied separately from the device and that is intended to drive, monitor the performance of or influence the performance or the use of a medical device – for example, pacemaker programming software or imaging software for use with X-ray machines or ultrasound systems.
- Stand-alone software applications that are able to perform their intended (medical) purpose without being embedded in a hardware medical device or being dependent on specific or proprietary medical purpose hardware – for example, data analysis software for the purpose of directly aiding in the diagnosis or treatment of a patient or replacing a diagnostic or treatment decision made by a physician.

Medical apps are stand-alone (medical) software applications that can be executed on a mobile platform such as iPhone, Android or Blackberry smartphones, tablet computers or other personal digital assistant devices or a web-based software application that is tailored to a mobile platform but is run on a server.

Examples of software that do not fall under the definition of medical devices/IVDs:

- Software that is not a computer program according to the ISO/IEC 2382-1:1993 standard, *Information technology – Vocabulary – Part 1: Fundamental terms,* and does not contain instructions or sub-routines in a particular programming language
- Stand-alone software intended solely for data storage, archival, lossless compression or communication or simple search (e.g., clinical trial data registries)
- Software tools used for production or other process controls such as testing, source code management or servicing

Because embedded software is considered an intrinsic part of the medical device, the risk classification and regulatory controls are applied to both hardware and software together according to existing regulations and guidelines.

For stand-alone software it is not as straightforward, though, as the existing regulatory framework does not address the latest developments in software technology. At a granular level there is significant divergence across jurisdictions regarding classification and regulatory controls for stand-alone software.

So far there is consensus that only the intended use as declared by the manufacturer is relevant for the qualification and classification of medical device software and that none of the following criteria are relevant for the qualification of stand-alone software as medical devices or for their risk classification:

- Operating systems or virtual environments on which the software may run;
- Whether the software is used in a healthcare environment;
- The engineering definition of software functionality; and
- The means by which the software is delivered to the end user: embedded, factory installed, field installed, downloaded from the Internet, installed from a CD, etc. [32].

Useful standards assisting manufacturers with establishing design and development processes for medical device software include:

- EN/IEC 62304:2006, *Medical device software – Software life cycle processes* – This standard is both an FDA Recognized Consensus Standard and an EN Harmonised Standard.
- AAMI TIR32:2004, *Medical Device Software Risk Management.*
- AAMI TIR36:2007, *Validation of Software for Regulated Processes* – an FDA Recognized Consensus Standard.
- AAMI TIR45:2012, *Guidance on the Use of Agile Practices in the Development of Medical Device Software* – an FDA Recognized Consensus Standard.
- AAMI ANSI SW87:2012, *Application of Quality Management System Concepts to Medical Device Software* – an FDA Recognized Consensus Standard.

According to the EN/IEC 62304:2006 standard, *Medical device software: Software life cycle processes*, software is classified according to the severity of possible effects on the patient, operator or other people resulting from a hazard to which the software system can contribute:

- Class A – no injury or damage to health is possible.
- Class B – non-serious injury is possible.
- Class C – death or serious injury is possible.

This classification, however, may be revised in the future to align it with regulations for medical device software (see Section 2.5.1.4, "International Regulatory Harmonization for Stand-Alone Medical Software").

Surprisingly, the standard includes the following statement that appears to contradict basic principles of risk classification of medical devices (emphasis added):

> If the risk of death or serious injury arising from a software failure is subsequently reduced to an acceptable level (as defined by ISO 14971) by a hardware risk control measure, either by reducing the consequences of the failure or by reducing the probability of death or serious injury arising from that failure, *the software safety classification may be reduced* from C [high risk] to B [moderate risk]; and if the risk of non-serious injury arising from

> a software failure is similarly reduced to an acceptable level by a hardware risk control measure, the software safety classification may be reduced from B [moderate risk] to A [low risk] (EN IEC 62304:2006, Section 4.3, "Software Safety Classification").

The risk classification of a medical device (including software) depends on its intended purpose and *intrinsic* risk to the patient (refer also to Section 1.5, "Risk-Based Classification"). The purpose of risk mitigations and control measures is to reduce risk to acceptable levels by reducing either the severity of a particular harm or the frequency of occurrence of that harm but not to down-classify the device into a lower-risk category. If the software controls functionalities with an intrinsic high risk, that software is likely to be classified in a high-risk class.

Perhaps the statement in EN/IEC 62304 could be interpreted as follows: If a hardware risk control measure ensures that a software failure cannot result in death or serious injury, the software safety classification is not Class C. Moreover, if the software failure cannot result in non-serious injury, the software safety classification is not Class B either. Or, if a functionality of the medical device leading to potential death or serious injury is implemented in hardware rather than software, the potential hazardous functionality should not be considered when determining the software safety classification.

Some key points relevant to the regulatory framework for stand-alone software in established markets and ongoing international harmonization efforts are provided hereafter.

2.5.1.1 Software regulations: EU, Australia and Canada

Under the EU, Australian and Canadian regulations software as a medical device is considered to be an active medical device (i.e., driven by electrical energy). As such, the classification rules for active devices apply.

Software incorporated in a medical device is considered as an integral part of the medical device and classified together with the complete device.

Stand-alone software applications with a medical purpose and software as accessories to medical devices are classified on their own by applying these general principles:

- Software that is intended to drive, control or influence the functions of a medical device usually falls in the same classification as the device.
- Software intended as an accessory to a medical device and not essential to its function is usually classified separately from the device it is used with.

Important regulatory guidelines assisting manufacturers to correctly classify software in the EU, Australia and Canada are listed below:

- MEDDEV 2.1/6, *Qualification and classification of stand-alone software used in healthcare within the regulatory framework of medical devices* [33]
- MEDDEV 2.4/1, *Classification of medical devices* [34]
- *Australian Regulatory Guidelines for Medical Devices* (ARGMD) [35]
- TGA *Regulation of Medical Software and Mobile Medical "Apps"* [36]
- Health Canada *Guidance for the Risk-Based Classification System* (draft) [37]
- Health Canada *Guidance for the Risk-Based Classification System of in vitro Diagnostic Devices* (draft) [38]
- Health Canada *Software Regulated as a Medical Device – Frequently Asked Questions* [39]

2.5.1.2 Software regulations: United States

In the United States, any software that meets the legal definition of a medical device is considered a medical device and classified according to the FDA's nomenclature-based system. The regulatory controls applicable to these devices are specified in the relevant regulations (21 CFR Parts 862–892). For software intended as an accessory to a medical device the classification is the same as that of the parent device.

In September 2013 the FDA has released a guideline for mobile apps, clarifying which mobile apps are subject to regulatory controls [40]. In the guidance, the FDA distinguishes three categories of mobile apps and gives examples for each category:

- Mobile apps that are not medical devices and as are such not regulated by the FDA.
- Mobile apps for which the FDA intends to exercise enforcement discretion – they meet the legal definition of medical devices but are low risk.
- Mobile apps that are the focus of the FDA's regulatory oversight – these are treated like any other medical software devices.

Additional FDA guidance documents relevant to medical device software are listed below:

- *General Principles of Software Validation* [41]
- *Off-the-Shelf Software Use in Medical Devices* [42]
- *Guidance for the Content of Premarket Submissions for Software Contained in Medical Devices* [43]

For pre-market submissions of medical device software, including stand-alone software applications and hardware-based devices that incorporate software, the FDA requires manufacturers to determine the level of concern (LoC), which is an estimate of the severity of injury that a device could permit or inflict, either directly or indirectly, on a patient or operator as a result of device failures or design flaws or simply by virtue of employing the device for its intended use.

The LoC may be Major, Moderate or Minor:

- The LoC is Major if a failure or latent flaw could directly result in death or serious injury to the patient or operator or indirectly through incorrect or delayed information or through the action of a care provider.
- The LoC is Moderate if a failure or latent design flaw could directly result in minor injury to the patient or operator, or indirectly through incorrect or delayed information or through the action of a care provider.

- The LoC is Minor if failures or latent design flaws are unlikely to cause any injury to the patient or operator.

The LoC is determined by assessing the risks associated with the software device. In general, risk is the product of the severity of harm and the probability of occurrence of that harm, but there is a significant difference between determining risk for hardware and determining risk for software. Software failures are *systemic* in nature; hence if a software failure can occur the assumption is that it will occur – that is, the *probability of occurrence is always 100%*. The estimation of risk for software should therefore be based on the severity of the hazard resulting from failure.

Importantly, the FDA recommends that the LoC be determined *before* any mitigation of relevant hazards. In other words, the LoC should be driven by the hazard analysis in the absence of mitigations regardless of the effects of the mitigations on the individual hazards. This approach is aligned with the principles of risk classification of medical devices in general but seemingly in contradiction with the EN/IEC 62304 statement mentioned earlier in Section 2.5.1, "Software and Firmware".

The software risk classification is relevant because it determines the level of rigor required for the software development process and the required technical documentation (refer also to Section 3.3.8.4, "Software and Firmware"). In situations such as this, where regulatory requirements and guidelines are or appear to be in conflict with requirements defined in voluntary standards, the regulatory requirements and guidelines take precedence.

2.5.1.3 Software regulations: Japan

In Japan embedded software is considered as an integral part of the medical device in which it is incorporated, and as such existing risk classifications and regulatory controls for medical devices apply.

The recently enacted Pharmaceutical and Medical Device (PMD) Act requires pre-market certification for some stand-alone medical software. At the time of going to print Japanese Medical Device Nomenclature (JMDN) codes and specific guidelines for stand-alone software are yet to be established and developed.

2.5.1.4 International regulatory harmonization for stand-alone medical software

The International Medical Device Regulatory Forum (IMDRF) guidance WG/N10:2013, *Software as a Medical Device (SaMD)*, distinguishes two categories of software with a medical purpose:

- Software in a medical device (sometimes referred to as embedded or part of)
- Software as a medical device (SaMD) – defined as software intended to be used for one or more medical purposes that perform these purposes without being part of a hardware medical device [44]

The IMDRF Working Group on Stand-Alone Medical Device Software Harmonization (SaMD) has also put forward a proposal intended to form the basis for the future harmonized regulations for medical software [45]. The goal is to classify medical software devices into four risk classes – from type I low risk to type IV very high risk – and define regulatory controls that ensure their safety and effectiveness.

The four risk classes are determined relative to the three levels of criticality for the state of the healthcare situation or condition and three main categories for the SaMD's intended purpose (see Fig. 2.5).

There are three proposed levels of criticality for the state of the healthcare situation or condition:

- Critical – where accurate and/or timely diagnosis or treatment action is vital to avoid death, long-term disability or other serious deterioration of the health of an individual patient or to mitigate the impact to public health;
- Serious – where accurate diagnosis or treatment is of vital importance to avoid unnecessary interventions; and
- Non-serious – where inaccurate diagnosis and treatment are important but not critical for interventions.

The intended purpose of the SaMD can be grouped into three main categories:

- Treat or diagnose – to provide therapy to a human body or to diagnose/screen/detect a disease or condition;

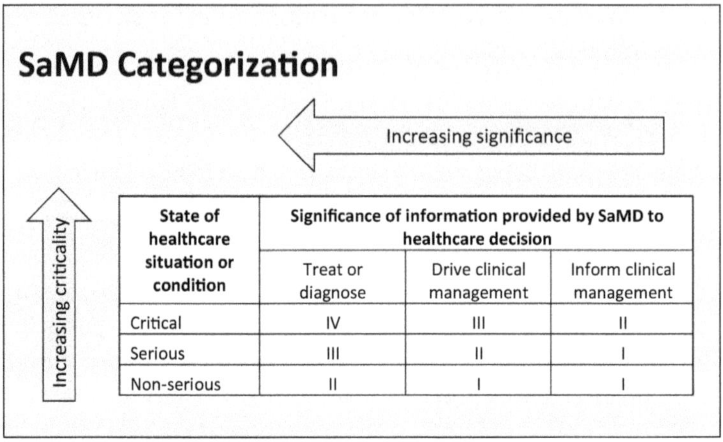

Figure 2.5 Risk classification for software as medical devices (SaMD) according to criticality of healthcare condition and significance of information managed by the SaMD. *Source*: Bakul Patel, IMDRF.

- Drive clinical management – to aid in treatment by providing enhanced support to safe and effective use of medicinal products or a medical device or to aid in making a definitive diagnosis or to triage or identify early signs of a disease or condition; and
- Inform clinical management – to inform of options or to provide clinical information by aggregating relevant information.

2.5.2 *RF Wireless Devices*

An increasing number of medical devices incorporate RF wireless technology. To ensure the safe and effective use of RF wireless devices specific aspects related to the incorporation and integration of this technology must be addressed.

According to the FDA guidance *Radio Frequency Wireless Technology in Medical Devices* [46] the hazards analysis needs to cover the following aspects, as applicable, at a system level:

- Poorly characterized or poorly utilized wireless systems (e.g., wireless networks);

- Lost, corrupted or time-delayed transmissions and degradations in wireless transmissions, including when caused by competing wireless signals or electromagnetic interference to the medical device or its wireless transmissions;
- Lack or compromise of wireless security; authentication and wireless encryption are typical means to prevent unauthorized access to patient data or hospital networks and to ensure that information and data received by a device are intended for that device; and
- Potential misuse of a wireless medical device because of lack of or inadequate instructions for use.

The wireless quality of service (QoS), that is, the level of service and performance needed for the wireless functions of the medical device, should be defined and related risks assessed, for example, connection loss without service, failure to establish connections or degradation of service.

If the wireless medical device is part of a network, a risk approach should be used for the deployment, security and maintenance of the QoS and the following aspects should be considered:

- Acceptable latency;
- Acceptable level of probability for loss of information within the network;
- Accessibility; and
- Signal priorities of the network.

Where applicable, manufacturers need to address requirements related to EMC, wireless networks and telecommunication defined in standards and regulations, including:

- IEC 60601-1-2:2014/EN 60601-1-2:2007, *Medical electrical equipment – Part 1-2: General requirements for basic safety and essential performance – Collateral standard: Electromagnetic disturbances – Requirements and tests.*
- EN/IEC 61326 series – *Electrical equipment for measurement, control and laboratory use – EMC requirements*: The EN/IEC 61326-2-6 standard covers particular EMC requirements for IVDs.

- IEC TR 80001-1:2010, *Application of risk management for IT-networks incorporating medical devices – Part 1: Roles, responsibilities and activities.*
- IEC TR 80001-2-1:2012, *Application of risk management for IT-networks incorporating medical devices – Part 2-1: Step by step risk management of medical IT-networks; Practical applications and examples.*
- IEC TR 80001-2-2:2012, *Application of risk management for IT-networks incorporating medical devices – Part 2-2: Guidance for the communication of medical device security needs, risks and controls.*
- IEC TR 80001-2-3:2012 *Application of risk management for IT-networks incorporating medical devices – Part 2-3: Guidance for wireless networks.*
- IEC TR 80001-2-4:2012 *Application of risk management for IT-networks incorporating medical devices – Part 2-4: General implementation guidance for healthcare delivery organizations.*
- ISO TR 16056:2004 *Health informatics – Interoperability of telehealth systems and networks.*
- ISO TR 21730:2007 *Health informatics – Use of mobile wireless communications and computing technology in healthcare facilities – Recommendations for the management of unintentional electromagnetic interference with medical devices.*
- US Federal Communications Commission (FCC) – Title 47 of CFR Parts 2, 15, 18 and 95.
- EU Radio Equipment Directive 2014/53/EU, which replaces the Radio and Telecommunications Terminal Equipment (R&TTE) Directive 1999/5/EC.
- Other national regulations for RF wireless equipment – Canada, China, Japan and Korea.

2.5.3 *Cybersecurity*

In an increasingly connected world, there is a need to ensure that electronic exchange of medical device–related health information via wireless-, Internet- and network-connected devices is secure.

The FDA recommends that manufacturers develop a set of security controls to ensure medical device cybersecurity to maintain information confidentiality, integrity and availability. Failure to maintain cybersecurity can result in compromised device functionality, loss of data availability or integrity or exposure of other connected devices or networks to security threats. These, in turn, have the potential to result in patient illness, injury or death [47].

Confidentiality means that data, information or system structures are accessible only to authorized persons and entities and are processed at authorized times and in the authorized manner, thereby helping ensure data and system security. Confidentiality provides the assurance that no unauthorized users (i.e., only trusted users) have access to the data, information or system structures.

Integrity means that data and information are accurate and complete and have not been improperly modified.

Availability means that data, information and information systems are accessible and usable on a timely basis in the expected manner (i.e., the assurance that the information will be available when needed).

Appropriate security control measures for networked medical devices include, but are not limited to:

- Limiting access to trusted users only – for instance, through authentication of users (e.g., user ID and password, smartcard, biometrics), automatic timed user session log-offs or different levels of access privileges
- Ensuring trusted content – for instance, by restricting software or firmware updates to authenticated code or using systematic procedures for authorized users to download version-identifiable software and firmware from the manufacturer
- Implementing fail-safe and recovery features to protect the device's critical functionality, even when the device's security has been compromised, and to allow for security compromises to be recognized, logged and acted upon

Many medical devices designed to be connected to computer networks incorporate off-the-shelf software that is vulnerable to cybersecurity threats such as viruses and worms. These vulnerabilities may represent a risk to the safe and effective operation of networked medical devices and typically require an ongoing maintenance effort throughout the product life cycle to ensure an adequate degree of protection. The FDA guidance *Cybersecurity for Networked Medical Devices Containing Off-the-Shelf (OTS) Software* clarifies how existing regulations apply to cybersecurity maintenance activities, such as validating software changes made to address cybersecurity vulnerabilities and reporting of software patches [48].

In addition, the IEC/IEC TR 80001 standard series, *Application of risk management for IT-networks incorporating medical devices*, provides detailed, practical guidance with regard to the roles, responsibilities and activities that are necessary for risk management of IT networks incorporating medical devices to address safety, effectiveness and data and system security (the key properties).

2.5.4 *Hazardous Substances Contained in Electronic Devices*

Environmental protection regulations exist in all established markets – for instance, those in the EU and the United States mentioned in this sub-section – and they may affect medical devices. The risk management must include an adequate analysis and assessment of the risks associated with hazardous substances, if applicable.

Since 2002 the EU has restricted the use of certain hazardous substances in electrical and electronic equipment: lead (Pb), mercury (Hg), cadmium (Cd) and hexavalent chromium (Cr^{6+}), as well as flame retardants polybrominated biphenyls (PBBs) and polybrominated diphenyl ethers (PBDEs). EU Directive 2002/95/EC on restricted hazardous substances (RoHS) requires that manufacturers replace, or for certain applications limit, the concentration of these chemicals in their products with less hazardous alternatives [49].

The RoHS directive was recast by EU Directive 2011/65/EU, also known as RoHS II. The restrictions regarding the use of hazardous substances apply as of July 2014 for medical devices and as of July 2016 for IVDs. At the time of going to print AIMDs were exempt from compliance to the RoHS requirements [50].

In addition to the requirements of RoHS II, medical device manufactures may be subject to other EU directives and regulations addressing the disposal of electronic waste, including batteries and the use of hazardous substances, such as:

- EU Directive 2012/19/EC on Waste Electrical and Electronic Equipment (WEEE II) [51]
- EU Regulation 1907/2006 concerning the Registration, Evaluation, Authorisation and Restriction of Chemicals (REACH) [52]
- EU directives on the disposal of batteries (53) and on product packaging and packaging waste [54]

In the United States, the Environmental Protection Agency (EPA) is authorized by Congress to issue regulations regarding environmental protection, including hazardous substances. These can be found under Title 40 of the CFR. Additional state environmental regulations may apply [55].

2.5.5 *Medicines and Biologics*

Medicines (or drugs, according to US terminology) are chemical substances (small molecules) that achieve their therapeutic effect via pharmacological, chemical, immunological or metabolic means in or on the body of a human. Examples include antibiotics (kill bacteria), antiseptics (inhibit or kill microorganisms within a wound), antipyretics (reduce fever), analgesics (reduce pain) and statins (lower cholesterol).

Biologics (or biopharmaceuticals) are therapeutic products, the active substance of which is a biological substance (large molecules) produced by or extracted from a biological source – human, animal or microorganism such as a virus, a therapeutic serum, a toxin, an antitoxin, or an analogous product. Examples of biologics include vaccines, human blood and blood products (plasma); recombinant proteins (insulin); allergenic extracts used for both diagnosis and treatment (e.g., allergy shots); human cells and tissues used for transplantation (tendons, ligaments and bone); gene therapies; cellular therapies; and tests to screen potential blood donors for infectious agents such as human immunodeficiency virus (HIV).

In contrast to drugs that are usually synthetic, organic compounds, relatively stable, with well-defined structures, biologics are usually protein or carbohydrate based and heat sensitive, with complex physico-chemical characteristics [56, 57]. Immunogenicity represents a key issue for biologics, as highlighted by the high-profile case of TeGenero's TGN 1412 compound, which caused severe adverse effects during a first-in-human (FIH) clinical trial in 2006 [58].

Medical devices can be combined with medicines or biologics to achieve therapeutic effects through controlled and targeted delivery of the medicinal substance. Some of the best-known drug–device and biologic–device combinations include insulin injector pens, drug-eluting vascular stents, pacemaker leads with steroid-coated tips, antimicrobial wound dressings, catheters with antimicrobial coating, protein-eluting scaffolds for tissue re-generation and condoms with spermicides.

The risk management of a combination product will have to cover known hazards and adverse effects for both the device and the drug components. In addition, specific hazards related to the delivery of the drug or biologic need to be considered, such as:

- Usability of drug delivery;
- Drug-eluting profile;
- Interaction between the drug and device components, degradation, particulate release;
- Performance of therapeutic coatings; and
- Stability of medicine or biologic incorporated into a device during manufacturing, transport and storage [59–61].

2.5.6 *Tissues of Animal Origin Susceptible to TSE*

Tissues of animal origin can be used in a medical device either as an integral part of the medical device or as an aid to the manufacturing process.

Medical devices incorporating tissues of animal origins include bovine and porcine heart valves, bone substitutes and bone filler materials, vascular grafts impregnated with bovine gelatin that seals the prosthesis without the need of pre-clotting, and haemostatic devices intended to produce haemostasis by accelerating the clotting process of blood during surgical procedures. Tissues of animal origin used in the manufacturing process, for instance, as mould release agents during silicone moulding, include tallow derivatives like glycerol and fatty acids.

Certain tissues, cells and substances of animal origin are susceptible to TSE, including:

- Bovine spongiform encephalopathy (BSE) in cattle
- Scrapie in sheep and goats
- Chronic wasting disease (CWD) in deer
- Kuru, Creutzfeldt–Jakob disease (CJD)

BSE and CJD are believed to be caused by a prion, an infectious, abnormally shaped, self-replicating protein that is much smaller than viruses or bacteria. Scientific evidence supports a link between the agent responsible for BSE in cattle and variant Creutzfeldt–Jakob disease (vCJD) in humans. Furthermore it is generally accepted that BSE may be transmitted from animals to humans by consumption of contaminated materials of ruminant origin. Therefore it is important to minimize the potential for this agent to be transmitted to humans [62].

Prions cannot be rendered non-viable by any of the known sterilization methods; therefore manufacturers using tissues of animal origins must ensure they are sourced from disease-free animals.

In the EU, Regulation 722/2012 effective from August 29, 2013 [63], replaces Directive 2003/32/EC [64] and defines requirements related to risk management, sourcing of materials and safety regarding the use of tissues from TSE-susceptible animals in medical devices.

EU Regulation 722/2012 currently applies to animal tissues, as well as their derivatives, originating from bovine, ovine and caprine species, deer, elk, mink and cats. Collagen, gelatine and tallow used for the manufacturing of medical devices must meet at least the requirements as fit for human consumption laid down in Regulation 1069/2009.

Important changes from the previous Directive 2003/32/EC include replacing the geographical BSE risk system with three risk categories related to the country of sourcing of the tissue of animal origin and mandating that for starting materials already certified by the European Directorate for the Quality of Medicines and Healthcare (EDQM), previously exempted from consultation with all EU member states, by subject to a mandatory, albeit expedited (four weeks), consultation procedure [65].

The FDA (draft) guidance *Medical Devices Containing Materials Derived from Animal Sources (Except for In Vitro Diagnostic Devices)* updates the policy regarding the use of animal-derived material in medical device manufacturing [66].

Other TSE- relevant regulations, standards and guidelines include:

- Australia: *Transmissible Spongiform Encephalopathies (TSE): TGA Approach to Minimising the Risk of Exposure* [62];
- Canada: *Guidance Document on the Regulation of Medical Devices Manufactured from or Incorporating Viable or Non-Viable Animal Tissue or their Derivative(s)* [67];
- Japan Pharmaceuticals and Medical Devices Agency (PMDA) guidance: *Some aspects of development, evaluation and control of biologics in Japan* [68]; and
- ISO/TR 22442-4:2010, *Medical devices utilizing animal tissues and their derivatives – Part 4: Principles for elimination and/or inactivation of transmissible spongiform encephalopathy (TSE) agents and validation assays for those processes.*

2.5.7 *Phthalates*

Phthalates are a group of chemicals widely used as plasticizers for rigid compounds such as polyvinyl chloride (PVC) to soften them and make them more malleable. Examples of medical devices containing phthalate-plasticized PVC include blood bags and tubing, intravenous bags and tubing, umbilical artery catheters, respiratory tubing and nasogastric feeding tubes [69]. Phthalates are also used in cosmetic products such as nail polish, hair spray, aftershave lotions, soaps, shampoos, perfumes and other fragrance preparations [70].

These are some of widely used plasticizers:

- *Bis*(2-ethylhexyl)phthalate, or DEHP;
- Dibutyl phthalate, or DBP; and
- Benzyl butyl phthalate, or BBP.

There has been an ongoing debate over the safety of phthalates. On one side, consumer safety and environmental groups argue that the incineration of PVC products produces dioxin, a toxic chemical with carcinogenic effects on humans. On the other side, industry representatives disagree, claiming that the currently available data on the effects on humans of DEHP when compared to alternative materials remain inconclusive.

In 2002 the FDA published a report stating that "children undergoing certain medical procedures may represent a population at increased risk for the effects of DEHP". The report also found that "the ability of DEHP to alter the hemocompatibility of PVC tubing or result in adsorption of drugs to PVC tubing may be the most clinically important endpoints to consider in the risk management phase of the assessment, depending on the device" [71].

In the same year the FDA issued a public health notification identifying two main risk factors related to PVC devices containing DEHP: "The first is the patient's sensitivity to DEHP. Based on the evidence cited above, the male fetus, male neonate, and peripubertal male would appear to be high-risk groups. The second factor is the dose of DEHP received by the patient. This is determined largely by the type of procedure performed, as well as the frequency and duration of these procedures." In its recommendation though, the FDA was adamant that "the risk of not doing a needed procedure is far greater than the risk associated with exposure to DEHP" [72].

To address community concerns in Europe, the 2007 revision of EU Directive 93/42/EEC introduced a requirement to label medical devices containing phthalates:

> If parts of a device (or a device itself) intended to administer and/or remove medicines, body liquids or other substances to or from the body, or devices intended for transport and storage of such body fluids or substances, contain phthalates which are classified as carcinogenic, mutagenic or toxic to reproduction, of

category 1 or 2, according to Annex I of Directive 67/548/EEC, these devices must be labelled on the device itself and/or on the packaging for each unit or, where appropriate, on the sales packaging as a device containing phthalates.

The actual symbols required for medical devices containing phthalates are defined in the European standard EN 15986:2011, *Symbol for use in the labelling of medical devices – Requirements for labelling of medical devices containing phthalates*.

In 2014 the European Scientific Committee of Emerging and Newly Identified Health Risks (SCENIHR) published an update to its previous 2008 opinion on the safety of medical device DEHP or alternative plasticizers for their PVC-based components. It states, "DEHP has been classified as possibly carcinogenic to humans (Group 2B)", but "there was no effect of DEHP and DBP (di-n-butyl phthalate) metabolites on testosterone production in human foetal testis tissue".

The SCENHIR report concludes: "It should be realised that the benefit of medical devices has also to be considered: the survival of premature infants often depends on the availability of the same medical devices which result in a relatively high DEHP exposure due to treatment. Whenever possible, material with low release potential should be used. The potential for replacement of DEHP in these products should be considered against their efficiency in the treatment, as well as the toxicological profile and leaching properties of the alternative materials. There is a strong need to develop and collect data on the toxicological profile and exposure of alternative materials" [73].

2.5.8 *Allergens*

Some materials and substances used in medical devices, such as latex (natural rubber) and nickel (used in stainless-steel surgical tools and some implants), may cause allergic reactions in patients and users. To avoid adverse reactions, the most common mitigation is to clearly label the existence of these materials in the accompanying documentation of a medical device and use alternatives, if available and practicable [74, 75].

2.6 Clinical Evaluation

Clinical evaluation is the ongoing assessment and analysis of clinical data pertaining to a medical device in order to establish the clinical safety and performance of the device throughout its life cycle. It represents a critical aspect of the conformity assessment process and serves to substantiate manufacturer's claims about the device and the benefit–risk determination. The clinical evaluation must be updated at regular intervals according to a pre-defined plan (six-monthly or yearly, as necessary) and must include all relevant evidence - favourable and unfavourable - required to support conclusions of safety and effectiveness.

Clinical data is generated from the actual use of a medical device under controlled and/or real-life conditions. Clinical data can be obtained from the manufacturer's own pre-market clinical investigations and post-market surveillance of the device concerned or from the scientific literature and published articles of clinical investigations and adverse event reports for the device in question or for equivalent devices.

For lower-risk devices and generic ("me too") devices, most or all clinical data is generated through literature search, which may relate directly to the device in question, for instance, from clinical investigations performed by third parties and adverse event reports, or to equivalent devices.

For higher-risk, novel and innovative devices the clinical data needs to be generated from pre-market clinical trials (also referred to as clinical investigations or studies) and also through post-market surveillance of the device in question and equivalent devices, if available.

The following standards and guidelines should be followed when performing clinical evaluations for medical devices and IVDs:

- GHTF SG5/N1R8:2007, *Clinical evidence* [76];
- GHTF SG5/N2R8:2007, *Clinical evaluation* [77];
- EU MEDDEV 2.7.1:2009, *Clinical evaluation: A guide for manufacturers and notified bodies* [78];
- NBOG CL 2010-1, *Checklist for audit of notified body's review of clinical data/clinical evaluation* - provides some insight

into how the EU notified bodies approach evaluation of clinical data [79];

- EN 13612:2002 *Performance evaluation of in vitro diagnostic medical devices*;
- GHTF SG5/N6:2012, *Clinical evidence for IVD medical devices* [80];
- GHTF SG5/N7:2012, *Clinical evidence for IVD medical devices – Scientific validity determination and performance evaluation* [81]; and
- GHTF SG5/N8:2012, *Clinical evidence for IVD medical devices – Clinical performance studies for IVDs* [82].

2.6.1 *Clinical Literature Review*

The literature search must be comprehensive and unbiased, with a well-defined strategy around carefully formulated review questions. The literature search protocol should identify, select and collate relevant published articles and data that address the review questions. A literature search protocol should include:

- The sources of data that will be used and a justification for their choice;
- The extent of any searches of scientific literature databases (the database search strategy);
- The selection criteria to be applied to published literature and justification for their choice; and
- Strategies for addressing the potential for duplication of data across multiple publications.

The literature search should be conducted by information retrieval experts to ensure it is effective and thorough. The results of the literature search should be analyzed and documented in a report, with enough details so that the methods can be appraised critically, the results verified and the search re-produced, if necessary.

A proposed format for a literature search report and methodology for documenting the screening and selection of literature is provided in Appendix A and B, respectively, of the MEDDEV 2.7.1 guidance *Clinical evaluation: A guide for manufacturers and notified bodies*.

The literature-based evidence may also be accepted as the sole basis for a regulatory approval of a significant change of a higher-risk medical device if the literature is sufficient, detailed, objective and directly applicable to the subject device.

There are, however, limitations when relying entirely on literature-based data. According to the FDA:

> Experience has shown that the published literature do not always contain a complete, or entirely accurate, representation of the device design, performance, manufacture, clinical study plans, conduct, accountability, and outcomes. Incompleteness, lack of clarity, failure to identify deviations from prospectively planned statistical analyses, use in a different setting from the intended use, and inadequate descriptions of how critical outcome measurements or assessments were made are common problems. These inadequacies associated with published reports are due to a variety of factors. For some peer reviewed articles, peer reviewers may have access only to a limited data set and analyses. Such reviewers ordinarily do not see the original protocol and amendments, and thus may lack sufficient information to detect critical omissions and problems in the reported data. The peer review process also may be affected by variability in the relevant experience and expertise of the peer reviewer. In a relatively small number of cases, omissions in published reports may be due to careless reporting or intentional fraud [83].

2.6.2 *Clinical Trials*

A clinical trial is a systematic investigation in one or more human subjects, undertaken to assess the safety and/or performance of a medical device. The terms "clinical investigation" and "clinical study" are synonymous with "clinical trial".

Regulators in established markets require that marketing applications for higher-risk, novel and innovative devices be supported by clinical data generated through clinical trials. Clinical investigations must follow scientific principles underlying the collection of clinical data, along with accepted ethical standards surrounding the use of human subjects.

The Declaration of Helsinki, first adopted in June 1964 and subsequently amended on a number of occasions, lays down the ethical principles for medical research involving human subjects and forms the basis for regulations of clinical trials worldwide. The Declaration of Helsinki was developed by the World Medical Association (WMA), an international organization representing physicians. It states that:

> Medical progress is based on research that ultimately must include studies involving human subjects.
>
> The primary purpose of medical research involving human subjects is to understand the causes, development and effects of diseases and improve preventive, diagnostic and therapeutic interventions (methods, procedures and treatments). Even the best proven interventions must be evaluated continually through research for their safety, effectiveness, efficiency, accessibility and quality [. . .]

While the primary purpose of medical research is to generate new knowledge, this goal can never take precedence over the rights and interests of individual research subjects [84].

Adherence to the principles of good clinical practices (GCPs), including adequate human subject protection, is universally recognized as a critical requirement to the conduct of research involving human subjects. Many countries have adopted GCP principles as laws and/or regulations. Sponsors must obtain approval from an Ethics Committee or an institutional review board, and, in some jurisdictions, also the approval from the relevant regulatory authority, before starting a clinical trial.

There are different types of clinical study designs – the most commonly used are listed hereafter, from the most to the least methodologically rigorous [85, 86].

2.6.2.1 Clinical study designs

Randomized controlled trials are interventional studies considered to be the gold standard for evaluating a given therapy and its causal impact on an outcome. Study subjects are randomly allocated either to the experimental group to receive the treatment being

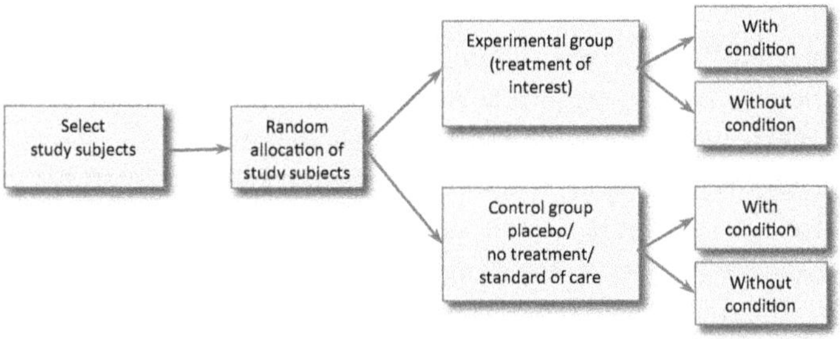

Figure 2.6 Randomized controlled study design.

investigated or to the control group, typically a placebo or standard of care (see Fig. 2.6). Randomization (allocation of study participants to the experimental or control group using chance) provides a sound statistical basis for the quantitative evaluation of the evidence relating to treatment effect.

When combined with blinding (i.e., when either the subject or the investigator or both are not aware of the allocation of treatment), randomization helps to avoid bias (systematic error resulting in an incorrect estimate of the association between a treatment and an outcome). For most clinical trials involving medical devices, however, blinding may not be feasible.

Furthermore, clinical effectiveness of a medical device depends not only on the device design itself but also on the skills and experience of the surgeons and other medical practitioners using the device.

Medical devices in the same category but from different manufacturers will have different properties, materials and specifications; hence, when comparing their safety and effectiveness, the criteria for comparison need to be carefully defined. The design and manufacturing processes of medical devices also evolve in time, so comparisons will have to factor in incremental improvements as well.

There are two types of errors that can occur during clinical investigations, type 1 errors and type 2 errors.

Type 1 errors occur when investigators reject, or do not accept, something that is true. For example, if the null hypothesis is that there is no difference between two treatments, then a type 1 error would occur if investigators concluded that the two treatments produced different effects when in fact there was no such difference. A type 1 error is generally seen as failing to accept the null hypothesis when the null hypothesis is in fact true.

Type 2 errors occur when investigators accept something that is false. For example, if the null hypothesis is that there is no difference between two treatments, then a type 2 error would occur if investigators concluded that there was no difference between the two treatments when in fact they produced different outcomes. A type 2 error is generally regarded as the probability of failing to reject the null hypothesis when the null hypothesis is in fact false. The larger the type 2 error, the weaker the statistical power of the clinical study. Type 2 errors occur when the sample size is too small.

Non-randomized controlled trials are interventional studies in which study subjects are allocated to different treatments using methods that are not random.

Prospective cohort studies are observational studies used to determine the causes and incidence of a medical condition, as well as identify risk factors. Study participants who do not have the condition of interest are followed over time to see whether they develop the condition or not. The investigator measures the predictor variables (risk factors) that might be relevant to the development of the condition (see Fig. 2.7).

Retrospective case control studies are observational studies comparing persons with the condition of interest with a control group without the condition but who are similar with respect to a

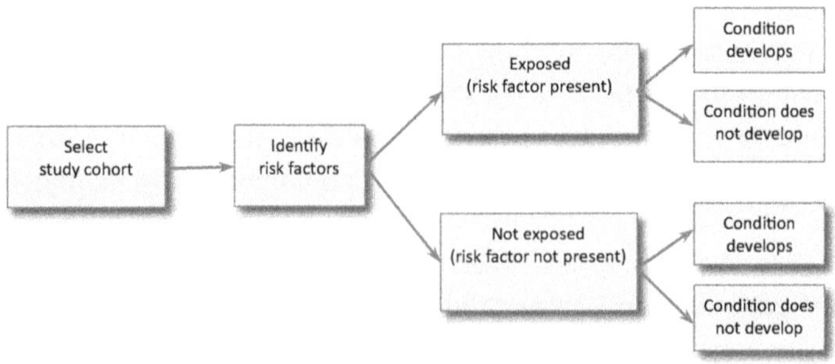

Figure 2.7 Cohort study design.

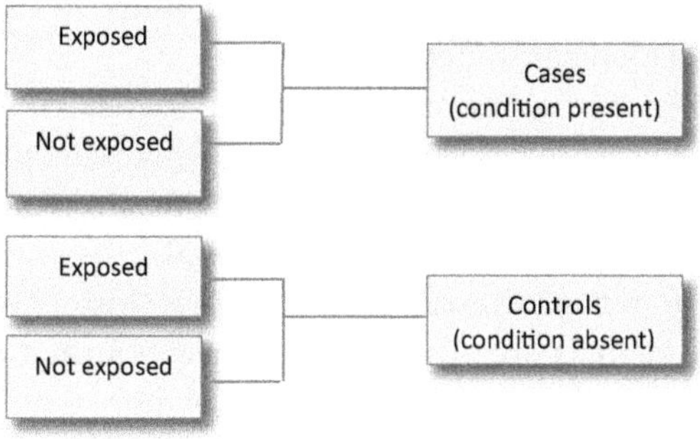

Figure 2.8 Case–control study design.

predictor variable (known risk factor). The investigator determines which individuals were exposed to the risk factors in each of the study groups. The frequency or levels of past exposure are measured to show the statistical (not causal) relationship between cases that develop the condition and controls that do not have the condition (see Fig. 2.8).

Cross-sectional studies are observational studies used to determine prevalence of a medical condition across a whole population by providing a snapshot of that population at a single point in time. The investigator looks whether study participants were exposed to the risk factors and whether they have the condition of interest, as well as whether there are any other health-related variables such as socio-economic status and geographic location (see Fig. 2.9).

Surveillance studies (e.g., using registries or surveys) are observational studies using previously collected data. They can be used to construct a cohort, to produce a sample for a cross-sectional study or

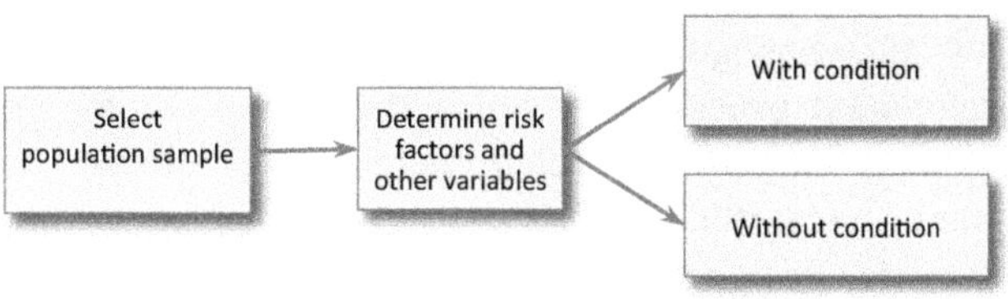

Figure 2.9 Cross-sectional study design.

to identify people with certain conditions or outcomes and produce a sample for a case-controlled study.

Consecutive case series are descriptive studies consisting of a collation of consecutive cases of a medical condition, usually originating from the practice of one or more healthcare professionals or a defined healthcare setting such as a hospital.

Single-case reports describe the medical history of a single patient. Case reports are often run together to form a consecutive case series, in which the medical histories of more than one patient with a particular condition are described to illustrate an aspect of the condition.

2.6.2.2 Feasibility and first-in-human studies

In some situations, a smaller feasibility or pilot study may be required for significant risk devices before embarking on a larger-scale pivotal study.

An early feasibility study is a limited clinical investigation of a device early in development, typically before the device design has been finalized, for a specific indication (e.g., innovative device for a new or established intended use, marketed device for a novel clinical application). When the study objective is to evaluate a specific device indication for the first time in human subjects the early feasibility study is also referred to as an FIH study.

An early feasibility study is mainly intended to evaluate the device design concept with regard to initial clinical safety and device functionality in a small number of patients (generally fewer than 10 initial subjects) when this information cannot practically be provided through additional nonclinical assessments or appropriate nonclinical tests are unavailable. Information obtained from an early feasibility study may guide design modifications and help optimize the development process by refining the indications for use and intended use, adjust the surgical or operator technique and develop subsequent clinical study protocols.

If the device design is finalized or almost finalized, a traditional feasibility study, which is focused on providing initial clinical safety and effectiveness information for a near-final or final device design or capturing data to guide the development of a pivotal study, may be more appropriate.

It is not required to perform exhaustive pre-clinical bench testing prior to embarking on a feasibility study; however, the basic safety tests (sterility, biocompatibility, electrical safety, EMC and chemical compatibility with concomitant drugs, chemicals or cleaners) should be completed with positive results before using the device on humans. The risk analysis should be mature enough so that catastrophic failure modes are identified and risk mitigation approaches implemented.

It is widely accepted that changes to the design are necessary during this phase so that performance can be improved through iteration before finalizing the design. As long as the intended use and principle of operation remain the same, changes to the device design do not require pre-approval from an Ethics Committee and/or regulatory authorities before implementation.

The FDA document *Investigational Device Exemptions (IDEs) for Early Feasibility Medical Device Clinical Studies, Including Certain First in Human (FIH) Studies* provides detailed guidance on the preparation of applications for early feasibility studies [87].

2.6.2.3 Pivotal studies

A pivotal study is a clinical investigation designed to collect definitive evidence of the safety and effectiveness of a device for a specified intended use, in a large enough number of patients so that the outcomes are statistically significant and not due to chance. A pivotal study may or may not be preceded by a feasibility study.

A pivotal clinical trial must have a clear objective supported by a scientific rationale for why the study is being performed. Clinical outcomes are expressed as primary and secondary endpoints. For example, the primary endpoint of an investigation involving a novel therapeutic device may be to demonstrate superior safety and effectiveness compared to the standard therapy, and the secondary endpoint may be to improve patients' quality of life.

The study protocol needs to describe the method used for subject selection, which must ensure that patients enrolled for the study adequately reflect the target population for the device (i.e., the population for whom the device is intended). The enrollment criteria must be specific and based on confirmatory laboratory or other testing.

The rationale for the selection of clinical study design, methods used for observing and recording results, including the variables measured, and steps taken to minimize any possible bias of subjects and observers must be documented. The clinical trial report must also include a statistical analysis of the primary endpoints and an evaluation of the data derived from the study [88].

Clinical trials can be very expensive to run. Qualified investigators and experts in clinical research, biostatistics and science are needed to design and manage a study, as well as to analyze and interpret the collected data. These international standards and guidelines are widely recognized as best practices and form the basis for national regulations on clinical trials involving human subjects:

- International Conference on Harmonization (ICH) guidance documents [89];
- EN/ISO 14155: 2011, *Clinical investigation of medical devices for human subjects – Good clinical practice*;
- GHTF guidance SG5/N3:2010, *Clinical investigations* [90]; and
- GHTF guidance SG5/N5:2012, *Reportable events during pre-market clinical investigations* [91].

An overview of regulations and guidelines for running clinical trials in the established jurisdictions – the EU, the United States, Australia, Canada and Japan – is provided in Chapter 5.

2.6.3 *Clinical Data from Post-Market Surveillance*

After obtaining marketing authorization, manufacturers must continue to collect and evaluate data on clinical safety and effectiveness throughout the life cycle of the medical device. Regulations require that manufacturers establish and maintain a systematic procedure for collecting feedback from the field, known as post-market surveillance, to provide early warning of product-related problems and for input into corrective and preventive action processes.

Clinical trials in the pre-market phase are not sufficient to provide information on the long-term safety and performance of medical devices, but on the other hand very large pre-market trials would unnecessarily delay patient access to new or improved medical technologies. According to the FDA:

> Getting the right balance between premarket and post-market data collection—specifically, where appropriate, a greater reliance on post-market collection—can reduce the extent of premarket data submission and directly impact when patients will have access to high-quality, safe and effective medical devices. But, greater reliance on post-market data collection could undermine patient safety if the necessary and timely data collection does not occur [92].

Clinical data in the post-market phase comes from two main sources:

- Vigilance and reporting system, which is reactive in nature, whereby data from complaints and adverse events is gathered, analyzed and reported to the relevant authorities.
- Post-market clinical follow-up (PMCF) studies, which are proactive in nature, carried out after a device has been placed on the market to answer specific questions relating to clinical safety or performance (i.e., residual risks) of a device when used in accordance with its approved intended purpose. For high-risk devices, performing PMCF studies may be a condition of approval.

Regulations and regulatory guidelines for post-market surveillance are covered in Chapter 6.

2.7 Case Study: Deficient Clinical Data

A company developing AIMDs for the hearing impaired submitted a pre-market application to the FDA, seeking approval for its innovative sound-processing algorithm used with the device. The algorithm represented a significant change from the previously approved version, with new claims of clinical performance added to the device labelling. The clinical data section of the submission included a review of the scientific literature as well as performance data from a clinical investigation.

After completing the review the agency sent a letter of deficiencies to the manufacturer, listing numerous problems with the clinical section of the submission. They included:

- Clinical performance data did not cover the modifications to the device design, and there was no justification to explain why clinical performance data was not required; hence the reviewer could not make a determination regarding the effectiveness of the proposed modifications.
- The new algorithm functionalities were not tested outside of a controlled clinical environment.
- The clinical performance data that was included had been collected using only experienced, adult implant patients at the same study site, whereas the claims in the proposed labelling referred to the "general population", implying applicability to the paediatric population as well.
- The investigational study report did not include a breakdown on the gender of the study subjects.
- The clinical investigational plan stated that analysis on up to 100 patients would be performed, but the clinical study report included only data from less than 50 study participants, with no justification explaining the reduced sample size.
- Data on certain new algorithm functionalities was collected using only a small number of patients (less than 10).
- The submission included claims that the new algorithm introduced other minor improvements, but with no clinical performance data to substantiate the claim.

The manufacturer faced a choice between re-running the clinical trial and removing the claims about the new algorithm from its labelling. Due to timelines and budget pressures the company decided to remove the claims from the labelling, which resulted in only a marginally improved version of the device being launched in the United States. In the next months the sales dropped by almost

70%, as the market did not receive the highly anticipated new, fully featured version of the device.

2.8 Concluding Summary

Chapter 2 discusses concepts and requirements related to safety and effectiveness of medical devices and IVDs:

- Definitions and terminology – safety, effectiveness, efficacy, intended use and indications for use;
- The two main areas of compliance: – [1] product compliance with the Essential Requirements or Essential Principles (ERs/EPs) of safety and effectiveness and [2] QMS compliance with relevant standards and regulations related to development, manufacturing and post-market surveillance of the device;
- Statutory ERs/EPs defined in established markets regulations, the GHTF guidance and the ASEAN MDD;
- QMS processes and related requirements defined in FDA quality system regulations and the ISO 13485 standard;
- The use of standards in demonstrating compliance with regulatory requirements;
- Risk management methodology and some of the specific risks associated with medical devices; and
- Clinical evaluation, including literature review, clinical trials and post-market surveillance.

References

1. ISO/IEC. ISO/IEC Guide 51:2014 Safety aspects – Guidelines for their inclusion in standards, Section 3 Terms and definitions. *www.iso.org.* [Online] April 1, 2014. [Cited: August 10, 2014.] http://www.iso.org/iso/catalogue_detail.htm?csnumber=53940.
2. Food and Drug Administration. 21 CFR 860.7 Determination of safety and effectiveness. *www.accessdata.fda.gov.* [Online] June 1, 2013.

[Cited: August 30, 2014.] http://www.accessdata.fda.gov/scripts/cdrh/cfdocs/cfCFR/CFRSearch.cfm?FR=860.7.

3. Global Harmonization Taskforce. GHTF SG1/N68:2012 Essential Principles of Safety and Performance of Medical Devices. *www.imdrf.org.* [Online] November 2, 2012. [Cited: April 28, 2014.] http://www.imdrf.org/docs/ghtf/final/sg1/technical-docs/ghtf-sg1-n68-2012-safety-performance-medical-devices-121102.pdf.
4. IEC. IEC 60601-1 Medical electrical equipment – Part 1: General requirements for basic safety and essential performance – Edition 3.1 Consolidated with Amendment 1, Section 3 Terminology and definitions. *webstore.iec.ch.* [Online] August 20, 2012. [Cited: August 10, 2014.] http://webstore.iec.ch/webstore/webstore.nsf/Artnum_PK/46826.
5. Food and Drug Administration. Guidance for Industry – Providing Clinical Evidence of Effectiveness for Human Drug and Biological Products. *www.fda.gov.* [Online] May 1998. [Cited: August 10, 2014.] http://www.fda.gov/downloads/drugs/guidancecomplianceregulatory information/guidances/ucm078749.pdf.
6. Food and Drug Administration. 21 CFR 814 Premarket Approval of Medical Devices, Section 814.20 Application. *www.accessdata.fda.gov.* [Online] June 1, 2013. [Cited: August 10, 2014.] http://www.accessdata.fda.gov/scripts/cdrh/cfdocs/cfcfr/cfrsearch.cfm?fr=814.20.
7. ISO. ISO 14971:2007 Medical devices – Application of risk management to medical devices, Section 2 Terms and definitions. [Online] October 1, 2007. [Cited: August 10, 2014.] http://www.iso.org/iso/catalogue_detail?csnumber=38193.
8. Food and Drug Administration. The 510(k) Program: Evaluating Substantial Equivalence in Premarket Notifications [510(k)]. *www.fda.gov.* [Online] July 28, 2014. [Cited: August 10, 2014.] http://www.fda.gov/downloads/MedicalDevices/DeviceRegulationand Guidance/GuidanceDocuments/UCM284443.pdf.
9. European Commission. New Legislative Framework – Blue Guide 2014. *ec.europa.eu.* [Online] April 2, 2014. [Cited: August 30, 2014.] http://ec.europa.eu/enterprise/policies/single-market-goods/documents/internal-market-for-products/new-legislative-framework/index_en.htm#h2-3.
10. European Commission. Council Directive 90/385/EEC of 20 June 1990 on the approximation of the laws of the Member States relating to active implantable medical devices. *eur-lex.europa.eu.* [Online]

[Cited: April 28, 2014.] http://eur-lex.europa.eu/legal-content/en/ALL/?uri=CELEX:31990L0385.

11. European Commission. Council Directive 93/42/EEC of 14 June 1993 concerning medical devices. *eur-lex.europa.eu.* [Online] [Cited: April 28, 2014.] http://eur-lex.europa.eu/legal-content/en/ALL/?uri=CELEX:31993L0042.
12. European Commission. Directive 98/79/EC of the European Parliament and of the Council of 27 October 1998 on in vitro diagnostic medical devices. *eur-lex.europa.eu.* [Online] [Cited: April 28, 2014.] http://eur-lex.europa.eu/legal-content/en/ALL/?uri=CELEX:31998L0079.
13. Therapeutic Goods Administration. Therapeutic Goods (Medical Devices) Regulations 2002, Part 2 Essential Principles. *www.comlaw.gov.au.* [Online] November 5, 2014. [Cited: November 18, 2014.] http://www.comlaw.gov.au/Details/F2014C01238/Html/Text#_Toc403049923.
14. Health Canada. Medical Devices Regulations SOR/98-282, Part 1 GENERAL – Safety and Effectiveness Requirements. *laws-lois.justice.gc.ca.* [Online] 12 16, 2011. [Cited: August 30, 2014.] http://laws-lois.justice.gc.ca/eng/regulations/SOR-98-282/FullText.html.
15. Regulatory Affairs Professionals Society. *Fundamentals of Japanese Regulatory Affairs, First Edition.* Regulatory Affairs Professionals Society, Rockville, MD, 2010.
16. ASEAN. ASEAN Agreement on Medical Device Directive. *www.hsa.gov.sg.* [Online] May 8, 2012. [Cited: April 28, 2014.] http://ec.europa.eu/enterprise/policies/european-standards/standardisation-policy/index_en.htm.
17. Food and Drug Administration. Content of a 510(k). *www.fda.gov.* [Online] [Cited: April 28, 2014.] http://www.fda.gov/MedicalDevices/DeviceRegulationandGuidance/HowtoMar-ketYourDevice/PremarketSubmissions/PremarketNotification510k/ucm142651.htm.
18. Food and Drug Administration. PMA Application Contents. *www.fda.gov.* [Online] [Cited: April 28, 2014.] http://www.fda.gov/MedicalDevices/DeviceRegulationandGuidance/HowtoMar-ketYourDevice/PremarketSubmissions/PremarketApprovalPMA/ucm050289.htm.
19. Theisz, V. Essential principles of safety and efficacy – Streamlining design and documentation processes for global compliance of medical devices. February, s.l.: *JMDR*, February 2009, Vol. Supplement.
20. Food and Drug Administration. Medical Devices; Current Good Manufacturing Practice (CGMP) Final Rule; Quality System Regulation.

www.fda.gov. [Online] [Cited: April 28, 2014.] http://www.fda.gov/MedicalDevices/DeviceRegulationandGuidance/PostmarketRequirements/QualitySystemsRegulations/ucm230127.htm.

21. Food and Drug Administration. What is the relationship between FDA's Quality System Regulation for Devices, Part 820, and ISO 9001:2000? *www.fda.gov.* [Online] [Cited: August 30, 2014.] http://www.fda.gov/downloads/MedicalDevices/DeviceRegulationandGuidance/PostmarketRequirements/QualitySystemsRegulations/UCM134625.pdf.
22. European Commission. Harmonised Standards. *ec.europa.eu.* [Online] February 4, 2014. [Cited: September 1, 2014.] http://ec.europa.eu/enterprise/policies/european-standards/harmonised-standards/index_en.htm#h2-3.
23. Food and Drug Administration. FDA Recognized Consensus Standards. *www.accessdata.fda.gov.* [Online] [Cited: September 1, 2014.] http://www.accessdata.fda.gov/scripts/cdrh/cfdocs/cfstandards/search.cfm.
24. Therapeutic Goods Administration. Standards orders and medical devices. *www.tga.gov.au.* [Online] December 15, 2008. [Cited: September 1, 2014.] http://www.tga.gov.au/industry/devices-standards-orders.htm#.VCO21vmSx8F.
25. Health Canada. Standards. *www.hc-sc.gc.ca.* [Online] October 28, 2013. [Cited: September 1, 2014.] http://www.hc-sc.gc.ca/dhp-mps/md-im/standards-normes/index-eng.php.
26. Pharmaceuticals and Medical Devices Agency. List of Certification Standards. *www.std.pmda.go.jp.* [Online] [Cited: September 1, 2014.] http://www.std.pmda.go.jp/scripts/stdDB/pubeng/stdDB_pubeng_stdlist.cgi?displist=1.
27. Pharmaceuticals and Medical Devices Agency. List of Approval Standards. *www.std.pmda.go.jp.* [Online] [Cited: September 1, 2014.] http://www.std.pmda.go.jp/scripts/stdDB/pubeng/stdDB_pubeng_stdlist.cgi?displist=2.
28. Food and Drug Administration. FDA guidance – Recognition and Use of Consensus Standards. *www.fda.gov.* [Online] September 17, 2007. [Cited: September 1, 2014.] http://www.fda.gov/MedicalDevices/DeviceRegulationandGuidance/GuidanceDocuments/ucm077274.htm.
29. Zentralstelle der Länder für Gesundheitsschutz (ZLG) bei Arzneimitteln und Medizinprodukten. Antworten und Beschlüsse EK-Med. *www.zlg.de.* [Online] October 2005. [Cited: September 1, 2014.] https://

www.zlg.de/index.php?eID=tx_nawsecuredl&u=0&file=fileadmin/downloads/ab/305-1004-A01.pdf&hash=ec5b912f41f615bc2b3fdc18975dc43eeac67061.

30. Theisz, V. RF focus – Risk management for medical devices – A practical approach. *www.certificationbody.com.au.* [Online] June 2012. [Cited: August 10, 2014.] http://www.certificationbody.com.au/documents/RF201206RiskMgmt.pdf.
31. Asian Harmonization Working Party (AHWP). White Paper on Medical Device Software Regulation – Software QWualification and Classification (draft). *www.ahwp.info.* [Online] May 22, 2014. [Cited: September 1, 2014.] http://www.ahwp.info/index.php?q=node/413.
32. European Commission. MEDDED 2.1/6 Guidelines on the qualification and classification of stand-alone software used in healthcare within the regulatory framework of medical devices. *ec.europa.eu.* [Online] January 2012. [Cited: September 1, 2014.] http://ec.europa.eu/health/medical-devices/files/meddev/2_1_6_ol_en.pdf.
33. European Commission. MEDDEV 2.4/1 Rev 9 June 2012 – Classification of medical devices. *ec.europa.eu.* [Online] June 2012. [Cited: April 28, 2014.] http://ec.europa.eu/health/medical-devices/files/meddev/2_4_1_rev_9_classification_en.pdf.
34. Therapeutic Goods Administration. Australian Regulatory Guidelines for Medical Devices (ARGMD), Section 13 Active medical devices. *www.tga.gov.au.* [Online] May 2011. [Cited: September 1, 2014.] http://www.tga.gov.au/pdf/devices-argmd-01.pdf.
35. Therapeutic Goods Administration. Regulation of medical software and mobile medical 'apps'. *www.tga.gov.au.* [Online] September 13, 2013. [Cited: September 1, 2014.] http://www.tga.gov.au/industry/devices-software-mobile-apps.htm#.VA0Zm_m1bYg.
36. Health Canada. Guidance for the risk based classification system (Draft). *www.hc-sc.gc.ca.* [Online] May 4, 1998. [Cited: April 28, 2014.] http://www.hc-sc.gc.ca/dhp-mps/md-im/applic-demande/guide-ld/risk5_risque5-eng.php.
37. Health Canada. Guidance for the risk based classification system of in vitro diagnostic devices (Draft). *www.hc-sc.gc.ca.* [Online] April 24, 1998. [Cited: May 10, 2014.] http://www.hc-sc.gc.ca/dhp-mps/alt_formats/hpfb-dgpsa/pdf/md-im/ivd-rsk_idiv-rsq-eng.pdf.
38. Health Canada. Software Regulated as a Medical Device – FAQ. *www.hc-sc.gc.ca.* [Online] January 24, 2011. [Cited: September 1, 2014.] http://www.hc-sc.gc.ca/dhp-mps/md-im/activit/announce-annonce/md_qa_software_im_qr_logicels-eng.php.

39. Food and Drug Administration. FDA Guidance – Mobile Medical Applications. *www.fda.gov.* [Online] September 25, 2013. [Cited: September 1, 2014.] http://www.fda.gov/downloads/MedicalDevices/DeviceRegulationandGuidance/GuidanceDocuments/UCM263366.pdf.
40. Food and Drug Administration. FDa Guidance – General Principles of Software Validation. [Online] January 11, 2002. [Cited: September 1, 2014.] http://www.fda.gov/medicaldevices/deviceregulationand guidance/guidancedocuments/ucm085281.htm.
41. Food and Drug Administration. FDA Guidance – Off-The-Shelf Software Use in Medical Devices. *www.fda.gov.* [Online] September 9, 1999. [Cited: September 1, 2014.] http://www.fda.gov/medicaldevices/deviceregulationandguidance/guidancedocuments/ucm073778.htm.
42. Food and Drug Administration. Guidance for the Content of Premarket Submissions for Software Contained in Medical Devices. *www.fda.gov.* [Online] May 11, 2005. [Cited: May 31, 2014.] http://www.fda.gov/MedicalDevices/DeviceRegulationandGuidance/GuidanceDocuments/ucm089543.htm.
43. IMDRF. IMDRF/SaMD WG/N10:2013 Software as a Medical Device (SaMD): Key Definitions. *www.imdrf.org.* [Online] December 9, 2013. [Cited: August 30, 2014.] http:// www.imdrf.org/docs/imdrf/final/technical/imdrf-tech-131209-samd-key-definitions-140901.pdf.
44. Patel, B. Software as a medical device (SaMD): Possible framework for risk categorization and corresponding considerations. *www.imdrf.org.* [Online] August 15, 2014. [Cited: September 1, 2014.] http://www.imdrf.org/docs/imdrf/final/meetings/imdrf-meet-140829-washington-presentation-samd.pdf#search="software".
45. Food and Drug Administration. Radio Frequency Wireless Technology in Medical Devices – Guidance for Industry and FDA Staff. *www.fda.gov.* [Online] August 13, 2013. [Cited: May 31, 2014.] http://www.fda.gov/medicaldevices/deviceregulationandguidance/guidancedocuments/ucm077210.htm.
46. Food and Drug Administration. FDA Guidance (draft) – Content of Premarket Submissions for Management of Cybersecurity in Medical Devices. *www.fda.gov.* [Online] June 14, 2013. [Cited: September 1, 2014.] http://www.fda.gov/medicaldevices/deviceregulationandguidance/guidancedocuments/ucm356186.htm.
47. Food and Drug Administration. FDA Guidance – Cybersecurity for Networked Medical Devices Containing Off-the-Shelf (OTS) Software. *www.fda.gov.* [Online] January 14, 2005. [Cited: September 1, 2014.]

http://www.fda.gov/medicaldevices/deviceregulationandguidance/guidancedocuments/ucm077812.htm.

48. European Commission. Directive 2002/95/EC on the restriction of the use of certain hazardous substances in electrical and electronic equipment. *eu-lex.europa.eu.* [Online] January 27, 2003. [Cited: September 1, 2014.] http://eur-lex.europa.eu/legal-content/EN/ALL/?uri=CELEX:32002L0095.
49. European Commission. Directive 2011/65/EU on the restriction of the use of certain hazardous substances in electrical and electronic equipment. *eu-lex.europa.eu.* [Online] June 8, 2011. [Cited: September 1, 2014.] http://eur-lex.europa.eu/legal-content/en/ALL/?uri=CELEX:32011L0065.
50. European Commission. Directive 2012/19/EU on waste electrical and electronic equipment (WEEE). *eur-lex.europa.eu.* [Online] July 4, 2012. [Cited: September 1, 2014.] http://eur-lex.europa.eu/legal-content/EN/TXT/?uri=CELEX:32012L0019.
51. European Agency for Safety and Health at Work. Regulation (EC) 1907/2006 – REACH. *osha.europa.eu.* [Online] December 18, 2006. [Cited: September 1, 2014.] https://osha.europa.eu/en/legislation/directives/exposure-to-chemical-agents-and-chemical-safety/osh-related-aspects/regulation-ec-no-1907-2006-of-the-european-parliament-and-of-the-council.
52. European Commission. Directive 2066/66/EC on batteries and acumulators and waste batteries and accumulators. *eur-lex.europa.eu.* [Online] September 6, 2006. [Cited: September 1, 2014.] http://eur-lex.europa.eu/legal-content/EN/ALL/?uri=CELEX:32006L0066.
53. European Commission. Directive 94/62/EC on packaging and packaging waste. *eur-lex.europa.eu.* [Online] December 20, 1994. [Cited: September 1, 2014.] http://eur-lex.europa.eu/legal-content/EN/ALL/?uri=CELEX:31994L0062.
54. Environmental Protection Agency. EPA Regulations. *www2.epa.gov.* [Online] March 13, 2014. [Cited: September 1, 2014.] http://www2.epa.gov/laws-regulations/regulations.
55. Valentin, J.-P., PhD. Pharmacological characteristics of biologics and large molecules. *www.hesiglobal.org.* [Online] [Cited: October 3, 2014.] http://www.hesiglobal.org/files/public/Committees/CV/June%2009%20Workshop/Day%202%20Presentations/01ValentinBiologics.pdf.
56. Biotechnology Industry Organization. How Do Drugs and Biologics Differ? *www.bio.org.* [Online] November 10, 2010. [Cited: October 3, 2014.] http://www.bio.org/articles/how-do-drugs-and-biologics-differ.

57. Mitchell, P. Critics pan timid European response to TeGenero disaster. *www.nature.com.* [Online] April 30, 2007. [Cited: September 1, 2014.] http://www.nature.com/nbt/journal/v25/n5/full/nbt0507-485.html.
58. Story, M.F., PhD. Human factors considerations for combination products. *www.fda.gov.* [Online] October 24, 2011. [Cited: September 1, 2014.] http://www.fda.gov/downloads/MedicalDevices/Device RegulationandGuidance/HumanFactors/UCM282338.pdf.
59. Klepper, M.J., MD. Risk considerations for combination drug-device products. *www.rti.org.* [Online] 2005. [Cited: September 1, 2014.] https://www.rti.org/pubs/risk_considerations.pdf.
60. Lockwood, N., PhD. Therapeutic coatings for medical device implants. *www.mdtmag.com.* [Online] January 10, 2013. [Cited: September 1, 2014.] http://www.mdtmag.com/articles/2013/10/therapeutic-coatings-medical-device-implants.
61. Therapeutic Goods Administration. Transmissible spongiform encephalopathies (TSE): TGA approach to minimising the risk of exposure. *www.tga.gov.au.* [Online] April 2, 2014. [Cited: September 1, 2014.] http://www.tga.gov.au/industry/tse-approach.htm#.VBZYq_mSx8E.
62. European Commission. Regulation (EU) No 722/2012 concerning particular requirements as regards the requirements laid down in Council Directives 90/385/EEC and 93/42/EEC with respect to AIMDs and MDs manufactured utilising tissues of animal origins. *eur-lex.europa.eu.* [Online] August 8, 2012. [Cited: September 1, 2014.] http://eur-lex.europa.eu/legal-content/EN/TXT/?qid=14107597090 02&uri=CELEX:32012R0722.
63. European Commission. Directive 2003/32/EC on the requirements with respect to medical devices manufactured utilising tissues of animal origin. *eur-lex.europa.eu.* [Online] April 23, 2003. [Cited: September 1, 2014.] http://eur-lex.europa.eu/legal-content/HR/TXT/?uri=CELEX: 32003L0032.
64. TÜV SÜD. BSE symposium – Everything about the new Regulation (EU) No. 722/2012. *www.tuv-sud.com.* [Online] [Cited: September 1, 2014.] http://www.tuv-sud.com/home-com/resource-centre/publications/e-ssentials-newsletter/mhs-e-ssentials/issue-1-march-2013/bse-symposium-everything-about-the-new-regulation-eu-no.-722-2012.
65. Food and Drug Administration. FDA Guidance (draft) – Medical Devices Containing Materials Derived from Animal Sources (Except for In Vitro Diagnostic Devices). *www.fda.gov.* [Online] January 23, 2014. [Cited: September 1, 2014.] http://www.fda.gov/medicaldevices/deviceregulationandguidance/guidancedocuments/ucm381379.htm.

66. Health Canada. Guidance Document on the Regulation of Medical Devices Manufactured from or Incorporating Viable or Non-Viable Animal Tissue or their Derivative(s). *www.hc-sc.gc.ca.* [Online] July 12, 2004. [Cited: September 1, 2014.] http://www.hc-sc.gc.ca/dhp-mps/md-im/applic-demande/guide-ld/anim_tiss-eng.php.
67. Hayakawa, T., Pharmaceuticals and Medical Devices Agency. Some aspects of development, evaluation and control of biologics in Japan. *www.pmda.go.jp.* [Online] February 15, 2007. [Cited: September 1, 2014.] http://www.pmda.go.jp/english/events/pdf/1-hayakawa.pdf.
68. Food and Drug Administration. DEHP in Plastic Medical Devices. *www.fda.gov.* [Online] January 28, 2014. [Cited: September 1, 2014.] http://www.fda.gov/medicaldevices/resourcesforyou/consumers/choosingamedicaldevice/ucm142643.htm.
69. Food and Drug Administration. Phthalates. *www.fda.gov.* [Online] March 19, 2014. [Cited: September 1, 2014.] http://www.fda.gov/cosmetics/productsingredients/ingredients/ucm128250.htm.
70. Food and Drug Administration. Safety Assessment of Di(2-ethylhexyl)phthalate (DEHP) Released from PVC Medical Devices. *www.fda.gov.* [Online] September 2001. [Cited: October 3, 2014.] http://www.fda.gov/downloads/MedicalDevices/DeviceRegulationandGuidance/GuidanceDocuments/UCM080457.pdf.
71. Food and Drug Administration. FDA Public Health Notification: PVC Devices Containing the Plasticizer DEHP. *www.fda.gov.* [Online] July 12, 2002. [Cited: October 3, 2014.] http://www.fda.gov/MedicalDevices/Safety/AlertsandNotices/PublicHealthNotifications/ucm062182.htm.
72. Scientific Committee on Emerging and Newly-Identified Health Risks (SCENIHR). Scientific opinion on the safety of medical devices containing DEHP-plasticized PVC or other plasticizers on neonates and other groups possibly at risk. *ec.europa.eu.* [Online] September 24, 2014. [Cited: October 3, 2014.] http://ec.europa.eu/health/scientific_committees/emerging/docs/scenihr_o_047.pdf.
73. European Commission. MEDDEV 2.5/9 Implications of the MDD (93/42/EEC) in relation to medical devices containing natural rubber latex. *ec.europa.eu.* [Online] February 2004. [Cited: September 1, 2014.] http://ec.europa.eu/health/medical-devices/files/meddev/2_5_9rev_latex_en.pdf.
74. Food and Drug Administration. FDA draft guidance – Recommendations for Labeling Medical Products to Inform Users that the

Product or Product Container is not Made with Natural Rubber Latex. *www.fda.gov.* [Online] March 11, 2013. [Cited: September 1, 2014.] http://www.fda.gov/medicaldevices/deviceregulationandguidance/guidancedocuments/ucm340972.htm.

75. Global Harmonization Taskforce. GHTF SG5/N1R8:2007 Clinical Evidence. *www.imdrf.org.* [Online] May 2007. [Cited: September 1, 2014.] http://www.imdrf.org/docs/ghtf/final/sg5/technical-docs/ghtf-sg5-n1r8-clinical-evaluation-key-definitions-070501.pdf.
76. Global Harmonization Taskforce. GHTF SG5/N2R8:2007 Clinical Evaluation. *www.imdrf.org.* [Online] May 2007. [Cited: September 1, 2014.] http://www.imdrf.org/docs/ghtf/final/sg5/technical-docs/ghtf-sg5-n2r8-2007-clinical-evaluation-070501.pdf.
77. European Commission. MEDDEV 2.7.1 Clinical evaluation: A guide for manufacturers and notified bodies. *ec.europa.eu.* [Online] December 2009. [Cited: September 1, 2014.] http://ec.europa.eu/health/medical-devices/files/meddev/2_7_1rev_3_en.pdf.
78. NBOG. NBOG documents. *www.nbog.eu.* [Online] [Cited: May 31, 2014.] http://www.nbog.eu/2.html.
79. Global Harmonization Taskforce. GHTF SG5/N6:2012 Clinical Evidence for IVD medical devices. [Online] November 2, 2012. [Cited: September 1, 2014.] http://www.imdrf.org/docs/ghtf/final/sg5/technical-docs/ghtf-sg5-n6-2012-clinical-evidence-ivd-medical-devices-121102.pdf.
80. Global Harmonization Taskforce. GHTF SG5/N7:2012 Clinical Evidence for IVD medical devices – Scientific Validity Determination and Performance Evaluation. [Online] November 2, 2012. [Cited: September 1, 2014.] http://www.imdrf.org/docs/ghtf/final/sg5/technical-docs/ghtf-sg5-n7-2012-scientific-validity-determination-evaluation-121102.pdf.
81. Global Harmonization Taskforce. GHTF SG5?N8:2012 Clinical Evidence for IVD medical devices – Clinical Performance Studies for IVDs. *www.imdrf.org.* [Online] November 2, 2012. [Cited: September 1, 2014.] http://www.imdrf.org/docs/ghtf/final/sg5/technical-docs/ghtf-sg5-n8-2012-clinical-performance-studies-ivd-medical-devices-121102.pdf.
82. Food and Drug Administration. Supplements to Approved Applications for Class III Medical Devices: Use of Published Literature, Use of Previously Submitted Materials, and Priority Review. *www.fda.gov.* [Online] May 20, 1998. [Cited: September 1, 2014.] http://

www.fda.gov/medicaldevices/deviceregulationandguidance/guidance-documents/ucm080183.htm.

83. WMA. WMA Declaration of Helsinki – Ethical Principles for Medical Research Involving Human Subjects. *www.wma.net.* [Online] October 2013. [Cited: September 1, 2014.] http://www.wma.net/en/30publications/10policies/b3/.
84. Clinical Information Access Portal (CIAP) eLearning. Module 4: Integrating Evidence into Practice, Section 3: Selecting the evidence. *www.ciap.health.nsw.gov.au.* [Online] [Cited: September 1, 2014.] http://www.ciap.health.nsw.gov.au/education/learning/module4/section_3_7.html.
85. The McGraw-Hill Companies. Basic and Clinical Biostatistics – Chapter 2. Study Designs in Medical Research. *www.people.vcu.edu.* [Online] [Cited: September 1, 2014.] http://www.people.vcu.edu/_albest/DENS580/DawsonTrapp/Chap2.htm.
86. Food and Drug Administration. Investigational Device Exemptions (IDEs) for Early Feasibility Medical Device Clinical Studies, Including Certain First In Human (FIH) Studies. *www.fda.com.* [Online] October 1, 2013. [Cited: September 1, 2014.] http://www.fda.gov/downloads/MedicalDevices/DeviceRegulationandGuidance/GuidanceDocuments/UCM279103.pdf.
87. Food and Drug Administration. Design Considerations for Pivotal Clinical Investigations for Medical Devices. *www.fda.com.* [Online] November 7, 2013. [Cited: September 1, 2014.] http://www.fda.gov/medicaldevices/deviceregulationandguidance/guidancedocuments/ucm373750.htm#s6.
88. International Conference on Harmonization (ICH). ICH Guidelines. *www.ich.org.* [Online] 2014. [Cited: September 1, 2014.] http://www.ich.org/products/guidelines.html.
89. Global Harmonization Taskforce. GHTF SG5/N3:2010 Clinical Investigations. *www.imdrf.org.* [Online] February 12, 2010. [Cited: September 1, 2014.] http://www.imdrf.org/docs/ghtf/final/sg5/technical-docs/ghtf-sg5-n3-clinical-investigations-100212.pdf.
90. Global Harmonization Taskforce. GHTF SG5?N5:2012 Reportable Events During PreMarket Clinical Investigations. *www.imdrf.org.* [Online] August 10, 2012. [Cited: September 1, 2014.] http://www.imdrf.org/docs/ghtf/final/sg5/technical-docs/ghtf-sg5-n5-2012-reportable-events-120810.pdf.

91. Food and Drug Administration. FDA draft guidance – Balancing Premarket and Postmarket Data Collection for Devices Subject to Premarket Approval. *www.fda.gov.* [Online] April 23, 2014. [Cited: September 22, 2014.] http://www.fda.gov/medicaldevices/device-regulationandguidance/guidancedocuments/ucm393882.htm.
92. IMDRF. About IMDRF. *www.imdrf.org.* [Online] [Cited: April 28, 2014.] http://www.imdrf.org/about/about.asp.

Chapter 3

Technical Documentation

This chapter describes the technical documentation that manufacturers need to generate and maintain and the sub-set required for regulatory submissions, including an example of product-specific documentation (Design History File) with modular content and structure that can be used to meet requirements in all major markets. The chapter also discusses trends in harmonizing the content and structure of regulatory applications and transitioning to electronic submissions.

3.1 Technical Documentation Required by Regulators

Decisions by regulatory agencies on whether or not to grant marketing approvals are based solely on evidence. When making their determination agency reviewers rely on submitted technical documentation; hence one cannot emphasize enough its importance. Claims made by a manufacturer regarding the performance of a medical device must be supported by objective, scientific data presented in a structured and logical manner. The higher the risk classification of a medical device, the more information (and documentation) to be expected.

Medical Device Regulatory Practices: An International Perspective
Val Theisz

ISBN 978-981-4669-10-8 (Hardcover), 978-981-4669-11-5 (eBook)
www.panstanford.com

Overall, the documentation and records generated by the manufacturer need to provide evidence and reasonable assurance that:

- The design and manufacture of the medical device comply with the Essential Requirements or Essential Principles of safety and effectiveness (ERs/EPs) and/or other applicable regulations and guidelines; and
- The quality management system (QMS) under which the medical device is produced consistently meets applicable regulatory requirements such as FDA 21 CFR 820, *Quality System Regulation* (QSR), and the ISO 13485 standard, *Medical devices: Quality management systems – Requirements for regulatory purposes*.

For higher-risk devices information about the product design, labelling and manufacturing processes must be provided for assessment as part of applications for marketing approval, such as design examinations in the European Union (EU) and 510(k)s and Premarket Approvals (PMAs) in the United States.

For lower-risk devices the product technical documentation must be made available to the Regulatory Authorities on request; hence it must be generated and maintained by the manufacturer, even if it is not required for PMAs.

Regulations and guidelines specify the information required to be submitted with applications or made available upon request. The next sub-sections provide a high-level overview of the product-specific and QMS information required by regulations in the main jurisdictions, along with references to relevant guidance documents.

Overall, the volume of documentation a manufacturer must manage – product development history, design and manufacturing specifications, testing undertaken to demonstrate safety and effectiveness, QMS procedures and work instructions – can be considerable. Therefore the first thing to do is to organize all this information into three main categories:

- QMS documentation – quality manual, procedures, work instructions and templates;

- Project documentation - business strategy and planning documents, project plans and reports; and
- Product technical documentation, a sub-set of which is used for regulatory submissions (where applicable) - requirements, specifications and testing.

The way these three different categories of documents are related to each other is represented conceptually in Fig. 3.1.

Needless to say, a well-structured, clear, complete and accurate documentation will significantly increase chances of obtaining regulatory approvals in the shortest possible time and will also make maintenance in the post-market phase a lot easier. This will, in turn, allow a device manufacturer to allocate precious resources where they are most needed, such as technology and product innovation.

3.1.1 *Documentation Mandated by EU Regulations*

Documentation requirements are provided in the following EU regulations and guidelines:

- Active Implantable Medical Device (AIMD) Directive, AIMDD, 90/385/EEC, Section 4 of Annex 2 and Section 3 of Annex 3
- Medical Devices Directive (MDD) 93/42/EEC, Section 4 of Annex II and Section 3 of Annex III
- In Vitro Diagnostics (IVD) Directive, IVDD, 98/79/EC, Section 3 of Annex III, Section 4 of Annex IV and Section 3 of Annex V
- NBOG BPG 2009-1, *Guidance on design-dossier examination and report content* [1], applicable to conformity assessment procedures involving design examination and type examination
- NBOG BPG 2009-4, *Guidance on notified body's tasks of technical documentation assessment on a representative basis* [2], applicable to QMS conformity assessment procedures for Class IIa and Class IIb medical devices
- NB-MED *Recommendation 2.5.1 Technical Documentation* [3]

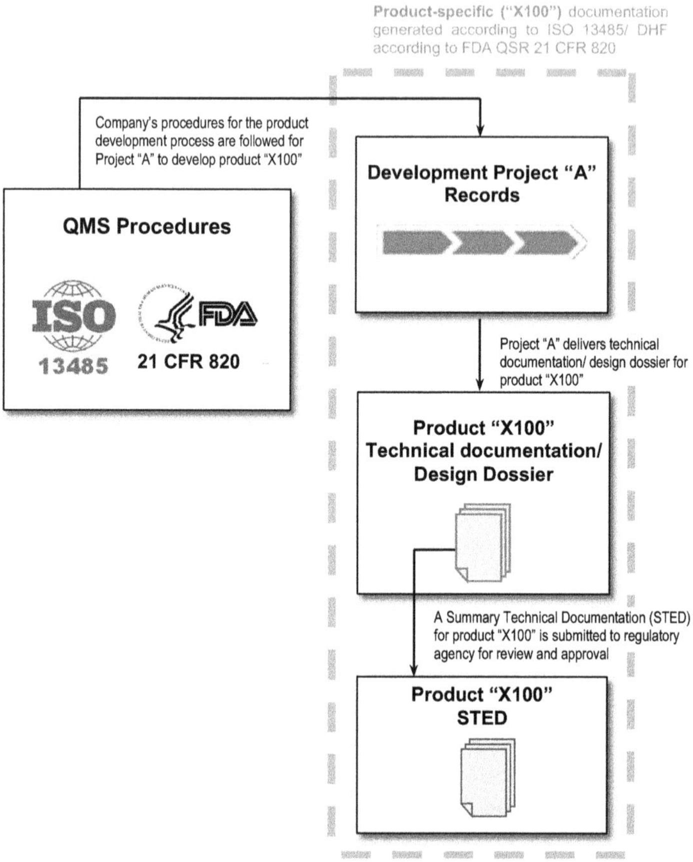

Figure 3.1 Overview of documentation and how it is structured.

The product-specific documentation mandated by EU regulations is referred to as a *design dossier* for Class III medical devices, AIMDs and IVDs and *technical documentation* for Class I, IIa and IIb medical devices. It represents a sub-set of the documentation required according to the standard EN ISO 13485, *Medical Devices – Quality management systems – Requirements for regulatory purposes*. It is not a separate document generated for the sole purpose of regulatory submissions.

Earlier versions of guidelines on technical documentation mentioned generating a technical file document, which many medical

Table 3.1 Information about the product and QMS required by EU regulations (high-level overview only)

Required information	AIMDD Annex 2 & 3	MDD Annex II & III	IVD Annex III & V
Description of design, including variants	√	√	√
Description of manufacturing process	√	√	√
Description and rationale of performance	√	√	√
QMS procedures and records, including design controls, process controls, sterilization (if applicable), product identification	√	√	√
Verification and validation (V&V)	√	√	√
Stability studies	-	-	√
Specifications, including standards applied	√	√	√
Risk analysis	√	√	√
Medicinal substances, human blood derivatives and tissues of animal origin	√	√	√
Connection to/combination with other devices	-	√	√
Clinical data/performance evaluation	√	√	√
Labelling	√	√	√

device manufacturers misinterpreted as being a separate, stand-alone document that had to be submitted for review to the notified body. In 1999 the notified bodies coordination group NB-MED replaced the term "technical file document" with "technical documentation", clarifying thus that a product *documentation system* rather than a document had to be generated and maintained (NB-MED/2.5.1, rationale for Rev 3, Meeting of NB-MED Brussels, Nov. 2 and 3, 1999: "The earlier concept to write a document on 'Technical file' was got away; not a technical file but a system/organisation of technical documentation is required.").

A high-level overview of the information required by EU regulations is presented in Table 3.1 (see also Section 1.7.3, "Regulatory Controls in Australia and the EU").

3.1.2 *Documentation Mandated by US Regulations*

Documentation requirements are provided in the following US regulations and guidelines:

- 21 CFR Part 814 Subpart B, *Premarket Approval (PMA)* Application [4];
- FD&C Act 520(h)(1)(A), Summary of Safety and Effectiveness Data (SSED) [5];
- Quality system information for certain PMA reviews [6];
- 21 CFR Part 807 Subpart E, *Premarket Notification Procedures (510k)* [7]; and
- Food and Drug Administration (FDA) *Design Control Guidance* March 11, 1997 [8].

Design controls defined in 21 CFR Part 820.30 are part of the quality system regulation (QSR) applicable to all medical devices. Virtually every section of the design control requirements specifies information which should be documented. The compilation of this information, required by the QSR to demonstrate that the design was developed in accordance with the approved design and development (D&D) plan, is referred to as the Design History File, or DHF.

Throughout the FDA *Design Control Guidance* suggestions are made as to the form and content of documents contained in the DHF. A sub-set of the DHF is required to be submitted with 510(k) and PMA applications. For certain PMAs information on the QMS (procedures, record) may be required as well.

The term "DHF" is unique to the US medical device regulations. There is no specific requirement in the International Organization for Standardization (ISO) 13485 standard or other medical device regulations for a DHF. However, the requirements for product-specific documentation in ISO 13485 and other jurisdictions overlap a great deal with the DHF.

A high-level overview of the information required by US regulations is presented in Table 3.2 (see also Section 1.7.1, "Regulatory Controls in the United States").

3.1.3 *Documentation Mandated by Australian Regulations*

Documentation requirements are provided in the following Australian regulations and guidelines:

Table 3.2 Information about the product and QMS required by US regulations (high-level overview only)

Required information	PMA, SSED	510(k)
Summary of:	√	√
Device description – design, performance, manufacturing; indications for use, contraindications, warning and precautions	√	√
Alternative practices and procedures/predicate device(s)	√	√
Marketing history	√	-
Summary of studies	√	√
Non-clinical laboratory studies summary	√	√
Clinical studies summary	√	√ (if applicable)
Conclusions drawn from the studies, risk–benefit analysis/substantial equivalence discussion	√	√
Details of:	√	√
Device description – design, functions, performance	√	√
Multiple components, accessories and/or part of a system	√	√
Manufacturing, process controls, sterilization	√	√
Performance standards applied	√	√
V&V data:	√	√
Non-clinical laboratory studies	√	√
Clinical studies	√	√ (if applicable)
Design changes	√ (if applicable)	√ (if applicable)
Relevant published literature	√	-
Labelling	√	√
Environmental assessment	√	-
QMS procedures and records, including design controls, process controls, sterilization (if applicable), product identification	√(if applicable)	-

- *Therapeutic Goods (Medical Devices) Regulations 2002*, Schedule 3 §1.4(5), §2.3(3)
- *Australian Regulatory Guidelines for Medical Devices* (ARGMD) (9 pp. 123–134; 181–187)

A high-level overview of the information required by Australian regulations is presented in Table 3.3 (see also Section 1.7.3, "Regulatory Controls in Australia and the EU").

Table 3.3 Information about the product and QMS required by Australian regulations (high-level overview only)

Required information	
Conformity assessment evidence for the medical device and/or manufacturer from third parties (if available and/or acceptable)	√
Device description, including intended purpose and principle of operation	√
Specifications	√
Labelling	√
Risk management	√
Clinical data	√
Summary of compliance with Essential Principles (EPs)	√
Compliance with applied standards, V&V	√
Materials of human blood or plasma derivatives, animal, microbial or recombinant origin; medicinal substances (if applicable)	√
Efficacy and performance data for medical devices that disinfect, including sterilization of other medical devices (if applicable)	√
Changes (if applicable)	√
QMS procedures and records, including critical suppliers, design and development (required for high-risk devices), production, sterilization (if applicable), post-market surveillance	√

3.1.4 *Documentation Mandated by Canadian Regulations*

Documentation requirements are provided in the following Canadian regulations and guidelines:

- Medical Device Regulations SOR/98-282 Section 32, Application for a Medical Device Licence
- Guidance on preparation of Summary Technical Documentation (STED)-based Class III and Class IV pre-market medical device license applications [10]
- Guidance on supporting evidence to be provided for new and amended licence applications for Class III and Class IV medical devices, not including IVDs [11]
- Guidance on preparation of STED-based Class III and IV pre-market IVD device licence applications and amendments (draft) [12]

Table 3.4 Information about the product and QMS required by Canadian regulations (high-level overview only)

Required information	Class II	Class III	Class IV
Intended purpose	√	√	√
List of standards complied with to satisfy safety and effectiveness	√	√	√
IVD performance data (if applicable)	√	√	√
QMS certification to CAN/CSA-ISO 13485	√	√	√
Device description, including principle of operation and functionalities	-	√	√
Marketing history, including a summary of reported adverse events and recalls	-	√	√
Sterilization method (if applicable)	-	√	√
V&V summary, list of published reports dealing with the use, safety and effectiveness of the device	-	√	√
Labelling	-	√	√
Risk assessment	-	-	√
Quality plan	-	-	√
Specifications	-	-	√
Manufacturing process	-	-	√
Details of V&V performed to demonstrate safety and effectiveness: pre-clinical and clinical studies, process validation, software validation (if applicable), literature studies	-	-	√
Materials of animal origin, human tissue or their derivatives	-	-	√

- Guidance on supporting evidence to be provided for Class III and IV IVD device licence applications and amendments (draft) [13]

A high-level overview of the information required by Canadian regulations is presented in Table 3.4 (see also Section 1.7.4, "Regulatory Controls in Canada").

3.1.5 *Documentation Mandated by Japanese Regulations*

Documentation requirements are provided in the following Japanese notifications and guidelines:

- *Handbook for Preparation of Summary Technical Documentation Submitted in Applications for Marketing Approval for*

Medical Devices (Yakushokukihatsu No. 0216003, February 16, 2005) [14]
- *Applications for Marketing Approval for Medical Devices* (Yakushokuhatsu No. 0216002, February 16, 2005) [15]
- *Points to Consider When Applying for Marketing Approval for Medical Devices* (Yakushokukihatsu No. 0216001, February 16, 2005) [16]
- *Medical Devices Which Need Registered Certification Bodies' Review: Designated Class II Medical Devices* (Yakushokukihatsu No. 0331008, 31 March 2005) [17]
- *Generic ("Me-Too") Medical Devices with Approval Standards* (Yakushokukihatsu No. 0401003, April 1, 2005) [18]
- *Generic ("Me-Too") Medical Devices without Approval Standards* (Yakushokukihatsu No. 0327004, March 27, 2009) [19]
- *Improved Medical Devices without Clinical Trial Data* (Yakushokukihatsu No. 0131-1, 31 January 2011) [20]

The recently enacted new Pharmaceutical and Medical Devices (PMD) Act of November 2014 introduced additional requirements for device package inserts or *Tenpubunsyo* (instructions for use [IFUs]). Manufacturers must prepare the device package inserts, taking into consideration the current scientific literature and safety data from the vigilance process, and include it in the regulatory submission. This applies to devices in all risk classes. In addition, package inserts for Class IV (high risk, specially controlled) medical devices must be provided to the Ministry of Health, Labor and Welfare (MHLW) and are published on the Pharmaceuticals and Medical Devices Agency (PMDA) website.

A high-level overview of the information required by Japanese regulations is presented in Table 3.5 (see also Section 1.7.2, "Regulatory Controls in Japan").

3.2 GHTF Summary Technical Documentation

As shown in the previous sub-sections, each established jurisdiction has its own requirements for documentation, and the level of

Table 3.5 Information about the product and QMS required by Japanese regulations (high-level overview only)

Required information	Generic ("me too") Class II, III, IV	Improved (innovative) Class II, III, IV	New (novel) Class II, III, IV
Development and marketing history, comparison with predicate devices	√ (if applicable)	√	√
Specifications	√	√	√
Stability and durability	√ (if applicable)	√ (if applicable)	√ (if applicable)
Conformity with ERs, applied standards	√	√	√
Performance, V&V, labelling	√	√	√
Risk analysis	√	√	√
Manufacturing process, sterilization (if applicable), quality control	√	√	√
Clinical data	-	√ (if applicable)	√

detail (summary or detailed device descriptions and reports) differs depending on the type of submission and risk classification of the medical device. The overall information that has to be covered, however, is largely the same.

Obviously, generating separate sets of documentation packages for each jurisdiction is laborious and difficult to maintain, incurring high administrative overheads. The industry prefers a standardized format for regulatory dossiers to reduce the burden on manufacturers who face conflicting pre-market submission formats and content requirements in different countries.

In 2008 the Global Harmonization Taskforce (GHTF) issued the guidance document N011:2008, *Summary Technical Documentation (STED) for Demonstrating Conformity to the Essential Principles of Safety and Performance of Medical Devices* [21], which provides a harmonized structure and content for documentation to be used both for regulatory submissions in the pre-market phase (refer to Fig. 3.2) and for demonstrating continued conformity in the post-market phase (refer to Fig. 3.3).

In 2011 a similar guidance document was generated for IVDs, the N063:2011, *Summary Technical Documentation (STED)*

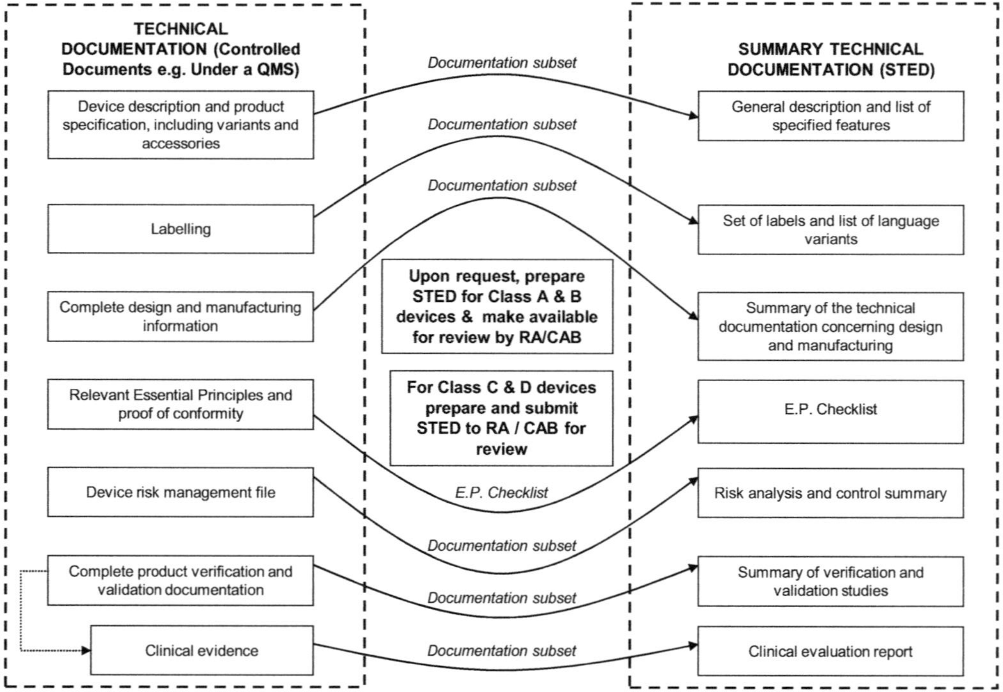

Figure 3.2 Pre-market use of the STED. *Source*: GHTF Guidance SG1/N011:2008.

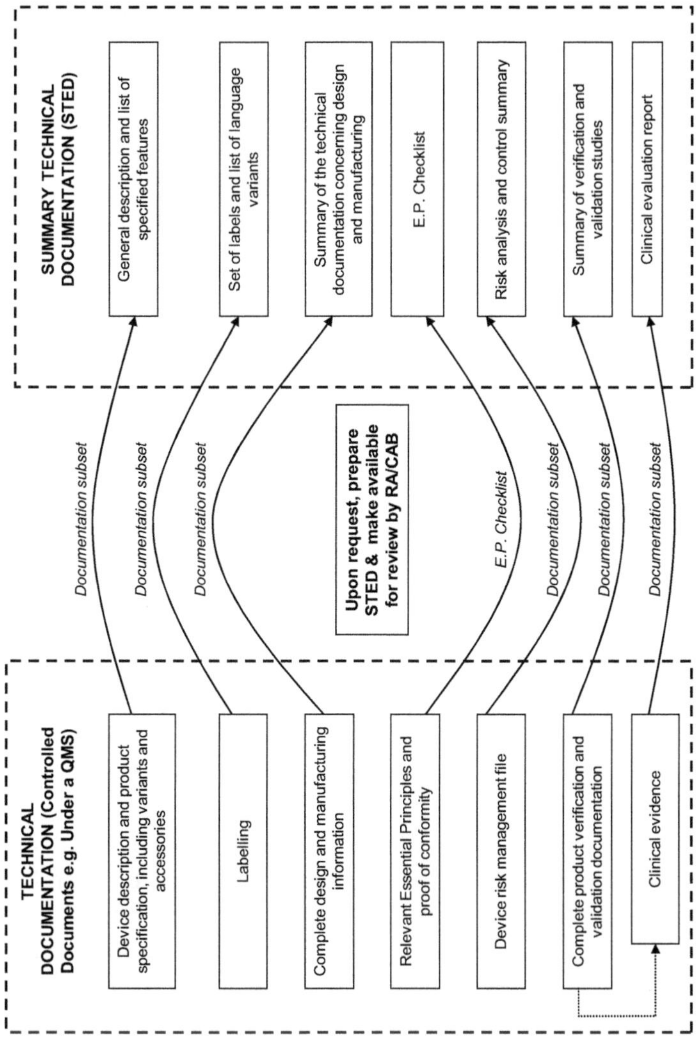

Figure 3.3 Post-market use of the STED. *Source:* GHTF Guidance SG1/N011:2008.

for Demonstrating Conformity to the Essential Principles of Safety and Performance of In Vitro Diagnostics Medical Devices [22]. The guidance provides a harmonized structure and content for documentation to be used both for regulatory submissions in the pre-market phase and for demonstrating continued conformity in the post-market phase in a similar way to the STED for medical devices other than IVDs (refer to Fig. 3.2 and Fig. 3.3).

Australia, Canada and Japan accept the STED format as is for their regulatory dossiers. More recent EU guidelines have partially aligned their recommended structure of a design dossier with the STED (1 p. 2), and notified bodies will accept a design dossier in STED format as long as the required information is included.

Since 2003 the FDA has been running a voluntary pilot pre-market review program to assess the feasibility of the STED format for PMAs and for traditional and abbreviated 510(k) submissions [23].

Using the GHTF STED model, the Association of Southeast Asian Nations (ASEAN) Medical Device Product Working Group (MDPWG) has developed its own Common Submission Dossier Template (CSDT) [24].

To ensure that documentation required for regulatory dossiers is generated during the product development stages and ready to be submitted as soon as the V&V is completed with positive results, the manufacturer's QMS should define a modular structure for the technical documentation, referred to henceforth only as the DHF, and define clear roles and responsibilities for authoring, review and approval of documents. It should be clear from the outset which DHF deliverables will form the STED.

Table 3.6 compares the documentation deliverables required for the DHF (left column) and the STED (right column). Greyed-out cells indicate that a particular document is not applicable for either the DHF or the STED. For example, legal and administrative documents for regulatory purposes such as application forms, Declarations of Conformity (DoCs), certificates, attestations and other statutory declarations, authorization letters, etc., are not part of the DHF; they should be kept in a dedicated regulatory submissions repository (explained in more detail in Section 3.3, "Example of STED-Aligned DHF"). Detailed procurement specifications for components,

Table 3.6 Comparative table indicating the content that is shared between the DHF and the STED

DHF	STED
1. Project Management	-
-	**1. Regulatory Administrative Information**
	1.1 Application forms, application fee payment receipts, correspondence
	1.2 Executive summary, development and marketing history, comparison with predicate devices
-	1.3 Declarations of Conformity (DoCs), certificates, attestations and other statutory declarations, authorization letters, etc.
2. Design Inputs	-
3. Design Outputs	-
3.1 Design description andproduct specifications	**2. Design Description and Product Specifications**
3.1.1 Design description	2.1 Design description
3.1.2 Detailed product specifications	-
3.1.3 Product codes	2.2 Product codes
3.1.4 System architecture and interoperability	2.3 System architecture and interoperability
3.2 Labelling and packaging	**3. Labelling and Packaging**
3.2.1 Labelling description	3.1 Labelling description
3.2.2 Labelling detailed specifications	-
3.2.3 Packaging description	3.2 Packaging description
3.2.4 Packaging detailed specifications	-
4. ERs/EPs Checklists	4. ERs/EPs Checklists
5. Risk Management	**5. Risk Management**
5.1 Risk Management Plan	-
5.2 Risk assessment	5.1 Risk assessment
5.3 *The Risk Management Summary Report*	5.2 *The Risk Management Summary Report*
5.4 Design failure modes and effects analysis (DFMEA)	-
5.4.1 *The DFMEA Summary Report*	5.3 *The DFMEA Summary Report*
5.4.2 Detailed DFMEAs	-
5.5 Process failure modes and effects analysis (PFMEA)	-
5.5.1 *The PFMEA Summary Report*	5.4 *PFMEA: Summary Report*
5.5.2 Detailed PFMEAs	-

(*Contd.*)

Table 3.6 (*Contd.*)

DHF	STED
6. Manufacturing Information	**6. Manufacturing Information**
6.1 Manufacturing process overview	6.1 Manufacturing process overview
6.2 Manufacturing Quality Plan	6.2 Manufacturing Quality Plan
6.3 Process characterization protocols and reports	-
6.4 Process validation protocols and reports	6.3 Process validation protocols and reports
6.5 Sterilization	6.4 Sterilization
6.5.1 Sterilization process	6.4.1 Sterilization process
6.5.2 Sterile packaging validation	6.4.2 Sterile packaging validation
7. Verification & Validation (V&V)	**7. Verification & Validation (V&V)**
7.1 *Traceability Report*	-
7.2 *V&V Summary Report*	7.1 *V&V Summary Report*
7.3 Design characterization protocols and reports	-
7.4 Firmware and software	7.2 Firmware and software
7.5 Usability	7.3 Usability
7.6 Animal studies	7.4 Animal studies
7.7 Other applicable regulations	-
8. Clinical Evaluation	**8. Clinical Evaluation**
8.1 *Clinical Evaluation Summary*	8.1 *Clinical Evaluation Summary*
8.2 Clinical investigations protocols and reports	8.2 Clinical investigations protocols and reports
8.3 Post-market surveillance	8.3 Post-market surveillance
QMS information required for audits and certain PMAs: quality manual, design controls, process controls, post-market surveillance	QMS information required for audits and certain PMAs: quality manual, design controls, process controls, post-market surveillance

materials and assemblies are part of the DHF but usually not required for the STED.

A DHF should be organized in sections and the documentation deliverables required for the STED identified upfront – see also Fig. 3.4.

The next section provides an example for DHF content and structure, with details describing the main documentation deliverables, which can be used for general medical devices, including complex, higher-risk devices.

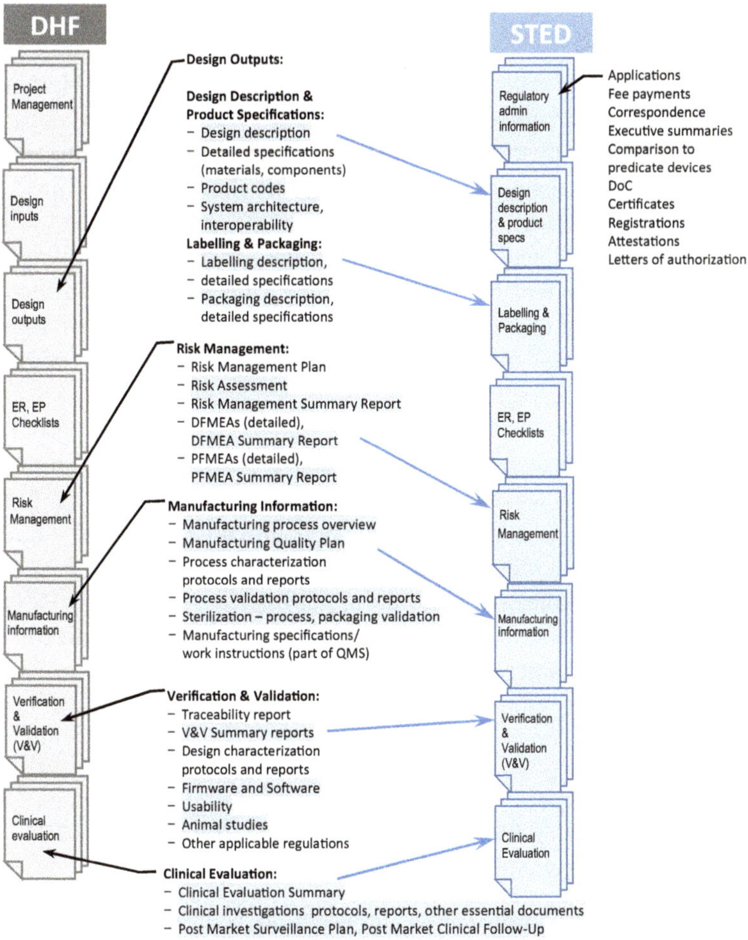

Figure 3.4 The STED (blue shading) is a sub-set of the DHF.

3.3 Example of STED-Aligned DHF

3.3.1 *Project Management*

The project management folder of the DHF contains all project management and planning documentation for a product or product family applicable throughout the entire product life cycle, such as:

- Market access strategy – clinical, regulatory and reimbursement strategies (an example of a market access strategy template is provided in Section 4.3.2, "Example of a Market Access Strategy Template");
- Marketing strategy – commercial product positioning and market segmentation (e.g., entry-level and premium product versions);
- D&D project plans – a D&D plan, including a software development plan (if applicable); labelling plan (expected labelling deliverables and translations); clinical trials, regulatory and reimbursement submissions planning (target countries/regions, timelines and application fees);
- Master V&V Plans listing the major V&V activities/group of activities, applicable standards, number of samples required for each V&V activity, cost and timelines (an example of a Master V&V Plan is provided in Section 4.5.2, "Software Identifiers");
- Design milestones (formal) reviews;
- Customer feedback, field data, project's lessons learned;
- Launch plans;
- Servicing plans; and
- Obsolescence plans.

3.3.2 *Regulatory Administrative Information (Regulatory Submissions Repository Only)*

The regulatory administrative information is probably the only product-specific documentation that does not belong in the DHF but rather in a dedicated regulatory submissions repository (detailed in Section 3.5, "Regulatory Submissions Repository"). It contains a record of applications submitted in various jurisdictions, including:

- Application forms (specific to each regulatory agency);
- Evidence of payment of relevant application fees;
- A list with all GMDN codes applicable to the company's products (and JMDN codes, if applicable) maintained by the Regulatory Affairs department;

- Executive summaries required for regulatory submissions with information on development and marketing history, comparison with predicate devices (if applicable);
- Correspondence, rounds of questions and answers with regulatory agencies;
- QMS certificates to ISO 13485; and
- DoCs, attestations, statutory declarations, authorization letters and other legal documents relevant to the country or region where the application for marketing approval is submitted.

3.3.3 *Design Inputs*

The design inputs folder of the DHF should contain the following information:

- User needs – clinical needs such as indications for use, intended use and expected clinical performance; user and marketing needs related to usability, ergonomics, comfort, esthetics and pricing; other stakeholder needs such as manufacturability; and technology and the principle of operation;
- Regulatory requirements – applicable ERs/EPs, standards and other statutory requirements; and
- Design input (engineering) requirements – defined for the product or product family and, if applicable, interfaces between main system components (e.g., implants, externals, software) defining compatibility/interoperability.

3.3.4 *Design Outputs*

3.3.4.1 Design description and product specifications

3.3.4.1.1 Design description

The design description should be a self-contained document, one per product or product family, without cross-references to other specifications and written at a level of detail that would not require the document to be revised if minor changes were made to the design. It should include:

- Indications for use, intended use, principle of function, contraindications, warnings and cautions.
- Lifetime and shelf life of the device, as applicable.
- A narrative description of the design with a rationale and justifications for functions, design features and materials chosen; within a product family, a clear delineation of what is common and what is different.
- Essential performance characteristics (specifications essential for the device to meet its intended purpose free from unacceptable risk).
- As applicable, it should also include exploded views, product images, block diagrams, firmware architecture diagrams, schematics, a table with list of components and materials and a list of accessories.
- If applicable, the firmware design description can be a section in this document or a separate document.
- For software, the software description is a summary overview of major or operationally significant software features and software operating environment (programming language, hardware platform, operating system, use of off-the-shelf software).
- Minor accessories and ancillary devices, for example, cables, power supplies, battery chargers, etc. – only a summary description for each, either as a section in this document or as a separate document.

3.3.4.1.2 Detailed product specifications

Specifications are a design output and cover the manufacturing and/or procurement specifications for the product, assemblies, subassemblies, materials and components. Specifications consist typically of mechanical drawings, electronic schematics and electronic circuit layout drawings, material specifications and binary images for software.

3.3.4.1.3 Product codes

This is a document that lists all model designations, catalogue numbers and part numbers relevant to the product or product family, including accessories, regional variants and configurations.

If products from other product families are used, the additional relevant product lists should be provided. Note that in this context, "product code" is different from the FDA's "Product Code" that is assigned to a device on the basis of the medical device product classification under 21 CFR Parts 862–892. The product codes document should include the GMDN and/or JMDN codes applicable to each saleable item identified by catalogue numbers.

3.3.4.1.4 System architecture and interoperability

Each product or product family that is part of a system (e.g., active implantable, external electronic controller, software application and accessories) must have a system architecture document that describes the interfaces - compatibility or interoperability - for that product or product family. For complex products and systems the interfacing information may need to be managed in a database that defines and tracks compatibility and interoperability between the various parts of the system.

3.3.4.2 Labelling and packaging

3.3.4.2.1 Labelling description

The labelling description is a document covering the labels (artworks) and IFUs of the product or product family. It should start with an overview of the device and its packaging system, for example:

- Sterile active implantable packed in inner Tyvek®, outer Tyvek® and sales packaging;
- External controller packed in sales packaging; and
- Software distributed as a compact disc (CD) or electronically via the Internet and its method of identification.

It should also include a list of labelling items identified by their part numbers. If there are any special arrangements, for instance, to ship externals separately to be packed in kits by a sub-contractor, this should be mentioned as well.

The label descriptions should cover markings on the device itself, on the sterile packs and on sales packaging, as applicable. The method of providing the labels (stickers, silk screening, etching) and the IFU formats (paper, electronic on CDs and/or on websites, audio format, Braille, etc.) should be specified.

The labelling description should include a list of languages in which the IFUs are to be translated; if no translations are provided for non-English-speaking countries, it should provide a justification why not and a reference to a translation SOP that indicates that only professional/certified translation offices are used.

No V&V information is needed in the labelling description document.

3.3.4.2.2 Labelling detailed specifications

The labelling specifications consist of the complete set of production and/or procurement specifications for labels and IFUs.

3.3.4.2.3 Packaging description

There should be one packaging description document per product or product family. The document should include or reference drawings of the sales packaging and, if applicable, the sterile packaging, together with information on environmental conditions for transport and storage and on the materials used.

If the manufacturer employs more than one configuration for the sterile packaging, the document should specify which sterilization product family is used for which products and the naming convention should be maintained consistent throughout the DHF, for example:

- EtO Sterilization Family 1 – list all implants and sterile accessories belonging to this family.
- EtO Sterilization Family 2 – list all implants and sterile accessories belonging to this family.

The document should include a summary description of the sterile barrier system used for each sterilization product family. For instance, one sterile barrier system can be comprised of an inner tray (holding the sterile product) heat-sealed with a lid, placed inside, and an outer tray that is also heat-sealed with a lid.

No V&V information is required in the packaging description document.

3.3.4.2.4 Packaging detailed specifications

Sterile packs and sales packaging specifications consist of the complete set of production and/or procurement specifications for all packaging items, including mechanical drawings and materials data.

3.3.5 *Essential Requirements/Principles Checklists*

There should be one ER/EP checklist for each product or product family and jurisdiction (Europe, Australia, Canada, ASEAN countries), as applicable. For each ER/EP the manufacturer should provide a short summary explaining how the ER/EP is met. Compliance with ERs/EPs requires a complete analysis, not just testing to standards. If standards don't cover an ER or only provide a partial solution, the manufacturer is still obliged to provide additional solutions to ensure compliance with ERs [25].

A recommended format for ER/EP checklists is shown in Table 3.7.

Some notified bodies and regulatory agencies still recommend the old ER/EP checklist format, which is nothing more than an itemization of standards and documents numbers. Such a checklist does not provide a complete picture because conformance with standards is not always sufficient to demonstrate compliance with statutory ERs/EPs (refer also to Section 2.4.1, "General Principles and the Use of Standards").

Without an explanation on how each individual ER/EP has been addressed agency reviewers need to delve deep into the individual documents referenced in the checklist just to try and piece the information together. By contrast, a clear and concise summary for each ER/EP (see third column in Table 3.7) helps reviewers to quickly understand the solutions adopted by the manufacturer and make a determination on whether the device is safe and effective, avoiding thus numerous rounds of questions and answers.

References to standards applied should be listed with the number and year of issue. For the EU ER checklist, the standards should be referenced using the European Norms (EN) Harmonised Standard, providing a presumption of conformity with the ERs [26].

Table 3.7 Recommended format for an ER/EP checklist, with examples of AIMDD ERs 8.ii, 9.v and 9.vii applied to a ventricular assist device (VAD)

ER/EP#	ER/EP requirements	Short summary of how ER/EP is met OR rationale for why ER/EP is not applicable	Standards applied	Documents providing evidence of compliance
...	...	...	...	...
8.ii	Risks connected with the use of energy sources with particular reference, where electricity is used, to insulation, leakage currents and overheating of the devices	The [VAD] is designed to ensure that the leakage currents from implantable and non-implantable parts do not exceed the safety limits, that the insulation has adequate dielectric strength and that the temperature of outer surfaces of the implanted parts does not exceed the normal surrounding body temperature by more than 2°C. The [controller], the battery receptacle and the mains power supply are designed with a degree of ingress protection of IP54. The user accessories include a shower protector to protect the controller, and the *Patient Handbook* and *Clinical Instructions for Use* (IFUs) include warnings against immersing the controller or percutaneous lead in water.	EN 45502-1:1997 (ISO 14708-1:2000) Sections 16.1, 16.2, 16.3, 17.1, 26.1 EN 60601-1: 2006+A1:2013 (IEC 60601-1:2014) EN 60529:2013 (IEC 60529:2013)	Report ### issued by [accredited test lab]

...	...	...	...	...
8.v	Risks connected with ionizing radiation from radioactive substances included in the device, in compliance with the protection requirements laid down in Council Directives 96/29 Euratom and 97/43/Euratom	N/A; the [VAD}does not incorporate any radioactive substances	N/A	N/A
...	...	...	...	...
9.v	Reliability of the source of energy	The [VAD] has a power source depletion indicator and built-in power redundancy, that is, there are two power sources at any one time (main and reserve battery or mains power supply and reserve battery); removal of one power source will automatically switch the controller to the other power source without interruption. Extra batteries are provided.	EN 45502-1:1997, section 19.2 EN ISO 14971:2012	*Risk Management Summary Report ###* Report ### issued by [accredited test lab]

(*Contd.*)

Table 3.7 (*Contd.*)

ER/EP#	ER/EP requirements	Short summary of how ER/EP is met OR rationale for why ER/EP is not applicable	Standards applied	Documents providing evidence of compliance
…	…	…	…	…
9.vii	Proper functioning of the programming and control systems, including software	The [controller] has built-in redundancy: if the main firmware fails, control is transferred automatically to the slave firmware, which runs on a different type of microprocessor than the main firmware and has different architecture. [Software application] is a customized software application used to set and view [VAD] programmable system parameters, monitor [VAD] performance and download data.	EN 45502-1:1997, section 19.3 EN ISO 14971:2012 EN IEC 62304:2006	*Risk Management Summary Report ###* Report ### issued by [accredited test lab] Controller design description ### [Software application] design description
…	…	…	…	…

For other countries such as Japan, China and Korea, reference to national standards may be required.

3.3.6 *Risk Management*

3.3.6.1 Risk Management Plan

Each product, product family or system should have a Risk Management Plan as per the EN/ISO 14971 standard.

3.3.6.2 Risk assessment

The *Hazards Analysis Report* is required as per the EN/ISO 14971 standard. This document should cover each product, product family or system, as defined in the Risk Management Plan. It should include:

- Descriptions of identified hazardous situations and sequence of events leading to harm in relation to hardware, software and use errors;
- Severity assessment;
- Probability of occurrence;
- Level of risk; and
- Mitigations and control measures.

For implants, a summary on the reliability performance should be included as a section of this document.

If applicable, the *Hazards Analysis Report* should also cover specific hazards in relation to:

- Software and firmware;
- Wireless technology using the radio frequency (RF) spectrum;
- Cybersecurity;
- Hazardous substances contained in electronic devices (lead, mercury, cadmium, hexavalent chromium, polybrominated biphenyls, or PBBs, and polybrominated diphenyl ethers, or PBDEs);
- Medicinal substances and biologics;

- Tissues of animal origin susceptible to transmissible spongiform encephalopathy (TSE);
- Phthalates; and
- Latex and other allergens.

3.3.6.3 The Risk Management Summary Report

The *Risk Management Summary Report* is required as per the EN/ISO 14971 standard. This document should cover each product, product family or system, as outlined in the Risk Management Plan.

It should include the risk classifications according to medical device regulations in major jurisdictions such as the EU, the United States, Australia, Canada and Japan. For software it should include the level of concern (LoC) – Minor, Moderate or Major. (This information is usually provided by the Regulatory function; refer to Section 4.3.2.7, "Medical Device Risk Classification and GMDN Code").

The *Risk Management Summary Report* should provide a summary of the currently known risks related to the use of the device, the main mitigation methods (e.g., adopted design solutions, provision of alarms, warnings and precautions in the labelling) and a discussion on the residual risks and their acceptability when compared to benefits.

3.3.6.4 Design failure modes and effects analysis

3.3.6.4.1 The DFMEA Summary Report

This document summarizes the design failure modes and effects analyses (DFMEAs) for a product, product family or system. It should include a table referencing all detailed DFMEAs performed during the D&D stage. The *DFMEA Summary Report* must be kept up to date and aligned with any design changes.

3.3.6.4.2 Detailed DFMEAs

Depending on a product complexity, it may be necessary to perform a number of DFMEAs: mechanical, electrical, for separate assemblies or for the finished product. All DFMEAs must be kept up to date and aligned with any design changes.

3.3.6.5 Process failure modes and effects analysis

3.3.6.5.1 The PFMEA Summary Report

This document summarizes the manufacturing process failure modes and effects analyses (PFMEAs) for a product, product family or system. It should include a table referencing all detailed PFMEAs performed during the D&D stage. The *PFMEA Summary Report* must be kept up to date and aligned with any changes in the manufacturing process.

3.3.6.5.2 Detailed PFMEAs

The number of detailed PFMEAs depends on the complexity of the product and its manufacturing process. All PFMEAs must be kept up to date and aligned with any process changes.

3.3.7 *Manufacturing Information*

3.3.7.1 Manufacturing process overview

A high-level manufacturing process description document should be generated for each product or product family that shares most or all production processes. It should be written at a level of detail that would not require the document to be revised if minor changes are made to the manufacturing processes. The document should include:

- A list of all manufacturing sites relevant for the product or product family;
- A high-level manufacturing flowchart identifying the major manufacturing steps and main quality control (QC) inspection steps;
- A high-level description of the special processes (those production processes requiring validation);
- Outsourced critical manufacturing operations, sub-assemblies, finished devices and accessories and the QCs applicable to outsourced products and services;
- A list of critical sub-contractors, their QMS certification status and supplier controls applied;
- In-house manufacturing facilities' layout plans; and
- Special environmental controls (e.g., clean rooms).

3.3.7.2 Manufacturing Quality Plan

The Manufacturing Quality Plan covers a product or product family and contains detailed manufacturing flowcharts, a list with or references to documents containing specifications, procedures and work instructions required to manufacture the product (e.g., bill of materials, or BOM, bill of operations, or BOO).

3.3.7.3 Process characterization protocols and reports

This section includes all characterization testing and references to test methods validations done as part of manufacturing validation activities. The purpose of the process characterization activities is to determine the capability of special processes, that is, setting the process capability indices, especially where there are no specific pass/fail criteria defined in standards or regulatory guidance documents [27].

Process validation protocols should reference the characterization reports that form the basis for selecting certain process capability limits.

3.3.7.4 Process validation protocols and reports

The *Process Validation Summary Report* should be generated for each product or product family. If applicable, this document should identify similarities and differences between the processes used for the various model numbers in the product family. It should summarize the validation activities and overall results for all special processes, with references to and attachments of detailed protocols and reports, such as installation qualification (IQ), operational qualification (OQ) and process qualification (PQ), as applicable. Note that sterilization requires a dedicated set of documents.

The *Process Validation Summary Report* and attachments should be kept up to date when revalidation activities are run as a result of significant changes in the manufacturing processes. There must be full correlation between the *Process Validation Summary Report* and any process flowchart and/or description.

3.3.7.5 Sterilization

3.3.7.5.1 Sterilization process

A sterilization product family definition document should list all medical devices, including surgical tools and accessories, if applicable, that are sterilized using the same sterile barrier system and master device. The document should include a detailed analysis of the selection of a master device and the rationale for adoption of additional devices to be included in the sterilization product family.

The sterilization process shall be validated for each sterilization product family. There should be a dedicated set of cleaning and sterilization validation protocols and reports for each sterilization process (autoclave, ethylene oxide [EtO], gamma) and sterilization product family, including related laboratory compliance with Good Laboratory Practices (GLPs) and/or the ISO/IEC 17025 standard.

For sterilization processes involving reprocessing of reusable devices, a comprehensive risk management assessment must be conducted and the outcomes documented in the product technical documentation.

The sterilization validation protocol and report should include information on:

- The sterilization equipment and controlled site;
- The sterilization cycle parameters – for example, for EtO: pre-humidification (if applicable), gas concentration, vacuum and gas pressure cycles, exposure time and temperature, humidity, degassing, aeration and determination of residuals;
- Specific procedures for routine monitoring and control of the sterilization process (e.g., selection of a process challenge device, location of biological indicators, type and duration of the sterilization cycle) to consistently meet the required sterility assurance level;
- Microbiological methods (growth medium, incubation temperature and time interval) for cultivating biological indicators used during validation and routine production monitoring; and

- The program for routine monitoring of the stability of packaging and the integrity of the sterile barrier system over the claimed shelf life.

The sterilization validation report should include:

- Information on IQ, OQ, physical and microbiological PQ;
- Confirmation that the sterilization process is effective at the most-difficult-to-sterilize location within the product;
- Confirmation that the product and its sterile packaging meet specified requirements for safety, quality and performance following the application of the defined sterilization process at the most challenging process parameters for the product and package, for the pre-defined number of sterilization cycles; and
- Evaluation of the biological safety of product following exposure to the sterilization process in accordance with EN/ISO 10993-1 and any subsequent parts of EN/ISO 10993 that apply (e.g., EtO residuals following EtO sterilization compliant with the requirements of EN/ISO 10993-7).

Requalification of the sterilization process should be performed at pre-defined intervals to demonstrate continuous compliance of the sterilization process with the initial validation and with the international standards' requirements. The requalification should be performed against specified acceptance criteria and in accordance with documented procedures. The requalification activities should be documented in a requalification report.

When new device models are added to the sterilization product family, or when there are design changes to the existing device models, a design analysis must be performed by comparing the new or modified device with the master device. Depending on the result of the detailed analysis one of the two options should be followed, as appropriate:

- The adoption of the new device/design to the sterilization product family on the basis of the design analysis and comparison with the master device; or
- A full PQ of the sterilization process using the new device/design.

3.3.7.5.2 Sterile packaging validation

There should be one sterile packaging validation summary document for each sterilization product family. The document should include a summary description of each sterile barrier system used for the sterilization product family including any special or critical processes used such as heat sealing. For instance, one sterile barrier system can be comprised of an inner tray (holding the sterile product) heat-sealed with a lid, placed inside and outer tray that is also heat-sealed with a lid.

The document should also include a validation summary report for each sterile barrier system, with references to and attachments of detailed reports, as applicable:

- Accelerated ageing;
- Dye migration;
- Bubble emission;
- Burst;
- Creep;
- Seal peel; and
- Aerosol challenge.

The validation reports should demonstrate maintenance of sterility for the specified shelf life.

This document should be kept up to date every time a new device is added to the sterile barrier system or when the master device is being changed.

3.3.8 *Verification and Validation*

3.3.8.1 Traceability Report

The *Traceability Report* is required to confirm that all design input requirements have been addressed, that is, that there is full traceability between requirements and V&V results and reports.

3.3.8.2 Overall V&V Summary Report

A high-level *Overall V&V Summary Report* should be generated for each product, product family or system to give an overview of all V&V activities and their outcomes. This high-level overview could use a similar format to a Master V&V Plan (refer also to Section 4.5.2, "Software Identifiers"), except that instead of the number of samples required, cost and timelines, it would contain the V&V results and references to individual summary reports, such as general safety to EN/IEC 60601-1, safety of implants to ISO 14708-1/EN 45502-1, electromagnetic compatibility (EMC) to EN/IEC 60601-1-2, biocompatibility to EN/ISO 10993 series, functional safety/performance, usability to EN/IEC 60601-1-6/-11, etc. (see Table 3.8).

Where EN and IEC/ISO standards are identical including the issue year the standard reference should be "EN IEC" or "EN ISO", as applicable. Where EN and IEC/ISO standards have differences in content or year of issue both references should be listed. Where the regional or national standards differ from their international counterparts, the Master V&V Plan should identify these. The V&V reports should have evidence of compliance with all applicable international, regional and national requirements. Results traceable to international, regional or national standard requirements should be documented in each summary report, as applicable.

Where testing to standards is performed, a summary report for each standard should be issued, preferably using professional templates such as the CB Scheme test report forms, or TRFs. The CB TRFs have a tabular format listing compliance with each clause in the standard and including a column for references to the test data for each individual test [28].

The *Biocompatibility Summary Report* according to Annex 1 of EN/ISO 10993-1 should contain a table with the materials used in the product or product family: parts and components in direct contact with the patient, type of contact, material, manufacturer, biocompatibility compliance status and references to individual biocompatibility reports. If a representative sample is used for the whole product or product family, the rationale for the selection should be included in the protocols.

Note that, when applicable, testing is done using a complete system. For instance, safety, EMC and performance testing must be performed on a complete system comprised of an active implantable device connected to an external electronic controller. If the system components have variants, instead of testing every

Table 3.8 Example of an Overall V&V Summary Report table (indicative only)

V&V activity	Overall result	Compliance to standards and regulatory guidelines	Comments/references
General safety requirements	Pass	EN 60601-1: 2006+A1:2013/IEC 60601-1:2014 Medical electrical equipment – Part 1: General requirements for basic safety and essential performance	CB Report ### Issued by [accredited test lab], accreditation #
AIMD general safety requirements	Pass	EN 45502-1:1997/ISO 14708-1:2000 Active implantable medical devices – General requirements for safety	Report ###
Specific safety and performance requirements	Pass	*Internal specifications* *Specific EN, IEC product standards, as applicable*	Report ### Report ###
Mechanical and environmental requirements	Pass	Environmental testing IEC 60068-2-1: Part 2-1:2007 Cold; Part 2-2:2007 Dry heat; Part 2-14:2009 Temperature change; Part 2-27:2008 Shock; Part 2-64:2008 Vibration; Part 2-75:2014 Hammer test	Summary report with references to individual reports: Report ### Report ###
EMC and RF wireless requirements	Pass	EN 60601-1-2: 2007/IEC 60601-1-2:2014 Medical electrical equipment – Part 1-2: General requirements for basic safety and essential performance – Collateral standard: Electromagnetic compatibility – Requirements and tests FDA guidance *RF Wireless Technology in Medical Devices: 2013* FDA guidance *Content of Premarket Submissions for Management of Cybersecurity in Medical Devices: 2014* FCC 47 Part 15 *List other EN, IEC, ETSI, CISPR standards, as applicable* *Declarations of Conformity/Attestations*	Summary report with references to individual reports: Report ### Report ### Report ###

(Contd.)

Table 3.8 *(Contd.)*

V&V activity	Overall result	Compliance to standards and regulatory guidelines	Comments/references
Labelling requirements	Pass	EN 980:2008, EN 1041:2008, ISO 15223-1:2012, EN 60601-1-2:2007/IEC 60601-1-2:2014, EN IEC 60601-1-11:2010 EU Radio Equipment Directive 2014/53/EU, Waste of Electrical & Electronic Equipment Directive 2002/96/EC FDA regulations and guidance for labelling *Other national labelling requirements, including compliance marks deriving from medical devices, EMC and RF wireless regulations (Australia, Canada, China, Japan, Korea)*	Report ###
Software/firmware	Pass	EN IEC 62304:2008, *Medical device doftware – Software life cycle processes* FDA guidance *Content of Premarket Submissions for Software Contained in Medical Devices*	Report ###
Usability	Pass	EN IEC 62366: 2008, EN IEC 60601-1-6: 2010 FDA guidance documents: *Design Considerations for Devices Intended for Home Use*; *Applying Human Factors and Usability Engineering to Optimize Medical Device Design*	Summary Report
Interoperability/backward compatibility	Pass	Interoperability matrix/database	Summary Report

Biocompatibility	Pass	EN ISO 10993, *Biological evaluation of medical devices* Statement concerning tissues of animal origin Statement concerning phthalates Statement concerning medicinal products Statement concerning human blood derivatives *The statements above should be based on information contained in specifications and/or received from suppliers. They must be kept up to date.*	Summary report with references to individual reports: Report ### Report ### Report ### Issued by [third-party lab], accreditation #
Environmental protection requirements	Pass	Statement concerning hazardous substances (EU RoHS Directive), electronic waste (EU WEEE Directive)	Summary reports
Sterility	Pass	EN ISO 11135-1:2007, *Sterilization of health care products – Ethylene oxide – Part 1: Requirements for development, validation and routine control of a sterilization process for medical devices* EN ISO 11138-2: 2009 Ed. 2.0, *Sterilization of health care products Biological indicators –Part 2: Biological indicators for ethylene oxide sterilization pro-cesses* EN ISO 11607-1:2009, *Packaging for terminally sterilized medical devices – Part 1: Requirements for materials, sterile barrier systems and packaging systems*	Summary report with references to individual reports: Report ### Report ### Report ###
Clinical data	Pass	EN ISO 14155:2011, *Clinical investigation of medical devices for human subjects – Good clinical practice* MEDDEV 2.7/1, *Clinical evaluation: guide for manufacturers and notified bodies* MEDDEV 2.7/4, *Guidelines on clinical investigations: A guide for manufacturers and notified bodies* FDA IDE guidance documents	Summary report with references to individual reports: Report ### Report ### Report ###
Process validation	Pass	As per internal process validation protocol ###	Report ###

possible permutation, select representative samples for each system component to ensure coverage for all variants. Document the rationale for sample selection in the protocols.

If interoperability requirements are covered in various individual V&V reports, the *Interoperability Verification Summary Report* can be a document listing the interoperability requirements including references to the relevant sections in the individual V&V reports where interoperability was tested. Ensure every combination in the interoperability matrix is covered (see also Section 3.3.4.1.1, "Design Description").

The V&V protocols should reference any test method validations performed for critical V&V activities, such as internally developed test methods for essential performance characteristics. Each test data set, including any re-test, should record the build standard (BOM version and revision), equipment used, who performed the test and the date of the test.

V&V testing should also be conducted to ensure that the product performs safely for the defined lifetime of the device under worst-case conditions (e.g., multiple sterilization cycles).

3.3.8.3 Design characterization protocols and reports

This section includes all characterization testing and test methods validations done as part of design verification activities. The purpose of the design characterization activities is to determine the limits of product design capabilities where no standards exist, and they are typically done by testing the device to failure and then determining the specifications limits and pass/fail criteria.

Design verification protocols should reference the characterization reports that form the basis for selecting certain design capability limits.

3.3.8.4 Software and firmware

The level of effort and rigor that is required during software development, as well as the documentation required, depends largely on the software risk classification or LoC – refer also to Section 2.5.1, "Software and Firmware".

The documentation required for each of the three software risk classes is shown in Table 3.9. The FDA LoC for software - minor, moderate and major – has been aligned with the classification in IEC 62304:2006 – Class A, B and C – for ease of reference.

3.3.8.5 Usability

Every product or product family should have a *Usability Summary Report.* For systems usability must be tested using a complete system (e.g., implant, externals and software applications). If the system components have design variants, select representative samples for each system component to ensure coverage for all combinations and variants. Document the rationale for sample selection in the protocols.

3.3.8.6 Animal studies

Where animal tests are carried out to validate certain requirements (e.g., biocompatibility, surgical procedure, etc.), the protocols and reports should be included in the V&V documentation and referenced in the ER/EP checklists in the relevant sections.

3.3.8.7 Other applicable regulations

This section typically covers compliance with additional regulations and regulatory guidelines, for example:

- Devices operating using RF;
- Medicinal substances;
- Human blood derivatives;
- Tissues of animal origin and protection against TSE;
- Phthalates;
- Latex and other allergens; and
- Environmental protection regarding electronic waste and hazardous substances.

Compliance is typically demonstrated by supplier declarations, protocols and reports demonstrating compliance with applicable standards and technical specifications. For devices incorporating blood derivatives or medicinal substances the quality, safety and

Table 3.9 Software documentation required for regulatory submissions

Software documentation	Minor LoC/Class A software	Moderate LoC/Class B software	Major LoC/Class C software
Software description, including software risk classification	Summary overview of the features and software operating environment		
Software hazards analysis	Tabular description of identified hardware and software hazards, including severity assessment and mitigations		
Software requirements specification (SRS)	Summary only	Complete requirements specification	
Software architecture design chart	–	Description of functional units and software modules, including state diagrams and flowcharts	
Software design specification (SDS)	–	Detailed design specification/description	
Traceability analysis	Traceability among requirements, specifications, identified hazards and mitigations and V&V testing		
Software development environment description	–	Summary of software life cycle development plan Summary of configuration management and maintenance activities	Summary of software life cycle development plan; Annotated list of documents generated during development process; Configuration management and maintenance plan

Software V&V	Software functional test plan, pass/fail criteria and results	Description of V&V activities at the unit, integration and system levels System-level test protocol, including pass/fail criteria and results	Description of V&V activities at unit, integration and system levels; Unit-, integration- and system-level test protocols, including pass/fail criteria, test report, summary and results
Revision level history	Revision history log, including release version number and date		
Unresolved anomalies (bugs and defects)	–	List of remaining software anomalies, annotated with an explanation of the impact on safety and effectiveness, including operator usage and human factors	

Source: FDA

usefulness of the blood derivatives or medicinal substances must be evaluated and approved according to relevant regulations.

3.3.9 *Clinical Evaluation*

3.3.9.1 Clinical Evaluation Summary

A *Clinical Evaluation Summary* report should be generated for each product or product family in accordance with regulatory guidelines. The report should summarize the available data, both favourable and unfavourable, from clinical experience with the device as well as from published literature on equivalent devices. The report must demonstrate objectively that the device is fit for purpose and that the benefits outweigh the risks when the device is used in accordance with its indications for use and intended purpose.

Where clinical evaluation is based on equivalence to predicate devices, the rationale for equivalence should be supported by a side-by-side comparison between the device and the predicate device(s), including comparative bench testing.

The clinical evaluation is first performed during the pre-market phase and then updated at regular intervals – six-monthly or yearly, as defined in the *Post-Market Surveillance Plan*. It must include any new safety and effectiveness information about the device obtained during its use, including post-market vigilance data (adverse events reporting) and the Post-Market Clinical Follow-Up (PMCF).

3.3.9.2 Clinical investigations essential documentation

Clinical investigational plans, trial protocols and reports should be included in this section, covering all the studies performed using the product or product family, as applicable:

- Early feasibility and first-in-human studies
- Feasibility studies
- Pivotal studies

If multiple studies support one regulatory submission a summary clinical report should provide an overview of all the studies conducted.

A Clinical Investigation Plan identifies the type of the clinical trial design (randomized or non-randomized controlled study, cohort study, case control study or case series study) and specifies the statistical methods to be used. It also includes the following information:

- Purpose – the name and intended use of the device and the objectives and duration of the investigation;
- Protocol – a description of the methodology to be used, including an analysis demonstrating its scientific soundness;
- Risk analysis – a description and analysis of all increased risks to the research subjects and how these risks will be minimized, a justification for the investigation and a description of the patient population, including the number, age, sex and condition;
- Description of the medical device – a description of each important component, ingredient, property and principle of operation of the device and any anticipated changes in the device during the investigation; and
- Monitoring procedures – the sponsor's written procedures for monitoring the investigation and the name and address of each monitor [29].

The statistical plan incorporated into the Clinical Investigation Plan needs to define:

- Primary and secondary endpoints to be assessed at a specified point in time;
- A testable hypothesis;
- Statistical significance levels and power;
- Justification for the selected sample size; and
- Method of analysis, including sensitivity and poolability of data [30].

A Clinical Trial Protocol describes:

- Patient selection, study inclusion and exclusion criteria;
- Measures for ensuring the quality and integrity of the data;

- Serious adverse event-reporting procedure in accordance with relevant regulatory requirements in the jurisdictions where the trial is being conducted; and
- Patient management and patient assessment.

The *Clinical Trial Report* documents the outcome of a clinical trial and its findings, including accountability of study subjects, a summary of all adverse events and any deviations to the protocol. Data should be presented in a structured manner using tables, where appropriate. A summary of the *Clinical Trial Report* data, including both favourable and unfavourable aspects, must be included in the *Clinical Evaluation Summary* report and must state explicitly whether the results support the claims made in relation to safety and effectiveness.

Other essential documentation relevant to clinical investigations include, but are not limited to:

- Ethics Committees' approvals;
- Regulatory approvals for clinical trials;
- Case report forms;
- Monitoring reports; and
- Information about the investigational device (design, manufacturing, identification and traceability, reconciliation of stock).

The EN/ISO standard 14155:2011, *Clinical investigation of medical devices for human subjects—Good clinical practice*, provides detailed information on the content and format of essential clinical trial documents: Clinical Investigation Plan (Annex A), the investigator's brochure (Annex B), case report forms (Annex C), *Clinical Investigation Report* (Annex D) and other essential clinical investigation documents (Annex E).

Templates for clinical research study documentation are also available from reputable governmental sources such as the US National Institutes of Health (NIH) [31].

3.3.9.3 Post-market surveillance

The Post-Market Surveillance Plan describes what information should be collected and how it should be generated during the

PMCF for each product or product family. The plan must define the time intervals for updating the *Clinical Evaluation Summary* report – typically every 6 or 12 months, depending on the device.

The *Post-Market Clinical Follow-Up Report* must summarize the clinical experience to date for a product or product family and must be kept up to date with any relevant new information that becomes available.

For high-risk devices such as implants reliability reports must be prepared and updated with a defined frequency (e.g., monthly). They should include a tally of device failures and malfunctions, listing the discreet failure modes and the number of devices that have been confirmed to have failed or malfunctioned. Data from the *Post-Market Clinical Follow-Up Report* should be used to provide an annual summary for trending purposes, taking into consideration:

- Complaints;
- Reliability reporting;
- Returned device analysis investigation results;
- User feedback; and
- Literature reviews.

The information obtained from the post-market surveillance activities must be fed back into the device risk analysis and may result in changes to the device design, manufacturing and/or IFUs.

3.4 Regulated Product Submission

The STED was an important step towards harmonization of submission content and formats; however, it only addressed the submission content that was common among the established jurisdictions. Regulatory Authorities recognized that a more comprehensive harmonized structure was needed to define the location of both common and regional content for all submission types.

In 2014 the International Medical Device Regulatory Forum (IMDRF) published two guidelines for an internationally harmonized, modular format for medical device and IVD submissions, known as Regulated Product Submission, or RPS:

- N9:2014, *Non–In Vitro Diagnostic Device Market Authorization Table of Contents* (nIVD MA ToC) [32] – see also Table 3.10.
- N13:2014, *In Vitro Diagnostic Medical Device Market Authorization Table of Contents* (IVD MA ToC) [33] – main differences between medical devices and IVD RPS are listed after Table 3.10.

At the time of going to print the STED was still the closest to an internationally accepted harmonized format for regulatory submissions. Once the RPS is adopted by Regulatory Authorities worldwide, applicants will be able to submit applications using the RPS format.

3.4.1 *RPS Structure and Content*

A hierarchical presentation of an RPS structure for medical devices is shown in Table 3.10, along with comparison and content alignment with the STED content introduced earlier in this chapter in Table 3.6.

The IVD RPS structure is similar to that of the medical device RPS structure, with some content that is specific to IVDs added to the IVD RPS (see Table 3.11) and other content that is specific to medical devices removed from the IVD RPS (see Table 3.12).

3.4.2 *Electronic Submissions*

Apart from the obvious advantage of having to manage only one structure and content for regulatory submissions internationally, another important benefit of having a harmonized submission format and content across jurisdictions is the ability to switch from paper to electronic medium.

Nowadays most Regulatory Authorities around the world accept duplicate copies of an application in electronic format but still request at least one paper copy. The submission of an additional electronic copy (or eCopy) has been mandatory in the United States since January 1, 2013. The eCopy is an exact duplicate of the paper

Table 3.10 RPS structure for medical devices

IMDRF, *Non–In Vitro Diagnostic Device Market Authorization Table of Contents* (nIVD MA ToC)		Corresponding STED content (Table 3.6)
CHAPTER 1: REGIONAL ADMINISTRATIVE		
CH1.01	Cover Letter	01. Administrative Information
CH1.02	Submission Table of Contents	
CH1.03	List of Terms/Acronyms	
CH1.04	Application Form/Administrative Information	
CH1.05	Listing of Device(s)	
CH1.06	Quality Management System, Full Quality System or Other Regulatory Certificates	
CH1.07	Free Sale Certificate	
CH1.08	User Fees	
CH1.09	Pre-Submission Correspondence and Previous Regulator Interactions	
CH1.10	Acceptance for Review Checklist	
CH1.11	Statements/Certifications/Declarations of Conformity	
CH1.11.1	Performance and Voluntary Standard	
CH1.11.2	Environmental Assessment	
CH1.11.3	Clinical Trial Certifications	
CH1.11.4	Indications for Use Statement with Rx and/or OTC Designation Enclosure	
CH1.11.5	Truthful and Accurate Statement	
CH1.11.6	USFDA Class III Summary and Certification	
CH1.11.7	Declaration of Conformity	
CH1.12	Letters of Reference for Master Files	
CH1.13	Letter of Authorization	
CH1.14	Other Regional Administrative Information	

(*Contd.*)

Table 3.10 *(Contd.)*

IMDRF, *Non–In Vitro Diagnostic Device Market Authorization Table of Contents* (nIVD MA ToC)		Corresponding STED content (Table 3.6)
CHAPTER 2: SUBMISSION CONTENT		
CH2.1	Chapter Table of Contents	-
CH2.2	General Summary of Submission	1.1 Executive Summary
CH2.3	Summary and Certifications for Premarket Submissions	
CH2.4	Device Description	2.1 Design Description and Product Specifications
CH2.4.1	Comprehensive Device Description and Principle of Operation	
CH2.4.2	Description of Device Packaging	
CH2.4.3	History of Development	
CH2.4.4	Reference and Comparison to Similar and/or Previous Generations of the Device	
CH2.4.5	Substantial Equivalence Discussion	
CH2.5	Indications for Use and/or Intended Use and Contraindications	2.1 Design Description and Product Specifications
CH2.5.1	Intended Use; Intended Purpose; Intended User; Indications for Use	
CH2.5.2	Intended Environment/Setting for Use	
CH2.5.3	Paediatric Use	
CH2.5.4	Contraindications for Use	
CH2.6	Global Market History	1.1 Marketing History 8.1 Clinical Evaluation Summary 8.3 Post-Market Surveillance
CH2.6.1	Global Market History	
CH2.6.2	Global Incident Reports and Recalls	

CH2.6.3	Sales, Incident and Recall Rates	
CH2.6.4	Evaluation/Inspection Reports	
CH2.7	Other Submission Context Information	–
CHAPTER 3: NON-CLINICAL EVIDENCE		
CH3.1	Chapter Table of Contents	–
CH3.2	Risk Management	5. Risk Management
CH3.3	Essential Principles (EP) Checklist	4. ER/EP Checklists
CH3.4	Standards	7.1 V&V Summary Reports
CH3.4.1	List of Standards	
CH3.4.2	Declaration and/or Certification of Conformity	
CH3.5	Non-clinical Studies	
CH3.5.01	Physical and Mechanical Characterization: Summary, Full Report, Statistical Data	
CH3.502	Chemical/Material Characterization: Summary, Full Report, Statistical Data	
CH3.5.03	Electrical Systems: Safety, Mechanical and Environmental Protection, and Electromagnetic Compatibility: Summary, Full Report, Statistical Data	
CH3.5.04	Radiation Safety: Summary, Full Report, Statistical Data	
CH3.5.05	Software/Firmware	4.7 Firmware and Software
CH3.5.05.01	SW/FW Description	
CH3.5.05.02	Hazard Analysis	
CH3.5.05.03	SW Requirement Specification	
CH3.5.05.04	Architecture Design Chart	
CH3.5.05.05	SW Design Specification	
CH3.5.05.06	Traceability Analysis	
CH3.5.05.07	SW Development Environment Description	
CH3.5.05.08	SW V&V: Summary, Full Report, Statistical Data	

(Contd.)

Table 3.10 (*Contd.*)

IMDRF, *Non–In Vitro Diagnostic Device Market Authorization Table of Contents* (nIVD MA ToC)		Corresponding STED content (Table 3.6)
CH3.5.05.09	Revision Level History	
CH3.5.05.10	Unresolved Anomalies (Bugs or Defects)	
CH3.5.06	Biocompatibility and Toxicology Evaluation: Summary, Full Report, Statistical Data	7.1 V&V Summary Reports
CH3.5.07	Non-Material-Mediated Pyrogenicity: Summary, Full Report, Statistical Data	
CH3.5.08	Safety of Materials of Biological Origin (Human/Animal): Certificates; Summary, Full Report, Statistical Data	
CH3.5.09	Sterilization Validation	6.4 Sterilization
CH3.5.09.1	End-User Sterilization Summary: Full Report, Statistical Data	
CH3.5.09.2	Manufacturer Sterilization Summary: Full Report, Statistical Data	
CH3.5.09.3	Residual Toxicity Summary: Full Report, Statistical Data	
CH3.5.09.4	Cleaning and Disinfection Validation Summary: Full Report, Statistical Data	
CH3.5.09.5	Reprocessing of Single-Use Devices (SUD) Validation Data: Summary, Full Report, Statistical Data	
CH3.5.10	Animal Testing: Summary, Full Report, Statistical Data	7.6 Animal Testing
CH3.5.11	Usability/Human Factors: Summary, Full Report, Statistical Data	7.5 Usability
CH3.6	Non-Clinical Bibliography	-
CH3.7	Expiration Period and Package Validation	6.4.2 Sterile Packaging Validation
CH3.7.1	Product Stability: Summary, Full Report, Statistical Data	
CH3.7.2	Package Validation: Summary, Full Report, Statistical Data	
CH3.8	Other Non-Clinical Evidence: Summary, Full Report, Statistical Data	–

CHAPTER 4: CLINICAL EVIDENCE		
CH4.1	Chapter Table of Contents	–
CH4.2	Overall Clinical Evidence Summary	8.1 Clinical Evaluation Summary
CH4.2.1	Clinical Evaluation Report	
CH4.2.2	Device Specific Clinical Trials: Clinical Trial Synopsis; Clinical Trial Report; Clinical Trial Data	8.2 Clinical Investigations Protocols and Reports
CH4.2.3	Clinical Literature Review and Other Reasonable Known Information	8.1 Clinical Evaluation Summary
CH4.3	Institutional Review Board (IRB)-Approved Informed Consent Forms	8.2 Clinical Investigations Protocols and Reports
CH4.4	Investigators Sites and IRB Contact Information	
CH4.5	Other Clinical Evidence: Summary, Full Report, Statistical Data	8.1 Clinical Evaluation Summary 8.3 Post-Market Surveillance
CHAPTER 5: LABELLING AND PROMOTIONAL MATERIAL		
CH5.01	Chapter Table of Contents	–
CH5.02	Product/Package Labels	3. Labelling and Packaging
CH5.03	Package Insert/Instructions for Use	
CH5.04	e-Labelling	
CH5.05	Physician Labelling	
CH5.06	Patient Labelling	
CH5.07	Technical/Operators Manual	
CH5.08	Patient File Stickers/Cards and Implant Registration Cards	
CH5.09	Product Brochures	
CH5.10	Other Labelling and Promotional Material	
CHAPTER 6A: QUALITY MANAGEMENT SYSTEM (QMS) PROCEDURES		
CH6A.1	Cover Letter	–

(Contd.)

Table 3.10 *(Contd.)*

IMDRF, *Non–In Vitro Diagnostic Device Market Authorization Table of Contents* (nIVD MA ToC)		Corresponding STED content (Table 3.6)
CH6A.2	Chapter Table of Contents	
CH6A.3	Administrative: Product Descriptive Information; General Manufacturing Information; Required Forms	
CH6A.4	QMS Procedures	
CH6A.5	Management Responsibilities Procedures	
CH6A.7	Product Realization Procedures: Design and Development Procedures; Purchasing Procedures; Production and Service Controls Procedures; Control of Monitoring and Measuring Devices Procedures	
CH6A.8	QMS Measurement, Analysis and Improvement Procedures	
CH6A.9	Other Quality System Procedures Information	
CHAPTER 6B: QMS DEVICE-SPECIFIC INFORMATION		
CH6B.1	Chapter Table of Contents	–
CH6B.2	QMS Information	1. Project Management: D&D Project Plan and Milestones Reviews (DHF) 6.2 Manufacturing Quality Plan
CH6B.3	Management Responsibilities Information	
CH6B.4	Resource Management Information	
CH6B.5	Device-Specific Quality Plan	
CH6B.6	Product Management Information: Design and Development Information; Purchasing Information; Production and Service Controls Information; Control of Monitoring and Measuring Devices Information	6.1 Manufacturing Process Overview
CH6B.7	QMS Measurement, Analysis and Improvement Information	
CH6B.8	Other Device-Specific QMS Information	

Table 3.11 IVD RPS: added content specific to IVDs

CHAPTER 2: SUBMISSION CONTEXT	
CH2.4.2	Material Specifications
CHAPTER 3: NON-CLINICAL EVIDENCE	
CH3.5	Analytical Performance
CH3.5.01	Stability of Sample(s): Summary, Full Report, Statistical Data
CH3.5.02	Validation of Samples: Summary, Full Report, Statistical Data
CH3.5.03	Metrological Traceability of Calibrator and Control Material Values: Summary, Full Report, Statistical Data
CH3.5.04	Accuracy of Measurement
CH3.5.04.1	Trueness
CH3.5.04.2	Precision (Repeatability and Reproducibility)
CH3.5.05	Analytical Sensitivity
CH3.5.06	Analytic Specificity: Summary, Full Report, Statistical Data
CH3.5.07	High-Dose Hook Effect: Summary, Full Report, Statistical Data
CH3.5.08	Measuring Range of the Assay: Summary, Full Report, Statistical Data
CH3.5.09	Validation of Assay Cut-Off: Summary, Full Report, Statistical Data
CH3.5.10	Validation of the Assay Procedure
CH3.6	Other Studies
CH3.6.5	Stability of the IVD
CH3.6.5.1	Claimed Shelf Life: Summary, Full Report, Statistical Data
CH3.6.5.2	In-Use Stability: Summary, Full Report, Statistical Data
CH3.6.5.3	Shipping Stability: Summary, Full Report, Statistical Data
CH3.7	Analytical Performance and Other Evidence Bibliography: Summary, Full Report, Statistical Data
CHAPTER 4: CLINICAL EVIDENCE	
CH4.2.1	Expected Values/Reference Ranges

submission, created and submitted on a CD, digital video disc (DVD) or flash drive [34].

Agencies will eventually transition to electronic-only submissions due to greater convenience in handling a large volume of documentation and cost savings in storing, transmitting and accessing information. To be able to electronically exchange regulated product information applicants and agencies need to use a harmonized submission structure and a standardized means for processing and reviewing electronic data (a messaging standard).

Table 3.12 IVD RPS – removed content specific to medical devices

CHAPTER 1: REGIONAL ADMINISTRATIVE	
CH1.11.6	USFDA Class III Summary and Certification
CHAPTER 3: NON-CLINICAL EVIDENCE	
CH3.5	Non-Clinical Studies
CH3.5.01	Physical and Mechanical Characterization
CH3.5.02	Chemical/Material Characterization
CH3.5.04	Radiation Safety
CH3.5.06	Biocompatibility and Toxicology Evaluation
CH3.5.07	Non-Material-Mediated Pyrogenicity
CH3.5.08	Safety of Materials of Biological Origin (Human/Animal)
CH3.5.09	Sterilization Validation
CH3.5.09.1	End-User Sterilization
CH3.5.09.2	Manufacturer Sterilization
CH3.5.09.3	Residual Toxicity
CH3.5.09.5	Reprocessing of SUD Validation Data
CH3.5.10	Animal Testing
CH3.6	Non-Clinical Bibliography
CH3.7.2	Package Validation
CHAPTER 5: LABELLING AND PROMOTIONAL MATERIAL	
CH5.05	Physician Labelling

The FDA has rolled out a voluntary electronic submissions program, whereby sponsors, manufacturers and importers use eSubmitter, a free stand-alone software application that allows the input of data and compilation of an FDA-compatible output submission file. Depending on the submission type data can be transmitted via a CD or through the Electronic Submissions Gateway, an agency-wide entry point for various electronic applications that enables the secure submission of regulatory information for review [35, 36].

In November 2014 Health Canada published the guidance for industry, *Formatting of Class III and Class IV Licence Applications (Electronic and Paper Formats)*, in which it announced that "Class III and IV medical device licence applications will now be accepted in electronic-only format if they meet the requirements of this notice, effective immediately." The guidance includes instructions for folder structures and naming conventions to be used in electronic applications, as well as acceptable media to use in submitting applications [37].

Effective December 1, 2014, paper-based applications will also be required to be structured in one of the formats described in the guidance in order to be accepted, namely:

- Health Canada's guidance on supporting evidence (see Section 3.1.4, "Documentation Mandated by Canadian Regulations");
- STED (see Section 3.2, "GHTF Summary Technical Documentation"); or
- The IMDRF's table of contents (see Table 3.10 for information on medical devices RPS table of contents and additionally Table 3.11 and Table 3.12 for information on IVDs RPS table of contents).

The acceptance of electronic-only submissions represents a step in Health Canada's long-term goal of accepting fully electronic applications structured in an international standard and submitted through a secure gateway [38]. A paper copy of the application form must also be included with each electronic submission; however, this is a temporary measure while Health Canada transitions to a fully electronic submission process.

An RPS standard for electronic submissions for all types of regulated products, including medical devices and IVDs, has been in development since 2006. Health Level Seven (HL7), a non-profit, US-based, American National Standards Institute (ANSI)-accredited standards development organization was tasked with the development of the RPS specification. RPS Release 1, restricted to the United States and applicable to medical devices and drugs for human use, became an ANSI normative standard in 2008. RPS Release 2, finalized in 2014, was expanded to include two-way communication between applicants and the agency [39, 40].

Companies switching from paper-based submissions to the RPS electronic format and messaging standard will be required to re-think their business processes and invest in their regulatory operations and IT infrastructure [41].

3.5 Regulatory Submissions Repository

Applications to regulators, deficiencies raised and responses addressing those deficiencies contain valuable information; therefore sponsors and manufacturers should keep records of applications and any related correspondence in a well-organized, controlled central repository, especially if they have to manage large product portfolios that are marketed worldwide.

Most medical device companies nowadays use electronic document management systems (EDMSs) to manage DHF documentation. Since regulatory submissions consist of STEDs, which are subsets of DHFs, the submissions repository can also be built on the same EDMS platform.

The DHF is constantly updated and maintained to include the latest changes to a product's design, labelling and manufacturing processes, including changes made in order to address deficiencies raised by regulators. Regulatory submissions on the other hand represent a snapshot in time. Hence the DHF is a "living" set of documents, whereas submissions are historical records.

The product technical documentation must be maintained so that information on what the product configuration was at any point in time can be easily retrieved, as well as re-constructing the complete history of changes made to the product design, labelling and manufacturing, if needed. It takes a solid understanding of submissions management best practices and considerable discipline to ensure that the company's view of the product (the DHF) remains in sync with the regulators' view of the same product (STED submissions).

3.5.1 *Structure of a Regulatory Submissions Repository*

An example of organizing the regulatory submissions repository is shown in Fig. 3.5. For each product or product family the regulatory submissions repository is structured as follows:

- The Submissions & Approvals directory containing records of applications for marketing approvals in various jurisdictions; they consist of protected copies of submitted

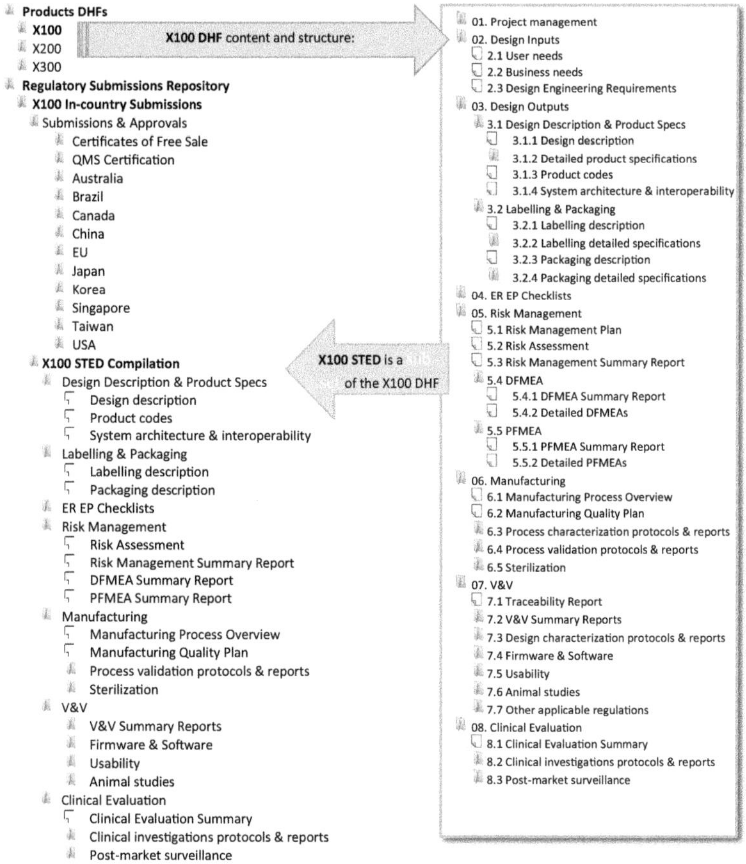
Products DHFs
X100
X200
X300
X100 DHF content and structure:
Regulatory Submissions Repository
X100 In-country Submissions
Submissions & Approvals
Certificates of Free Sale
QMS Certification
Australia
Brazil
Canada
China
EU
Japan
Korea
Singapore
Taiwan
USA
X100 STED Compilation
X100 STED is a
of the X100 DHF
Design Description & Product Specs
Design description
Product codes
System architecture & interoperability
Labelling & Packaging
Labelling description
Packaging description
ER EP Checklists
Risk Management
Risk Assessment
Risk Management Summary Report
DFMEA Summary Report
PFMEA Summary Report
Manufacturing
Manufacturing Process Overview
Manufacturing Quality Plan
Process validation protocols & reports
Sterilization
V&V
V&V Summary Reports
Firmware & Software
Usability
Animal studies
Clinical Evaluation
Clinical Evaluation Summary
Clinical investigations protocols & reports
Post-market surveillance
01. Project management
02. Design Inputs
2.1 User needs
2.2 Business needs
2.3 Design Engineering Requirements
03. Design Outputs
3.1 Design Description & Product Specs
3.1.1 Design description
3.1.2 Detailed product specifications
3.1.3 Product codes
3.1.4 System architecture & interoperability
3.2 Labelling & Packaging
3.2.1 Labelling description
3.2.2 Labelling detailed specifications
3.2.3 Packaging description
3.2.4 Packaging detailed specifications
04. ER EP Checklists
05. Risk Management
5.1 Risk Management Plan
5.2 Risk Assessment
5.3 Risk Management Summary Report
5.4 DFMEA
5.4.1 DFMEA Summary Report
5.4.2 Detailed DFMEAs
5.5 PFMEA
5.5.1 PFMEA Summary Report
5.5.2 Detailed PFMEAs
06. Manufacturing
6.1 Manufacturing Process Overview
6.2 Manufacturing Quality Plan
6.3 Process characterization protocols & reports
6.4 Process validation protocols & reports
6.5 Sterilization
07. V&V
7.1 Traceability Report
7.2 V&V Summary Reports
7.3 Design characterization protocols & reports
7.4 Firmware & Software
7.5 Usability
7.6 Animal studies
7.7 Other applicable regulations
08. Clinical Evaluation
8.1 Clinical Evaluation Summary
8.2 Clinical investigations protocols & reports
8.3 Post-market surveillance

Figure 3.5 Example of organizing a regulatory submissions repository.

documents, rounds of questions and answers with Regulatory Authorities, certificates and letters of approvals containing protected copies of application documents that were actually submitted.

- The STED Compilation directory, which is a working space for assembling the STED; the administrative sections containing cover letters, applications forms, etc., should be filed directly in the directories dedicated to national or regional jurisdictions in the Submissions & Approvals directory.

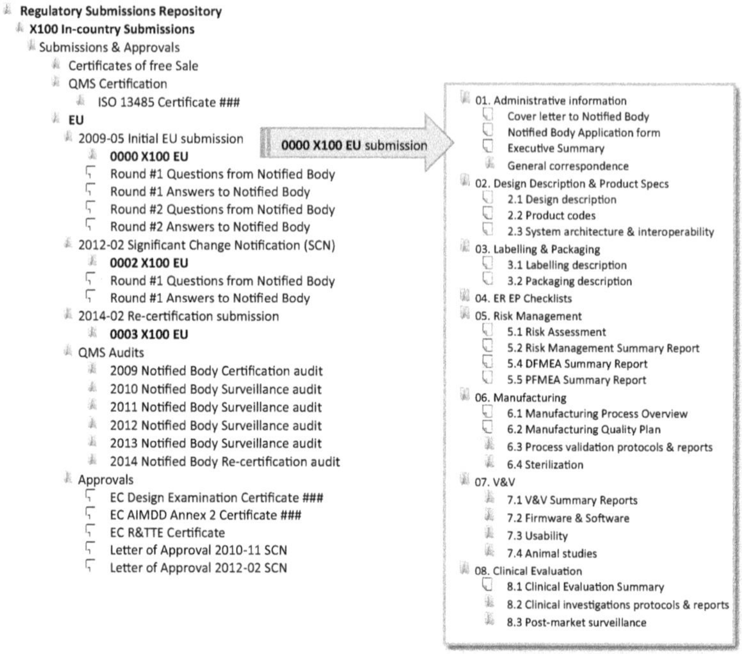

Figure 3.6 Example of organizing the EU repository.

The STED compilation files, once finalized and complete, are added to the administrative section of a particular jurisdiction, then printed and/or saved on electronic media (CDs or DVDs) to form the initial regulatory submission for that jurisdiction. This process is often referred to as *submission production*.

The rounds of questions and answers leading to the marketing approval, and any subsequent submissions and notifications of changes (also referred to as *variations*), should be saved chronologically under the relevant jurisdiction directory. Naming convention for files and directories should be intuitive and applied consistently (see examples in Fig. 3.6 and Fig. 3.7). It is expected though that once the RPS is adopted by Regulatory Authorities, the naming convention for files and directories will be mandated by the RPS standard.

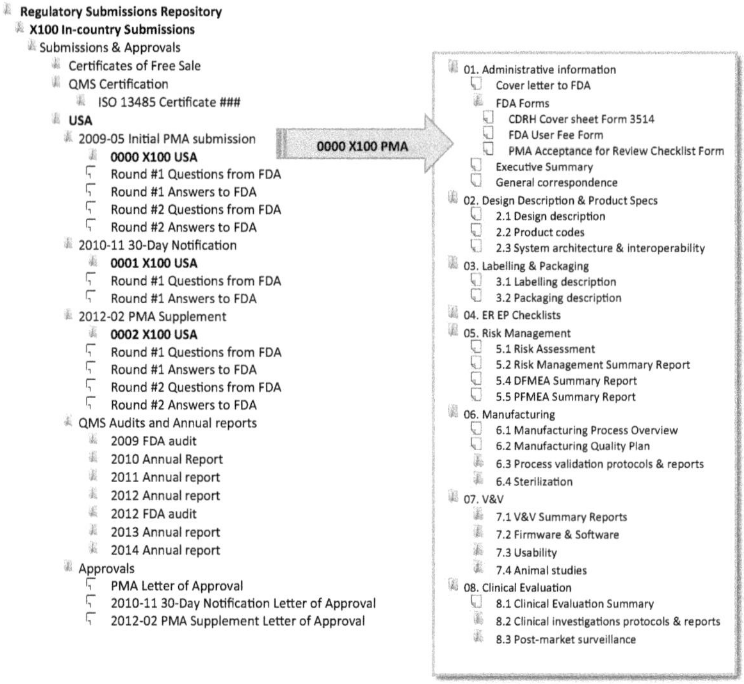

Figure 3.7 Example of organizing the US repository.

3.5.2 *Maintaining the Regulatory Submissions Repository*

A regulatory approval is granted for a particular product configuration and version of the design, labelling and manufacturing processes, as recorded in the regulatory submission documentation. Certain changes can be made by the manufacturer without notifying the regulatory agencies, but others cannot be implemented without proper notification or pre-approval from the authorities, in line with each jurisdiction's requirements and guidelines. Chapter 6 covers in more detail how changes are classified and what regulatory actions apply for those deemed to be significant.

As the product design and manufacturing processes evolve, the DHF is maintained by revising the documentation it is comprised of. For significant changes requiring regulatory action notifications and applications for change approval must be prepared and submitted

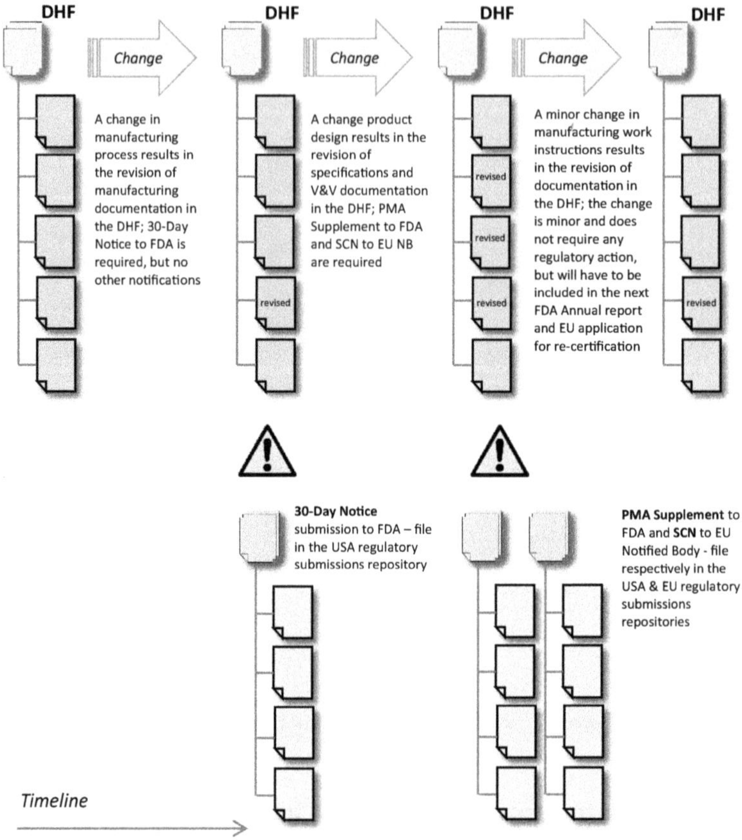

Figure 3.8 The DHF is maintained to reflect the latest product information; for changes requiring regulatory approval the submission records should be filed in the regulatory submissions repository.

in each jurisdiction, where required. The regulatory submissions repository should be maintained by filing these submissions in the appropriate locations – see Fig. 3.8 illustrating this concept.

Submissions for change notifications or approvals consist typically of a cover letter, a summary explaining what the changes are, the rationale for making the changes and the supporting verification and/or validation to demonstrate safety and effectiveness.

3.6 Case Study: The Scattered DHF

A medical device manufacturer rolled out quality system procedures that failed to define a clear structure for the company's technical documentation. Design control procedures also failed to define the content and structure for the DHF and how a DHF would be generated during the D&D phase.

Each D&D project team would create a *project space* on the company's EDMS. Project- and product-related documents would be generated and saved in folders created by individual project members. There would be a project with the initial design of a product, another project for design changes, then another project for adding features to the original product, as well as introducing a new variant of the product, and so on.

The DHF for one product family would end up scattered across many project folders, making it very difficult and time-consuming to find and retrieve information about the product design, existing product variants and latest manufacturing processes. This was exacerbated by the fact that each team member organized his or her project sub-folders according to his or her individual preferences. Some project teams did not generate certain important documents required for regulatory submissions at all.

The lack of well-organized DHFs for the company's products was causing ongoing inefficiencies, errors and documentation re-work for the D&D and regulatory affairs teams, resulting in lengthy regulatory review and approval times for most projects.

3.7 Concluding Summary

Chapter 3 discusses the technical documentation required for medical devices and IVDs. It covers the following topics:

- A high-level overview of documentation requirements in the established jurisdictions – the EU, the United States, Australia, Canada and Japan – with references to key regulations and regulatory guidance documents;

- A synopsis of the two main international initiatives to harmonize the structure and content of regulatory submissions:
  - The GHTF STED is currently the most widely accepted format for regulatory submissions internationally.
  - RPS: An RPS specification is currently being developed to enable the electronic exchange of submission information between applicants and Regulatory Authorities.
- An example of a STED-aligned DHF with a modular structure and identification of the documentation deliverables that form the STED, which reinforces the concept that the STED is a sub-set of the DHF; and
- An example of a regulatory submissions repository holding submission records for all countries and regions where the devices are being marketed and some basic maintenance requirements.

References

1. NBOG. NBOG BPG 2009-1 Guidance on Design-Dossier Examination and Report Content. *www.nbog.eu.* [Online] March 2009. [Cited: August 10, 2014.] http://www.nbog.eu/resources/NBOG_BPG_2009_1.pdf.
2. NBOG. NBOG BPG 2009-4 Guidance on Notified Body's Tasks of Technical Documentation Assessment on a Representative Basis. *www.nbog.eu.* [Online] July 2009. [Cited: August 10, 2014.] http://www.nbog.eu/resources/NBOG_BPG_2009_4_EN.pdf.
3. NB-MED. NB-MED 2.5.1/Rec5 Technical Documentation. *www.team-nb.org.* [Online] February 29, 2000. [Cited: August 10, 2014.] http://www.team-nb.org/documents/2010/Recommendation-NB-MED-R2_5_1-5_rev4_Technical_Documentation.pdf.
4. Food and Drug Administration. 21 CFR 814 Subpart B – Premarket Approval Application (PMA). *www.accessdata.fda.gov.* [Online] June 1, 2013. [Cited: August 10, 2014.] http://www.accessdata.fda.gov/scripts/cdrh/cfdocs/cfcfr/cfrsearch.cfm?fr=814.20.

5. Food and Drug Administration. Summary of Safety and Effectiveness Data. *www.fda.gov.* [Online] January 6, 2014. [Cited: August 10, 2014.] http://www.fda.gov/MedicalDevices/DeviceRegulationandGuidance/HowtoMarketYourDevice/PremarketSubmissions/PremarketApprovalPMA/ucm050289.htm#ssed.
6. Food and Drug Administration. Quality System Information for Certain Premarket Application Reviews – Guidance for Industry and FDA Staff. *www.fda.gov.* [Online] February 3, 2003. [Cited: August 10, 2014.] http://www.fda.gov/MedicalDevices/DeviceRegulationandGuidance/GuidanceDocuments/ucm070897.htm.
7. Food and Drug Administration. 21 CFR Part 807 Subpart E – Premarket Notification Procedures. *www.accessdata.fda.gov.* [Online] June 1, 2013. [Cited: August 10, 2014.] http://www.accessdata.fda.gov/scripts/cdrh/cfdocs/cfcfr/CFRSearch.cfm?CFRPart=807&showFR=1&subpartNode=21:8.0.1.1.5.5.
8. Food and Drug Administration. Design Control Guidance for Medical Devices. *www.fda.gov.* [Online] March 11, 1997. [Cited: August 10, 2014.] http://www.fda.gov/medicaldevices/deviceregulationandguidance/guidancedocuments/ucm070627.htm.
9. Therapeutic Goods Administration. Australian Regulatory Guidelines for Medical Devices (ARGMD). *www.tga.gov.au.* [Online] May 2011. [Cited: May 31, 2014.] http://www.tga.gov.au/pdf/devices-argmd-p2.pdf.
10. Health Canada. Guidance Document: Preparation of Summary Technical Documentation (STED)-based Class III and Clas IV Premarket Medical Device Licence Applications, not including IVDDs. *www.hc-sc.gc.ca.* [Online] November 2, 2011. [Cited: May 31, 2014.] http://www.hc-sc.gc.ca/dhp-mps/md-im/applic-demande/guide-ld/md_gd_im_ld_sted-eng.php.
11. Health Canada. Guidance Document: Guidance on supporting evidence to be provided for new and amended licence applications for Class III and Class IV medical devices, not including In Vitro Diagnostic Devices (IVDDs). *www.hc-sc.gc.ca.* [Online] July 5, 2012. [Cited: October 3, 2014.] http://www.hc-sc.gc.ca/dhp-mps/md-im/applic-demande/guide-ld/md_gd_data_im_ld_donnees_ciii_civ-eng.php.
12. Health Canada. Draft Guidance Document: Preparation of Summary Technical Document (STED)-based Class III and IV Premarket in vitro diagnostic device licence applications and amendments. *www.hc-sc.gc.ca.* [Online] August 22, 2012. [Cited: October 3, 2014.]

http://www.hc-sc.gc.ca/dhp-mps/consultation/md-im/md_gd_data_im_ld_donnees_ciii_civ_ivdd_sted-eng.php.

13. Health Canada. Draft Guidance Document: Guidance on supporting evidence to be provided for Class III and IV in vitro diagnostic device licence applications and amendments. *www.hc-sc.gc.ca.* [Online] August 22, 2012. [Cited: October 3, 2014.] http://www.hc-sc.gc.ca/dhp-mps/consultation/md-im/md_gd_data_im_ld_donnee_ciii_civ_ivdd-eng.php.
14. Pharmaceuticals and Medical Devices Agency. Yakushokuki No. 0216003 – Handbook for Preparation of Summary Technical Documentation Submitted in Applications for Marketing Approval for Medical Devices. *www.pmda.go.jp.* [Online] February 16, 2005. [Cited: August 10, 2014.] http://www.pmda.go.jp/english/service/pdf/notifications/PFSB-ELD-OMDE-0216003.pdf.
15. Pharmaceuticals and Medical Devices Agency. Yakushokuhatsu No. 0216003 Applications for Marketing Approval for Medical Devices. *www.pmda.go.jp.* [Online] February 16, 2005. [Cited: August 10, 2014.] http://www.pmda.go.jp/english/service/pdf/notifications/PFSB-0216002.pdf.
16. Pharmaceuticals and Medical Devices Agency. Yakushokukihatsu No. 0216001 Points to Consider When Applying for Marketing Approval for Medical Devices. *www.pmda.go.jp.* [Online] February 16, 2005. [Cited: August 10, 2014.] http://www.pmda.go.jp/english/service/pdf/notifications/PFSB-ELD-OMDE-0216001.pdf.
17. Pharmaceuticals and Medical Devices Agency. Yakushokukihatsu No. 0331008 – Points to Consider When Preparing Attachments for Applications for Manufacturing Approval for Medical Devices Which Need Registered Certification Bodies' Review. *www.pmda.go.jp.* [Online] March 31, 2005. [Cited: August 10, 2014.] http://www.pmda.go.jp/operations/notice/2005/file/0331008.pdf.
18. Pharmaceuticals and Medical Devices Agency. Yakushokukihatsu No. 0401003 – Points to Consider When Preparing Attachments for Applications for Manufacturing Approval for Generic ("Me-Too") Medical Devices with Approval Standards. *www.pmda.go.jp.* [Online] April 1, 2005. [Cited: May 31, 2014.] http://www.pmda.go.jp/operations/notice/2005/file/0401003.pdf.
19. Pharmaceuticals and Medical Devices Agency. Yakushokukihatsu No. 0327004 – Points to Consider When Preparing Attachments for Applications for Manufacturing Approval for Generic Medical Devices

without Approval Standards. *www.pmda.go.jp.* [Online] March 27, 2009. [Cited: May 31, 2014.] http://www.pmda.go.jp/operations/notice/2009/file/0327004.pdf.

20. Pharmaceuticals and Medical Devices Agency. Yakushokukihatsu No. 0131-1 – Points to Consider When Preparing Attachments for Applications for Manufacturing Approval for Improved Medical Devices without Clinical Trial Data. *www.pmda.go.jp.* [Online] January 31, 2011. [Cited: May 31, 2014.] http://www.pmda.go.jp/operations/notice/2011/file/20110131-1.pdf.
21. Global Harmonization Taskforce. GHTF SG1/N011:2008 Summary Technical Documentation for Demonstrating Conformity to the Essential Principles of Safety and Performance of Medical Devices (STED). *www.imdrf.org.* [Online] February 21, 2008. [Cited: May 31, 2014.] http://www.imdrf.org/documents/doc-ghtf-sg1.asp.
22. Global Harmonization Taskforce. GHTF SG1/N063:2011 Summary Technical Documentation (STED) for Demonstrating Conformity to the Essential Principles of Safety and Performance of In Vitro Diagnostic Medical Devices. *www.imdrf.org.* [Online] March 17, 2011. [Cited: May 31, 2014.] http://www.imdrf.org/docs/ghtf/final/sg1/technical-docs/ghtf-sg1-n063-2011-summary-technical-documentation-ivd-safety-conformity-110317.pdf.
23. Food and Drug Administration. Guidance for Industry and FDA Staff: A Pilot Program to Evaluate a Proposed Globally Harmonized Alternative for Premarket procedures. *www.fda.gov.* [Online] November 10, 2005. [Cited: May 31, 2014.] http://www.fda.gov/MedicalDevices/DeviceRegulationandGuidance/GuidanceDocuments/ucm071520.htm.
24. ASEAN. Common Submission Dossier Template. *www.asean.org.* [Online] October 21, 2010. [Cited: May 10, 2014.] http://www.asean.org/archive/SnC/ASEAN%20MDPWG%20CSDT_Final_21%20Oct%202010.pdf.
25. Selvey, P. MDD Essential Requirements. *www.medteq.info.* [Online] [Cited: August 10, 2014.] http://www.medteq.info/med/EU_ER.
26. European Commission. Harmonised Standards. *ec.europa.eu.* [Online] February 4, 2014. [Cited: September 1, 2014.] http://ec.europa.eu/enterprise/policies/european-standards/harmonised-standards/index_en.htm#h2-3.
27. Global Harmonization Taskforce. GHTF SG3/ N99-10:2004 Quality Management Systems – Process Validation Guidance. *www.imdrf.org.* [Online] January 2004. [Cited: September 1, 2014.] http://www.

imdrf.org/docs/ghtf/final/sg3/technical-docs/ghtf-sg3-n99-10-2004-qms-process-guidance-04010.pdf.

28. IECEE. IECEE Test Report Forms (TRFs). *www.iecee.org.* [Online] 2013. [Cited: May 31, 2014.] http://www.iecee.org/cbscheme/html/cbtrep.htm.
29. Food and Drug Administration. Investigational Device Exemptions (IDE) regulations – 21 CFR Part 812.25 Investigational plan. *www.accessdata.fda.gov.* [Online] September 1, 2014. [Cited: September 22, 2014.] http://www.accessdata.fda.gov/scripts/cdrh/cfdocs/cfcfr/CFRSearch.cfm?fr=812.25.
30. European Commission. MEDDEV 2.7/4 Guidelines on clinical investigation. [Online] December 2010. [Cited: September 1, 2014.] (a testable hypothesis, statistical significance levels and power, justification for the selected sample size clinically relevant, well-defined endpoints to be assessed at a specified point in time).
31. National Institutes of Health (NIH). Toolkit for Clinical Researchers. *www.nidcr.nih.gov.* [Online] [Cited: October 3, 2014.] http://www.nidcr.nih.gov/research/toolkit/#startup2.
32. IMDRF. Non-In Vitro Diagnostic Device Market Authorization Table of Contents (nIVD MA ToC). *www.imdrf.org.* [Online] June 30, 2014. [Cited: October 3, 2014.] http://www.imdrf.org/docs/imdrf/final/technical/imdrf-tech-140630-rps-nivd-toc.pdf.
33. IMDRF. In Vitro Diagnostic Medical device Market Authorization Table of Contents (IVD MA ToC). *www.imdrf.org.* [Online] June 30, 2014. [Cited: October 3, 2014.] http://www.imdrf.org/docs/imdrf/final/technical/imdrf-tech-140630-rps-ivd-toc.pdf.
34. Food and Drug Administration. eCopy Program for Medical device Submissions. *www.fda.gov.* [Online] September 29, 2014. [Cited: October 3, 2014.] http://www.fda.gov/MedicalDevices/Device RegulationandGuidance/HowtoMarketYourDevice/UCM370879.htm.
35. Food and Drug Administration. FDA eSubmitter. *www.fda.gov.* [Online] August 8, 2014. [Cited: October 3, 2014.] http://www.fda.gov/ forindustry/fdaesubmitter/default.htm.
36. Food and Drug Administration. Electronic Submissions Gateway. *www.fda.gov.* [Online] May 30, 2014. [Cited: October 3, 2014.] http://www.fda.gov/ForIndustry/ElectronicSubmissionsGateway/.
37. Health Canada. Guidance for Industry: Formatting of Class III and Class IV Licence Applications (Electronic and Paper Formats). *www.hc-sc.gc.ca.* [Online] November 10, 2014. [Cited: November

18, 2014.] http://www.hc-sc.gc.ca/dhp-mps/md-im/activit/announce-annonce/md_notice_im_avis_CIII_CIV_format_mise_en_forme-eng.php.

38. Health Canada. Common Electronic Submissions Gateway. *www.hc-sc.gc.ca.* [Online] May 23, 2014. [Cited: October 3, 2014.] http://www.hc-sc.gc.ca/dhp-mps/prodpharma/applic-demande/guide-ld/cesg-pcde/index-eng.php.

39. HL7. HL7 Regulated Product Submissions. *www.hl7.org.* [Online] January 3, 2012. [Cited: October 3, 2014.] http://wiki.hl7.org/index.php?title=Regulated_Product_Submissions.

40. Food and Drug Administration. Regulated Product Submission. *www.fda.gov.* [Online] July 29, 2009. [Cited: October 3, 2014.] http://www.fda.gov/ForIndustry/DataStandards/RegulatedProductSubmission/default.htm.

41. Theisz, V., Smith, T. Medical devices and the regulated product submission. 9(3), s.l.: *Journal of Medical Device Regulation*, Global Regulatory Press, 2012, Vols. 15-24.

Chapter 4

Pre-Market Phase

This chapter covers regulatory controls applicable to design and development (D&D) of medical devices in the pre-market phase, also known as design controls. It includes an example of a market access strategy template that can be used in the D&D planning stage. The fundamentals of design inputs, design outputs, verification and validation (V&V) and design transfer are explained. The chapter concludes with an overview of identification and traceability for medical devices and the Unique Device Identifier (UDI).

4.1 Design Controls

In a 1996 report the Food and Drug Administration (FDA) found that "approximately 44% of the quality problems that led to voluntary recall actions during 1983–1989 were attributed to errors or deficiencies that were designed into devices and may have been prevented by adequate design controls. These design-related defects involved non-critical devices (for example, patient chair lifts, in vitro diagnostics and administration sets) and critical devices (for example, pacemakers and ventilators). [...] With respect to software used to operate medical devices, the data were even more striking. A

Medical Device Regulatory Practices: An International Perspective
Val Theisz

ISBN 978-981-4669-10-8 (Hardcover), 978-981-4669-11-5 (eBook)
www.panstanford.com

study of software-related recalls for the period of fiscal years 1983 through 1991 indicated that more than 90% of all software-related device failures were due to design errors—generally, the failure to validate software prior to routine production" [1].

More than 10 years later, poor design controls, including for software, remain one of the major causes of device recalls in the United States. According to the FDA's *Medical Device Recall Report* for FY2003 to FY2012, "The most frequent causes for recalls are related to device design, software, and non-conforming material or component issues. If industry and CDRH [Center for Devices and Radiological Health] can address these problems jointly, we may be able to prevent as many as 400 recalls each year" [2].

This shows how important design controls are and explains why the US regulations mandate that medical device manufacturers, with very few exceptions, implement design controls. As mentioned in Chapter 1, the European Union (EU), Australian and to some extent Canadian regulations allow manufacturers to apply conformity assessment procedures whereby only a part of the quality management system (QMS) is certified (production quality assurance [QA], product QA or product verification). In Japan, the requirements for design controls apply to specially controlled medical devices (Classes III and IV) and to designated medical devices (Class II). However, it is highly recommended that a full QMS, including design controls, be always implemented, especially for complex, moderate and high-risk medical devices.

What are design controls? In a nutshell, design controls are a set of interrelated checks and balances that systematically assess the design of a product during the design and development (D&D) process. As a result, deficiencies in design input requirements, and discrepancies between the proposed designs and requirements, are made evident and corrected earlier in the development process. Design controls increase the likelihood that the design transferred to production will translate into a device that is appropriate for its intended use.

According to the FDA *Design Control Guidance*, "Design controls provide managers and designers with improved visibility of the design process. With improved visibility, managers are empowered to more effectively direct the design process—that is, to recognize

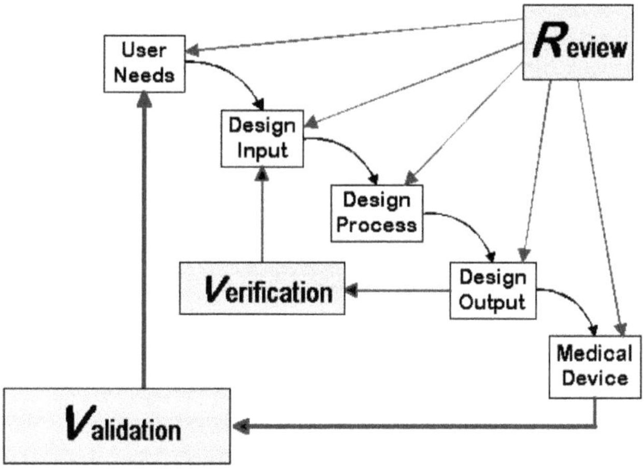

Figure 4.1 Application of design control to the waterfall design process. *Source*: FDA *Design Control Guidance.*

problems earlier, make corrections, and adjust resource allocations. Designers benefit both by enhanced understanding of the degree of conformance of a design to user and patient needs, and by improved communications and coordination among all participants in the process" (3 pp. Introduction - I. Purpose).

There are various models and representations of the D&D process and the application of design controls, such as the waterfall model (Fig. 4.1) and the V-model (Fig. 4.2).

When looking at the waterfall model and the V-model it is important to remember that the arrows represent relationships, not some sort of linear, rigid order that process steps have to follow. In reality the D&D process is iterative. Concurrent engineering methods can be used with both the waterfall model and the V-model. What does this mean? It means that user needs and design input requirements can be changed if during the design process new information comes to light or if the test results require that requirements be revised. It also means that the decision to proceed to the next step in the D&D process can be made as soon as *enough* information is available and if there is agreement among stakeholders that the company should commit to expensive or time consuming work activities associated with the next D&D stage.

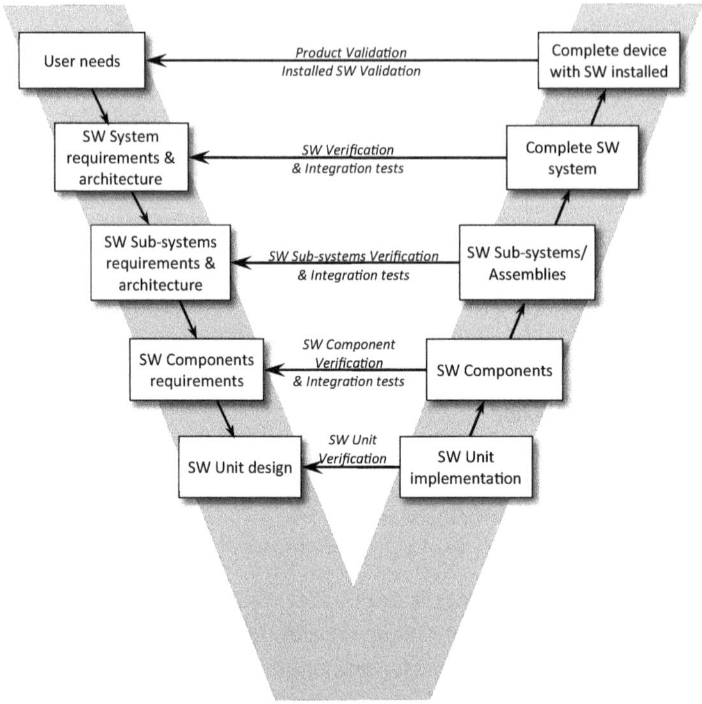

Figure 4.2 V-model process for software (SW). Based on Fig. C.2 of IEC 62304 and FDA *Guidance on General Principles of Software Validation* [4, 5].

For example, as soon as the clinical user needs (indications for use and intended use) and technology platform (principle of operation) are defined *well enough*, the D&D project can proceed to the next step and "translate" the user needs into design engineering requirements. No detailed design features need to be specified at this stage. Experienced systems engineering and regulatory experts should have a good understanding of what constitutes *enough* information when deciding whether to proceed or not to the next D&D phase and whether design control requirements have been met.

More recently, methodologies for rapid software development have emerged, such as the Agile model shown in Fig. 4.3. The Agile methodology defines an incremental, evolutionary life cycle, in which software development activities (defined in the international

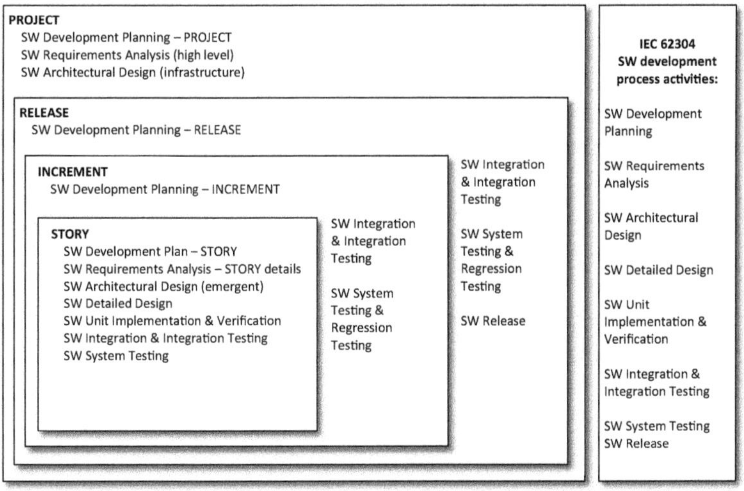

Figure 4.3 Software development activities defined in IEC 62304 mapped to the Agile incremental/evolutionary life cycle with four layers of abstraction. Based on Fig. 4 of AAMI TIR45 [6].

standard IEC 62304:2006, *Medical device software – Software life cycle processes)* are executed in four layers of abstraction:

- Project layer – consists of the complete set of activities needed to deliver a finished software product.
- Release layer – consists of activities to create a usable product; a project is made up of one or more releases.
- Increment layer – consists of activities to create a set of useful functionality; a release is made up of one or more increments.
- Story layer – consists of activities to create a small piece of functionality; an increment is made up of one or more stories [6].

Design control processes should be mapped and described in the QMS procedures. Depending on the type and complexity of the medical device the QMS procedures may need to address device quality aspects as well, such as:

- Risk management
- Device reliability

- Device durability
- Device maintainability
- Device serviceability
- Human factors engineering
- Software engineering
- Use of standards
- Configuration management
- Compliance with regulatory requirements
- Device evaluation (which may include third-party product certification or approval)
- Clinical evaluations
- Document controls
- Use of consultants
- Use of sub-contractors
- Use of company historical data (3 pp. Introduction - II. Scope)

4.2 Information Management During the Pre-Market Phase

Good information management is crucial throughout all D&D stages and it starts with the planning documentation. By following some basic principles project teams can avoid the usual pitfalls: incoherent, too much or not enough documentation leading to lack of clarity, and design errors.

The volume of information generated during D&D can be staggering; therefore it is important to manage it well by defining its structure and maintenance process. Information can be organized into three distinct categories:

- Product information about the medical device – includes design inputs (user needs, design input requirements), design outputs (design descriptions, drawings, schematics, components and materials specifications, software architecture and module specifications), risk management file, verification and validation (V&V) protocols and reports, clinical data;

- Project information – includes project plans and schedules for a particular project, D&D milestones review records; and
- QMS information – typically comprised of quality policy, quality manual, and procedures and work instructions that apply to any product or project, as well as manufacturing quality plans and work instructions for the mass production of medical devices.

Because their purpose is different, these three types of information should not be mixed in the same document. For instance, a D&D plan should contain only project type of information and should not be mixed with actual product requirements or test specifications.

When organizing information, firstly, map the content required (what), determine the folder structure and identify in which section each type of document belongs (where), what role or function is responsible for it (who) and at what stage in the process it is required (when). This structured approach should provide clarity to the various functions across the company and avoid duplicate, contradictory or missing information.

Secondly, define the required level of detail for each document: high-level documents (e.g., strategy documents, overall project plan), mid-level documents (e.g., project schedule, Master V&V Plan, summary V&V reports) and detailed-level documents (e.g., requirements, specifications, V&V protocols and reports).

As discussed in Chapter 3 manufacturers must put in place a Design History File (DHF) for each product or product family to demonstrate that the design was developed in accordance with the approved D&D plan. A DHF contains both product and project information. The sub-set of the technical documentation required for regulatory submissions is referred to as the Summary Technical Documentation (STED). By creating a STED-aligned DHF structure at the beginning of each project D&D project teams ensure that no required documentation deliverables will be left out and hence regulatory submissions will be practically written by the time the project is completed (see example in Fig. 4.4; refer also to Section 3.3, "Example of STED-Aligned DHF").

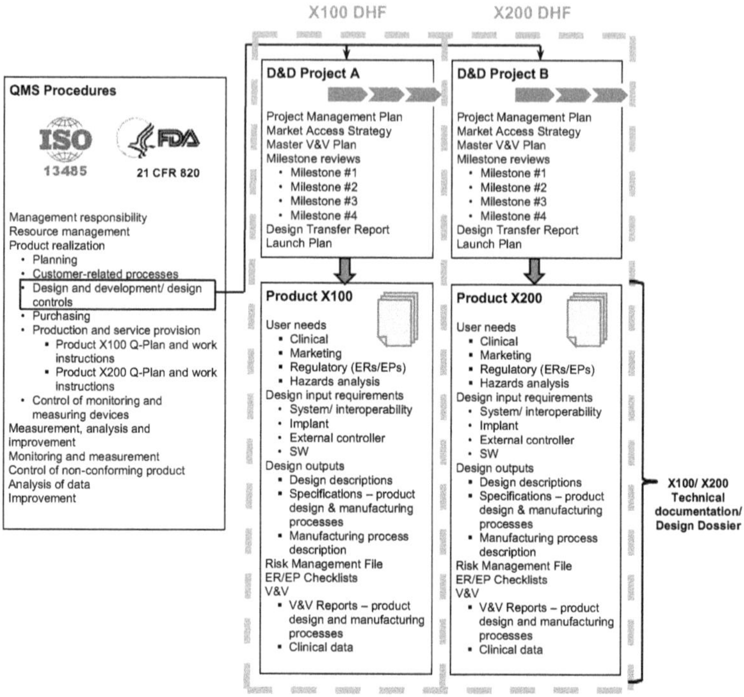

Figure 4.4 Example of information structured into QMS procedures, project documentation and (product-specific) technical documentation/ design dossier.

The QMS design control procedures are applied to the D&D projects A and B that deliver the DHF (including technical documentation) for the finished products X100 and X200, respectively.

4.3 D&D Planning Stage

During the D&D planning stage the following elements need to be defined and documented, typically in a Project Management Plan (PMP):

- What medical device will be developed, that is, the indications for use, intended use and other user needs, the technology and the principle of operation for the device;

- Risk management activities to be undertaken;
- Main tasks required to develop the medical device – from product definition through market launch;
- Key deliverables, including documentation required for each milestone, and the major reviews and decision points;
- Resources required for completing each task – personnel (internal staff, external contractors), budget and timelines;
- Individual and organizational responsibilities for each task;
- QMS procedures to be followed to ensure quality during the D&D stage;
- Applicable regulations, regulatory guidelines and standards; and
- Market access (clinical, regulatory, reimbursement) strategy.

This seems pretty straightforward, but often companies fall short of generating D&D planning documents that are clear and easy to follow, without contradictory information and with enough but not too much details or unnecessary information. If more than one planning document is needed, the PMP should provide the high-level view of the overall project and reference all other planning documents covering the constituent sub-projects.

In its *Design Control Guidance* the FDA gives some very useful advice to manufacturers trying to balance the need for documenting information with avoiding unnecessary bureaucracy:

> Design activities should be specified at the level of detail necessary for carrying out the design process. The extent of design and development planning is dependent on the size of the developing organization and the size and complexity of the product to be developed. Some manufacturers may have documented policies and procedures which apply to all design and development activities. For each specific development program, such manufacturers may also prepare a plan which spells out the project-dependent elements in detail, and incorporates the general policies and procedures by reference. Other manufacturers may develop a comprehensive design and development plan which is specifically tailored to each individual project....

> . . . Unless a manufacturer has experience with the same type of device, the plan will initially be limited in scope and detail. As work proceeds, the plan is refined. Lack of experience in planning often leads to optimistic schedules, but slippage may also occur for reasons beyond the control of planners, for example, personnel turnover, materiel shortage, or unexpected problems with a design element or process. Sometimes the schedule can be compressed by using additional resources, such as diverting staff or equipment from another project, hiring a contractor, or leasing equipment.
>
> It is important that the schedule be updated to reflect current knowledge. At all times, the plan should be specified at a level of detail enabling management to make informed decisions, and provide confidence in meeting overall schedule and performance objectives. This is important because scheduling pressures have historically been a contributing factor in many design defects which caused injury. To the extent that good planning can prevent schedule pressures, the potential for design errors is reduced.
>
> However, no amount of planning can eliminate all development risk. There is inherent conflict between the desire to maximize performance and the need to meet business objectives, including development deadlines. In some corporate cultures, impending deadlines create enormous pressure to cut corners. Planning helps combat this dilemma by ensuring management awareness of pressure points. With awareness, decisions are more likely to be made with appropriate oversight and consideration of all relevant factors. Thus, when concessions to the clock must be made, they can be justified and supported .(3 p. Section B. Design and Development Planning).

During the D&D planning stage the manufacturer needs to outline the strategy for placing the product on the market. Depending on the type of medical device and its risk classification the market access strategy will have to specify whether clinical trials are required, what regulatory controls apply and the applications that will be submitted to regulatory agencies and how the company will obtain reimbursement in the target markets.

4.3.1 *Regulatory Strategy and Planning*

The regulatory strategy identifies the regulatory controls or conformity assessment procedures applicable to a medical device for the target markets. The type and level of regulatory controls depend on the medical device risk classification. The risk class is determined on the basis of the indications for use, intended use and principle of operation using the available regulations and guidelines in each market (refer also to Section 1.5, "Risk-Based Classification").

The product does not have to be in an advanced D&D stage to be able to determine the risk class and thus define the regulatory strategy. A high-level User Needs Document, typically co-authored by the Clinical and Marketing functions, should define what medical device the company wants to develop, including its indications for use, intended use and the principle of operation.

The regulatory strategy is part of the wider market access strategy, which includes the clinical strategy that specifies what clinical trials are required, if any, in support of the regulatory submission, and the reimbursement strategy in markets where the purchase of the device can be covered by health insurance or other payer systems.

It is therefore advisable to have one Market Access Strategy document that covers clinical, regulatory and reimbursement strategies in the target markets. The owner of this deliverable can be the Regulatory function; however, the clinical specialist and health economist would have to contribute with information on the clinical and reimbursement strategies, respectively. Any changes to one area is likely to impact the other two, so having the information in one place will avoid discrepancies and ensure agreement across the three functions (an example of a Market Access Strategy template is provided in the next section).

Some regulatory strategy documents include scheduling information, such as estimated dates for submissions and approvals, and budgeting costs. This kind of information is captured anyway in project plans, schedules and milestone presentations. Some of it changes quite often, for instance, dates and timing. It makes more sense therefore to include regulatory planning information (such as budgeted costs, estimated and actual dates of applications and approvals in each country or region) in the PMP only.

Similarly, the company should maintain a separate list of standards applicable to the company's products rather than have each regulatory specialist make up his or her own list in the regulatory strategy for the project he or she is working on. This becomes especially important if the list of standards applicable to the company's products is very long or if it includes standards that tend to be revised often (see example in Section 2.4, "Standards"). Having one source of truth that project teams can refer to will avoid errors, omissions and unnecessary duplicate work.

4.3.2 *Example of a Market Access Strategy Template*

This is an example of a Market Access Strategy template that a medical device company might generate in the planning stage to articulate the clinical, regulatory and reimbursement strategies in the target markets. The text in each sub-section describes what information would typically be included and how it would be structured.

4.3.2.1 Purpose

Define the purpose of the Market Access Strategy, for example, "to define the clinical, regulatory and reimbursement strategies in the target markets – the EU, the United States, Australia, Canada, Japan and specified countries in Asia Pacific, Latin America and the Middle East".

4.3.2.2 Scope

Specify the [product, product family, system] – identified with model designation(s) – that is the subject of the market access strategy.

4.3.2.3 Indications for use and intended use

The "Indications for Use" statement is a general description of the disease or condition the device will diagnose, treat, prevent, cure or mitigate. It identifies the target population in a significant portion of which sufficient scientific evidence has demonstrated that the device as labelled will provide clinically significant results and at the same time does not present an unreasonable risk of illness or injury associated with the use of the device. The indications for use will determine whether a device is invasive or non-invasive, implanted or not, sterile or non-sterile. Any differences between indications for use in different markets should be identified.

Intended use refers to the general purpose for which the medical device is intended according to the specifications, instructions and information provided by the manufacturer. It includes the indications for use and any intended circumstances surrounding the distribution of the device, such as "reusable" versus "single use", "prescription" versus "over the counter" (OTC) and "healthcare facility environment" versus "home use".

4.3.2.4 Principle of operation

Principle of operation refers to the mode of operation or mechanism of action through which a device fulfils (or achieves) its intended use, such as electronic versus mechanical, controlled by software or other mechanism, incorporating a radio frequency (RF) or Bluetooth device or incorporating a medicinal product.

4.3.2.5 Marketing history

The provision of this information can be used toward the demonstration of safety and effectiveness of the device if the device has identical or substantial equivalent features or specifications with one or more predicate devices already marketed. A higher-risk novel device is likely to require clinical studies to support claims of safety and effectiveness. For already marketed (precursor) devices, a list of countries where the device is marketed and the year of marketing approvals should be included so that it can be used for regulatory submissions, if required.

Information on the product marketing history and/or current regulatory status is required with product submissions in the following jurisdictions:

- The United States: The FDA requirement for PMA submission contents: "Give a brief description of the foreign and U.S. marketing history, if any, of the device known to the applicant. At a minimum, include a list of all countries in which the device has been marketed and a list of all countries in which the device has been withdrawn from marketing for any reason related to the safety or effectiveness of the device" [7].

- Canada: Health Canada requirement for submissions for Class III and IV devices: "If predicate devices manufactured by the applicant are licensed in Canada and have identical features or specifications as the subject device, provision of this information may be used towards the demonstration of safety and effectiveness for this device and therefore should be provided. This subsection may also state the name of that predicate, its Canadian medical device license number and the number of units sold in Canada" [8].
- Japan: Pharmaceuticals and Medical Devices Agency (PMDA) Notifications Applications for Marketing Approval for Medical Devices and Handbook for Preparation of STED Submitted in Applications for Marketing Approval for Medical Devices: "Submissions must include sections on 'Origin or History of Discovery and History of Development' and 'Usage Conditions in Foreign Countries'" [9, 10].
- Association of Southeast Asian Nations (ASEAN): Common Submission Dossier template: "An executive summary shall be provided with the common submission dossier template, which shall include the following information: [...] commercial marketing history; [. . .] list of regulatory approval or marketing clearance obtained; status of any pending request for market clearance [...]" [11].
- Global Harmonization Taskforce (GHTF): STED guidance: "Where relevant to demonstrating conformity to the Essential Principles, and to the provision of general background information, the STED should contain an overview of: (a) the manufacturer's previous generation(s) of the device, if such exist; and/or (b) similar devices available on the local and international markets" [12].

4.3.2.6 Comparison to a predicate device, significant changes

This section applies when the regulatory submission requires a comparison to a predicate device, such as a 510(k) submission in the United States or a submission for an improved device in Japan –

Table 4.1 Comparison between [innovative/additional new model to product family/modified device] and [predicate device]

Comparison item	[Innovative/ additional new model/ modified device]	[Predicate device]	Substantially equivalent or major difference
Intended use			
Indications for use			
Contraindications			
Principle of operation			
Design features			
Materials			
Manufacturing technology			
Critical suppliers			
Sterilization method			
Other			

for instance, for an innovative device, or when adding a new model to an existing product family or for a significant change to an already approved device. The side-by-side comparison should be in tabular form, for example, using a table like Table 4.1.

4.3.2.7 Medical device risk classification and GMDN code

Determine how the product is regulated in each target market – as a medical device, drug, biologic or combination product. Establish the risk classification using the latest regulations and guidelines in each target market. Document the justification for the risk classification by referencing the classification rule applied – for the EU, Australia and Canada – and/or the applicable regulation number, classification or nomenclature code – for the United States and Japan (see example in Table 4.2).

Determine the Global Medical Device Nomenclature (GMDN) term, code and definition applicable to the medical device. For Japan, determine the Japanese Medical Device Nomenclature (JMDN) code.

For accessories, kits, systems or procedure packs, determine how they are regulated and classified in each target market. For parts that are made by other companies clarify any branding issues (model designation, commercial branding, sponsor or manufacturer) and

Table 4.2 Medical device risk classification and GMDN code (example for an anaesthesia gas machine)

Jurisdiction	Classification	Justification of classification (applied rule)
Nomenclature definition	CT250	Anaesthesia and respiratory gas supply equipment; GMDN Code ### JMDN Code ###
Australia	Class IIb	Classification rule 4.4
Canada	Class III	Classification rule 9
European Union	Class IIb	Classification rule 11
United States	Class II	21 CFR 868.5160 Gas machine for anaesthesia, Product Code BSZ
United States	Major level of concern (LoC) software	Software controls the delivery of anaesthetic gas such that an error or malfunction could result in death or serious injury.
Japan	Class II	Controlled medical device
GHTF/ASEAN Medical Devices Directive (AMDD)	Class C	Classification rule 5

identify any existing approvals, their scope and whether they can be used for the submission of the whole system.

For software, determine the risk classification in each target market according to the latest regulatory guidelines relevant to software (refer also to Section 2.5.1, "Firmware and Software").

4.3.2.8 Clinical strategy

Specify how the clinical evidence will be provided, for example, via a clinical trial or a clinical literature review. If a clinical trial is deemed necessary, indicate the type of the study (e.g., feasibility, pivotal), its purpose, the study design, its approximate size (e.g., up to 10 patients for a feasibility study, up to 150 patients for a pivotal study) and the location(s) where the study will be run and (see example in Table 4.3).

Table 4.3 Clinical investigations and clinical data registries

Study type	Objective	Study design	Population size	Number of sites and location
Feasibility, pilot, design validation	Safety for indication [*X*]; usability, consumer preference testing	Multi-centre sequential case series	No. of patients (##)	EU, United States, Australia
Feasibility, pivotal	Evaluate safety and effectiveness	Multi-centre, single blinded randomized controlled trial	## randomized; ## non-randomized	EU, United States (mandatory), Australia, UK
Continued access	Reimbursement	Single armed multi-centre study	–	EU, United States, Australia, UK
Registry	Post-market surveillance	–	–	–

Clinical studies should be scientifically rigorous and have sufficient statistical strength to support claims of safety and effectiveness and any other marketing claims made about the product.

The clinical strategy and planning should make provisions for gathering additional economic data required for obtaining reimbursement (see also Section 4.3.2.12, "Reimbursement Strategy").

4.3.2.9 Regulatory strategy

Specify the regulatory submissions types, approval paths in the target markets and whether any Mutual Recognition Agreements (MRAs) between regulatory agencies will be used. Mention if the intent is to submit applications in a staggered manner and/or in a particular order, for instance, to obtain approval in the country of origin required in emerging markets.

The planning details of multiple submissions (timelines, budget) should be included in the PMP because they need to be managed as part of the whole project anyway. The strategy document should only include a high-level overview of submissions (see example in Table 4.4) and a reference to the relevant PMP.

4.3.2.10 Other applicable regulations and guidelines

Medical devices may also be required to comply with other regulations, depending on their composition or technology used. Additional regulatory requirements that may apply include, but are not limited to:

- Radio communication regulations – EU Radio Equipment Directive RED 2014/53/EU, which replaces the Radio and Telecommunications Terminal Equipment (R&TTE) Directive 1999/5/EC; US FCC 47 CFR Part 15 – for devices using the RF spectrum (e.g., remote controls);
- Medicinal products for human use regulations – EU Directive 2001/83/EC; US 21 CFR Part 314 – for device drug combination products (e.g., implants with drug eluting components);
- Human blood derivatives;

Table 4.4 Example of regulatory submissions high level planning

Region/Country	Approval path	Typical approval timeline	Notes
		NORTH AMERICA	
United States	510(k) pre-market notification	90 days	From application date to first round of questions
Canada	Pre-market approval	3 months	From application date to first round of questions
		LATIN AMERICA	
Argentina	Country of origin approval/CE marking	6 months	Requires additional registration
Brazil	Country of origin approval/CE marking – with consular stamp	6 months	Requires additional registration
Chile	Unregulated	N/A	N/A
Colombia	Country of origin approval/CE marking	3–4 months	Requires additional registration
Mexico	Country of origin approval/CE marking	6–12 months	Requires additional registration
		EUROPE	
EU member states	MDD Annex II excluding Section II.4 (full QMS excluding design examination)	2 months to audit date; another 3 months to approval	EU member states requiring additional registration or notification: France (6 months) Germany (online registration via DIMDI) Italy (6 weeks) Poland (7 days) Spain (6 weeks)

(*Contd.*)

Table 4.4 (*Contd.*)

Region/Country	Approval path	Typical approval timeline	Notes
EU candidate and potential candidate countries	CE marking accepted	–	EU candidate and potential candidate countries requiring additional registration: Serbia (3 months) Turkey (3 months)
EFTA member states	CE marking accepted	–	Iceland, Lichtenstein, Norway, Switzerland
		MIDDLE EAST & CENTRAL ASIA	
Armenia	CE marking and registration	6 months	CE marking or similar approval will simplify registration.
Kazakhstan	CE marking and registration	6–9 months	CE marking or similar approval will simplify registration.
Moldova	CE marking and registration	2 months	CE marking or similar approval will simplify registration.
Russia	CE marking and registration	5–6 months	CE marking or similar approval will simplify registration.
Ukraine	CE marking and registration	3–6 months	CE marking or similar approval will simplify registration.
Uzbekistan	CE marking and registration	5–6 months	CE marking or similar approval will simplify registration.
Iran	CE marking and/or FDA accepted	–	–
Iraq	CE marking and/or FDA accepted	–	–
Israel	CE marking and registration	–	CE marking or similar approval will simplify registration.
Jordan	CE marking and/or FDA accepted	–	–
Kuwait	CE marking and/or FDA accepted	–	–
Lebanon	CE marking and/or FDA accepted	–	–
Oman	CE marking and/or FDA accepted	–	–
Palestine	CE marking and/or FDA accepted	–	–

Qatar	CE marking and/or FDA accepted	–	–
Saudi Arabia	CE marking and/or FDA accepted	–	Additional registration required
Syria	CE marking and/or FDA accepted	–	–
UAE	CE marking and/or FDA accepted	–	–
		AFRICA	
Egypt	CE marking and/or FDA accepted	–	–
Nigeria	Country of origin approval	Not known	Additional registration required
Kenya	CE marking and/or FDA accepted	Not known	Additional registration required
South Africa	CE marking and licence required for electronic medical devices	Not known	Licensing required for electronic medical devices
		ASIA PACIFIC (APAC)	
Australia	Schedule 3, Part 1 excluding Clause 1.6 (Full QMS excluding design examination) and inclusion onto ARTG	1 month	EC certificate accepted
China	Country of origin approval and registration	18 months	Requires type testing

(Contd.)

Table 4.4 *(Contd.)*

Region/Country	Approval path	Typical approval timeline	Notes
Hong Kong	Registration (optional)	12 months	Approvals from established jurisdictions are accepted.
India	Country of origin approval and registration	9 months	Approvals from established jurisdictions are accepted.
Indonesia	Country of origin approval and registration	6 months	–
Japan	Premarket certification by Registered Certification Body and registration	12 months	Supported by US FDA approval
Korea	Registration	4 months	–
Malaysia	Registration	6–12 months	Supported by approvals from established jurisdictions
New Zealand	Notification	Immediate	Therapeutic Goods Administration (TGA) approval in Australia (ARTG number)
Philippines	Country of origin approval and registration	10–12 months	–
Singapore	Registration	8–14 months	Approvals from established jurisdiction will allow for expedited evaluation.
Taiwan	Country of origin approval and registration	12 months	–
Thailand	Country of origin approval and registration	2–6 weeks	–
Vietnam	Country of origin approval and registration	6–8 weeks	–

- Tissues of animal origin – EU Regulation 722/2012, which replaces Directive 2003/32/EC – regarding protection against transmissible spongiform encephalopathy, or TSE;
- Phthalates;
- Latex and other allergens;
- Regulations restricting the use of certain hazardous substances in electric and electronic equipment – EU Directive RoHS 2002/95/EC; and
- Waste of Electrical and Electronic Equipment regulations (WEEE 2002/96/EC).

Specify any additional regulatory submissions types (e.g., for drug substances), certifications (e.g., for tissues of animal origins) and any significant regulatory challenges that may be expected. Specific labelling requirements may apply for these additional regulations.

4.3.2.11 Standards and guidelines

Compliance with published standards and regulatory guidelines should be the preferred method of demonstrating compliance with mandatory regulatory requirements for safety and effectiveness, in particular standards and guidelines referenced or published by Regulatory Authorities, such as:

- European Norms (EN) standards providing presumption of conformity with the Essential Requirements (ERs) of the medical devices directives listed in *Official Journal of the European Union*;
- The FDA's database with Recognized Consensus Standards, Blue Book Memos and guidance documents for medical devices;
- Australian medical device standards orders (MDSO) and conformity assessment standards orders (CASO) that can be used to demonstrate compliance with the Essential Principles (EPs) or Conformity Assessment Procedures;
- Health Canada's List of Recognized Standards for Medical Devices;

- Japan's Certification Standards, Approval Standards and Review Guidelines; and
- Other standards required for marketing authorizations or voluntary certification schemes – for example, YY, GB and T standards for China; International Electrotechnical Commission (IEC), International Organization for Standardization (ISO) standards required for Brazil INMETRO certification; or IEC, ISO standards for CB Scheme certification.

4.3.2.12 Reimbursement strategy

Define the reimbursement strategy in the (established/major) target markets, such as the United States, France, Germany, U.K., Italy, Japan and Spain. Since obtaining regulatory approval represents one of the conditions for obtaining reimbursement approval, the reimbursement application or tender should be timed closely to the date of regulatory approval in the market where reimbursement is sought.

Identify competing products in countries where reimbursement is being sought (see example in Table 4.5) or the current standard medical practice that the device is being compared with. For novel and innovative devices, reimbursement would typically be sought in countries where key opinion leaders (KOLs) and centres of excellence are located, as they would be more likely to adopt new technologies and support reimbursement processes.

Determine relevant reimbursement coverage, coding and payment applicable in each country where reimbursement is sought and

Table 4.5 Comparable competing products and their markets

Product	Manufacturer	Countries
Model 1	Manufacturer	United States, France, Germany, Italy, Spain, U.K., China, Japan, Korea, Australia
Model 2	Manufacturer	United States, France, Germany, Japan, U.K., Australia
Model 3	Manufacturer	United States, Canada, France, Germany, Italy, U.K.

Table 4.6 Reimbursement coverage, coding and payment

Country	Reimbursement coverage, coding and payment – official sources
Australia	Australian Refined Diagnostic Related Group (AR-DRG) classification codes [13] Devices approved for reimbursement included in the Prostheses List [14]
Canada	Health Technology Assessment (HTA) required in British Columbia, Ontario, Alberta and Quebec for new and existing technologies [15]
China	National Development and Reform Commission (NDRC), Ministry of Health (MOH) – provincial/municipal reimbursement schemes for implantables and disposables [16]
France	Diagnostic Related Group (DRG) tariffs apply [17]. The Economic Committee on Health Care Products (Comité Economique des Produits de Santé or CEPS) determines the price or the tariff. Union Nationale des Caisses d'Assurance Maladie (UNCAM) makes decisions on coding and tariffs on the basis of appraisals by the National Authority for Health (Haute Autorité de Santé, or HAS). Devices approved for reimbursement are listed in Liste des Produits et Prestations Remboursables (LPPR) [18].
Germany	Health Technology Assessment (HTA) required by the Joint Federal Committee (Gemeinsamer Bundesausschuss, or G-BA) – comprised of statutory health funds, hospital organizations, patient organizations (19). The Institute for Quality and Efficiency in Health Care (IQWiG) makes recommendations to approve reimbursement [20]. Reimbursement rates according to the German Diagnostic Related Group (G-DRG); devices approved for reimbursement included in the list of approved assistive technology products (Hilfsmittelverzeichniss) by the Central Federal Association of Health Insurance Funds (GKV-Spitzenverband) [21]
Italy	National/Regional DRG Hospital Tariffs and Regional Extra Tariff for some innovative and/or costly devices apply [22].
Japan	National Health Insurance (NHI), Diagnosis Procedure Combinations (DPC) [23]
Korea	Ministry of Health and Welfare (MoHW), Health Insurance Review and Assessment Services (HIRA) decide on reimbursement coverage, coding and pricing [24].
Spain	Health Technology Assessment (HTA) required by central and regional governments who make decisions on pricing, coverage and reimbursement decisions [25]
United States	Health Technology Assessment (HTA) by the Agency for Healthcare Research and Quality (AHRQ) provided to Centers for Medicare & Medicaid Services (CMS) who make decisions on National Coverage Determination (NCD) and Local Coverage Determination (LCD) [26] Coverage split into 4 parts:

(*Contd.*)

Table 4.6 Reimbursement coverage, coding and payment

Country	Reimbursement coverage, coding and payment – official sources
	• A – hospital coverage • B – medical coverage • C – Advantage Plans – managed care plans, usually a health maintenance organization (HMO) or a preferred provider organization (PPO) • D – prescription drug coverage
	Classification coding MS-DRGs converted to ICD-10-CM and ICD-10-PCS [27, 28]
U.K.	Payment-by-Result (PBR) – Healthcare Resource Groups HRG4 payment schedule; Primary Care Trust (PCT) contracts [29]

what the applicable reimbursement processes are using information from official sources and/or research organizations (see Table 4.6).

Determine what data – both clinical and economic – is required for reimbursement applications or tenders and what methodologies will be used for assessing the health technology. Health Technology Assessment (HTA) should compare the cost and benefit of *the care using the product* with *the care that is actually being delivered to the target population in healthcare facilities*, also taking into consideration staff training or changes to the current systems that may be required to adopt the new technology.

4.4 D&D Process Stage

4.4.1 *Design Inputs*

4.4.1.1 User needs

One of the first things a D&D project team needs to do is to define what product will be developed, that is, the intended purpose and main functional, safety and performance requirements.

For example, a ventricular assist device must be able to provide circulatory support safely and effectively, within a certain flow and pressure range and blood haematocrit values. Performance and reliability must be comparable with other marketed ventricular assist devices and known hazards identified and mitigated according to the state of the art.

If no comparable devices exist, the novel device must provide a level of safety and effectiveness at least as good as the existing standard of care (optimal therapy or method of diagnosis) for the same indications for use and intended use.

User needs are defined in terms of patient benefits and outcomes (not product features) during the D&D planning stage, using *medical, clinical and marketing terminology*. User needs are then "translated" into design input requirements using *engineering terminology and technical parameters.*

Defining the design input requirements may require considerable time and effort, especially for complex medical devices. Hence it is advisable to have a formal review to ensure the relevant stakeholders agree on the user needs and market access strategy before work on the design input requirements can start. As mentioned earlier, no specific methods of implementing user needs into design or any detailed design features need to be specified at this stage.

The first D&D project milestone review (define validatable user needs) – typical deliverables:

- A User Needs Document that defines clinical needs such as indications for use, intended use and expected clinical performance; user and marketing needs related to usability, ergonomics, comfort, aesthetics and pricing; other stakeholder needs such as manufacturability; and technology and the principle of operation, which can be either well established or, for novel devices, confirmed during the proof of concept stage
- Identified applicable ERs/EPs, standards and other statutory requirements
- Quality of user needs definition checked for:
  - √ Completeness – covers all stakeholders (Clinical, Marketing, Regulatory, other)
  - √ Clarity – requirements are validatable, that is, user needs can be tested and pass/fail criteria defined
  - √ Accuracy – no duplicate or conflicting requirements

- Preliminary hazards analysis
- Outputs from the preliminary hazards analysis identifying the (medical) risks to the patient and other users
- Market access strategy – clinical, regulatory and reimbursement – for the target markets, including medical device risk classification
- High-level project plan – major D&D activities, responsibilities, alignment to relevant QMS procedures, timelines for milestone reviews, budget, main deliverables

4.4.1.2 Common mistakes when defining user needs

Although it seems to be a fairly straightforward exercise, many companies struggle with the definition of user needs. Hereafter are some of the most common mistakes.

- The hodgepodge: A User Needs Document mixing clinical needs, detailed design specifications, regulatory requirements, project performance targets and aspirational statements lacks clarity and structure.
  Trying to manage this hodgepodge of requirements, some duplicating each other (different wording for the same thing), some duplicating ERs/EPs and some others duplicating requirements from applicable performance standards becomes confusing, unnecessarily cumbersome and time-consuming.
- Ambiguous definition: User needs must be expressed in validatable terms. It must be clear how the manufacturer will demonstrate that the user need was met, that is, the user need was validated; otherwise the product labelling will likely end up with claims that are not substantiated by any objective evidence. For example, the user need "[Device controller] presents the input processing features in a way that delivers competitive advantage" is at best ambiguous. What is it exactly that the engineers are expected to deliver? How will this requirement be validated and what will represent a pass validation result?

A more clearly written user need could be, for example, "[Device controller] has user-friendly means for the selection and display of [input parameters – specify!]." The usability of this functionality can be easily validated, for instance, in a small-size study with up to 20 patients in which the patients are asked to try the new device and rate its ease of use on a scale from 0 to 10. The validation criterion for this user need could be defined as follows: "At least 80% of interviewed users must score the ease-of-use of [device controller functionality] as 7 or higher."

- Design intent vs. pass/fail criteria: A project may start with overly idealistic pass/fail criteria for user needs and design specifications, only to find out during the verification and validation (V&V) phase that quite a few tests return fail results. The project team may decide that the results are acceptable anyway and includes justifications in the V&V reports ("no concern for safety or performance"). Leaving fail results in V&V reports, albeit with justifications, is not acceptable to regulatory agencies, resulting in lengthy rounds of questions and answers with agency reviewers.

  The project team is faced with a decision to either re-design and re-test until all results are pass or re-define the pass/fail criteria and re-do the technical documentation. Both options involve spending valuable time and effort on rework, delays in obtaining the approval and ultimately delay in the market launch.

  To avoid these situations, it is better to separate the aspirational design intent from the design pass/fail criteria. The very purpose of pass/fail criteria is to identify the design and performance limits that must be met to demonstrate device safety and effectiveness. If pass/fail limits are not met the device must be re-designed and re-tested. If a fail result is considered acceptable the question is whether the pass/fail limit was set correctly in the first place.

4.4.1.3 Design input requirements

After the first D&D milestone is completed and an agreement is reached on what product will be developed, the project team can proceed to the next stage and define the design inputs.

The FDA defines *design input* as "the physical and performance requirements of a device that are used as a basis for device design" (30 p. (f) Design input). According to Section 7.3.2 of the ISO 13485 standard, "Design and development inputs shall include:

(a) Functional, performance and safety requirements, according to the intended use,
(b) Applicable statutory and regulatory requirements,
(c) Where applicable, information derived from previous similar designs,
(d) Other requirements essential for design and development, and
(e) Output(s) of risk management."

The FDA requires that "each manufacturer shall establish and maintain procedures to ensure that the design requirements relating to a device are appropriate and address the intended use of the device, including the needs of the user and patient. The procedures shall include a mechanism for addressing incomplete, ambiguous, or conflicting requirements. The design input requirements shall be documented and shall be reviewed and approved by a designated individual(s). The approval, including the date and signature of the individual(s) approving the requirements, shall be documented" (31 p. (c) Design input).

A similar requirement is defined in Section 7.3.1 of the ISO13485 standard: "The organization shall establish documented procedures for design and development. The organization shall plan and control the design and development of product. During the design and development planning, the organization shall determine

(a) the design and development stages,
(b) the review, verification, validation and design transfer activities [. . .] that are appropriate at each design and development stage, and
(c) the responsibilities and authorities for design and development.

The organization shall manage the interfaces between different groups involved in design and development to ensure effective communication and clear assignment of responsibility."

A second D&D milestone review is needed to ensure the design input requirements are correctly defined before the team can move to the next D&D stage of implementing the design of the product. The role of the regulatory professional is to check that the applicable ERs/EPs and the performance user needs are adequately captured in the D&D inputs in order to ensure that the mandatory ERs/EPs and the claims made about the product will be addressed in the V&V stage of product development.

The second D&D project milestone review (define verifiable design input requirements) – typical deliverables:

- Design input requirements defined at system level, system main components, sub-systems and assemblies, as applicable;
- Product development plan, software development plan;
- Product/software requirements analysis report; quality of design input requirements definition checked for:

  √ Completeness – addressing all user needs, including applicable ERs/EPs;
  √ Clarity – requirements are verifiable, that is, requirements can be tested and pass/fail criteria are clear or can be characterized; and
  √ Accuracy – no duplicate or conflicting requirements.

- Master V&V Plan generated, with main V&V activities, applicable standards, required number of test samples, timing, budget.

Sometimes a project team may decide to build prototypes (a design output) and run some critical testing before the design input requirements are finalized, depending on the complexity and type of medical device and whether more than one design options are being explored. If managed well, this concurrent engineering approach can shorten the overall timeline for project delivery.

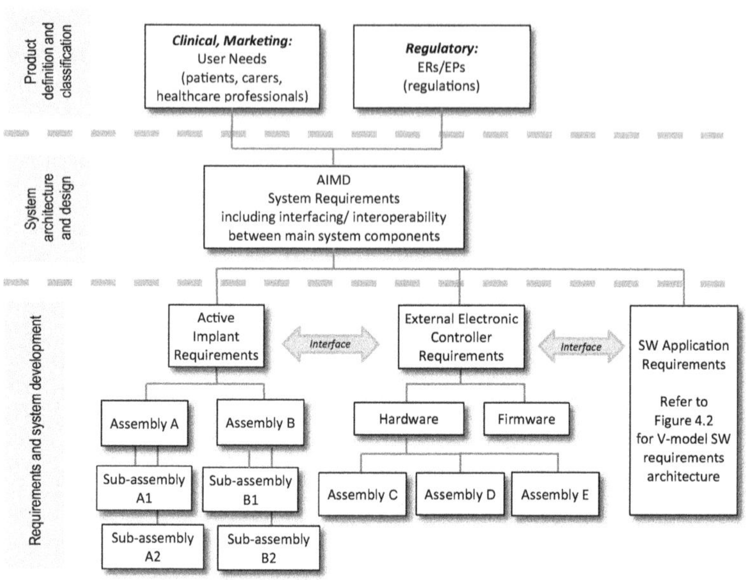

Figure 4.5 Example of requirements architecture for an active implantable medical device (AIMD) system (indicative only).

4.4.1.4 Multi-level requirements

Depending on the complexity of the product, design input requirements may need to be defined on multiple levels (see example in Fig. 4.5):

- System requirements are high-level design input requirements applicable to the whole system, including interfacing (interoperability) requirements between the main system components, for example, active implantable device, external electronic controller driving the implant and programming software application.
- Main system component (sub-system element) requirements define the requirements applicable to each main system component separately, including requirements for interfacing with the other main system components; for software applications Fig. 4.2 is a typical example of a software requirements architecture.

- Assembly and sub-assembly requirements identify the required functionalities of modules comprising a main system component.

4.4.1.5 Master V&V Plan

It is recommendable to generate a Master V&V Plan as soon as the design inputs are reviewed and approved to avoid missing testing that is required but also avoid performing tests that are not necessary. The Master V&V Plan belongs in the D&D planning documentation and needs to be re-visited if design inputs are revised or if new information comes to light during the D&D process.

A Master V&V Plan (see example in Table 4.7) would typically list the following items:

- *Major* V&V activities or modules (not the individual tests!).
- Number of test samples, budget and timelines required for each V&V module.
- Standards applied; if the company maintains a list of standards applicable to the company's products, the Master V&V Plan for every project should reference that document to ensure that all D&D project teams use the correct version of standards (see also Section 2.4.3, "Example of List of Standards Applicable to Medical Devices").

To rationalize testing efforts, the Master V&V Plan should identify applicable international standards (IEC, ISO) and any regional or national standards that differ from the international standards and that the company may have to comply with (e.g., EN Harmonised, Chinese or Japanese standards).

For instance, the protocol for testing to the IEC 60601-1 standard should cover all tests that are common between the IEC, EN and any other national versions of the standard and include at the end the national deviations, as applicable. Typical national deviations include markings on labels and labelling language. Accredited testing laboratories specializing in type testing to certain standards (safety, electromagnetic compatibility [EMC], RF wireless) should be able to assist with this task.

Table 4.7 Example of a Master V&V Plan

V&V major activity/ module	Test samples	Cost	Timeline	Notes – standards versions as per List of Standards document (###)
General safety requirements – electrical medical devices	3	$10,000	Results expected 3 months from application to [accredited test lab]	Type testing to EN IEC 60601-1 (coverage for Australia, Canada, EU, Korea and United States); plus national standards/deviations to IEC 60601-1 for: China: GB 9706.1-2007 Japan: JIS T 0601-1
AIMDs	3	$5000	Mechanical and environmental test results expected in 8 weeks from application to [accredited lab]	EN 45502-1:1997/ ISO 14708-1:2000 Performance – as per internal specifications document ###
Electromagnetic compatibility (EMC) and RF wireless requirements (remote control, Bluetooth)	3	$8000	Result expected 3 weeks from application to [accredited test lab]	EN IEC 60601-1-2 (covers EMC for Australia, Canada, EU, Korea and United States) EU: ETSI EN 300 328; ETSI EN 300 440-2; ETSI EN 301 489-3 Australia: AS/NZS 4268 Canada: RSS-210 China: YY 0505:2012 Japan: JIS T 0601-1-2; ARIB STD-T66 Korea: RRL Notice 90 United States: FCC 47 CFR Part 15 Subpart C

Labelling requirements	1	–	1 week	Internal verification to labelling requirements and compliance marks (medical devices, radio equipment, recycling and disposal) for: Australia, Canada, China, EU, Japan, Korea, United States
Software/firmware	–	–	4 weeks	Internal SW V&V as per SW specifications
Usability	20	$25,000	Results analysis within 2 weeks of completing consumer preference testing in 20 patients	EN IEC 62366 EN IEC 60601-1-6
Interoperability/backward compatibility	5	$10,000	2 months	As per functional requirements Internal type testing
Biocompatibility	10	$50,000	Results expected 4 months from application to [accredited test lab]	Type testing to standards: EN ISO 10993-1/-5/-6/-7/-11/-18
Environmental protection requirements	–	–	1 week	Documentation check – suppliers' Declaration of Conformity (DoC) and data
Sterilization validation	50	$20,000	3 months	EN ISO 11135-1, EN ISO 11138-2, AAMI TIR28, EN ISO 11607-1

(Contd.)

Table 4.7 (*Contd.*)

V&V major activity/ module	Test samples	Cost	Timeline	Notes – standards versions as per List of Standards document (###)
Clinical trials	150	$1.5 million	Results analysis within 3 months of completing clinical trial	As per the Clinical Strategy in the Market Access Strategy document ###, Clinical Investigation Plan ### and EN IEC 14155
Process validation	50	–	3 months	Internal process validation as per process validation protocol
…	…	…	…	…

In China, Class II and III devices are required to undergo type testing (testing on a representative sample for which certification of compliance with standards is sought) by a China Food and Drug Administration (CFDA)-accredited laboratory, even if test reports from a foreign accredited independent third-party laboratory are already available. The manufacturer is required to provide a Product Technical Requirements document (formerly known as Product Standard) detailing the specifications of its product and how to test for those specifications. Testing laboratories in China will then conduct the tests on samples based on the Product Technical Requirements (Product Standard) document. Obviously, it is important to choose a laboratory that has experience with the manufacturer's type of devices [32].

4.4.2 *Design Outputs*

Design outputs include the finished device and its labelling, drawings, schematics, components and materials specifications, software architecture and module specifications.

The FDA defines *design output* as the "results of a design effort at each design phase and at the end of the total design effort" (30 p. (g) Design output). Especially for complex devices the output of one design effort represents the input into another design effort; hence the D&D process may need to be divided into manageable modules, for instance, into main components of a complex medical device system; the main device and its accessories; and hardware and software.

The FDA regulation requires that "each manufacturer shall establish and maintain procedures for defining and documenting design output in terms that allow an adequate evaluation of conformance to design input requirements. Design output procedures shall contain or make reference to acceptance criteria and shall ensure that those design outputs that are essential for the proper functioning of the device are identified. Design output shall be documented, reviewed, and approved before release. The approval, including the date and signature of the individual(s) approving the output, shall be documented" (31 p. (d) Design output).

Similarly, Section 7.3.3 of the ISO 13485 standard stipulates that "design and development outputs shall:

(a) meet the input requirements for design and development,
(b) provide appropriate information for purchasing, production and for service provision,
(c) contain or reference product acceptance criteria, and
(d) specify the characteristics of the product that are essential for its safe and proper use".

The D&D process can be incremental and iterative, especially for complex medical devices, with partial or preliminary testing performed on intermediate design versions. Once the engineering team is closer to finalizing the design, a third D&D milestone review should check that the project has delivered the outputs as per the D&D plan, before comprehensive, final verification and validation are performed.

The third D&D project milestone review (deliver design outputs) – typical deliverables:

- Design descriptions;
- Product specifications (drawings, schematics, component and materials procurement specifications);
- Labelling and packaging specifications;
- Finished device (engineering prototypes for V&V);
- Risk management file – risk assessment, design failure modes and effects analyses (DFMEA), process failure modes and effects analyses (PFMEA);
- Design V&V plans and protocols;
- Manufacturing quality plan, manufacturing process overview/description; and
- Process validation plans and protocols.

The regulatory professional should check that the design outputs such as design descriptions, labelling and packaging descriptions and the risk management file are generated and that the V&V protocols address all applicable ERs/EPs.

4.4.3 *Verification & Validation*

Design outputs are verified against design inputs. The verification activities will answer the question, Have we designed the product right? The finished medical device is validated against the user needs. The validation will answer the question, Have we designed the right product? (See also Fig. 4.6.)

Early verification activities, sometimes referred to as *pre-testing*, can run concurrently using engineering prototypes while the design is being developed and refined. Intermediate test results can be documented in lab books or test data sheets and can be used to characterize the product design and manufacturing process, that is, to determine the V&V pass/fail criteria, especially if no standards exist.

For novel devices, clinical feasibility studies may be appropriate during this stage, provided the basic safety tests (sterility, biocompatibility, electrical safety, EMC and chemical compatibility with concomitant drugs, chemicals or cleaners) are completed with positive results before using the device on humans. A feasibility study:

- Provides support for a subsequent pivotal study or may be used to answer basic research questions;
- Is not intended to be the primary support for a marketing application;
- Is small in size - generally 10 to 40 patients - and its endpoints and sample size are generally not statistically driven; and
- Is often required by the FDA prior to a pivotal study to assess basic safety and potential for effectiveness.

The regulatory review of a feasibility study is primarily focused on safety and whether the potential benefit or value of the data justifies the risk. Questions being asked during the review of a feasibility study include:

- Is the study conceptually reasonable?
- Is the pre-clinical validation of the device adequate? Why is clinical investigation really the next necessary step?

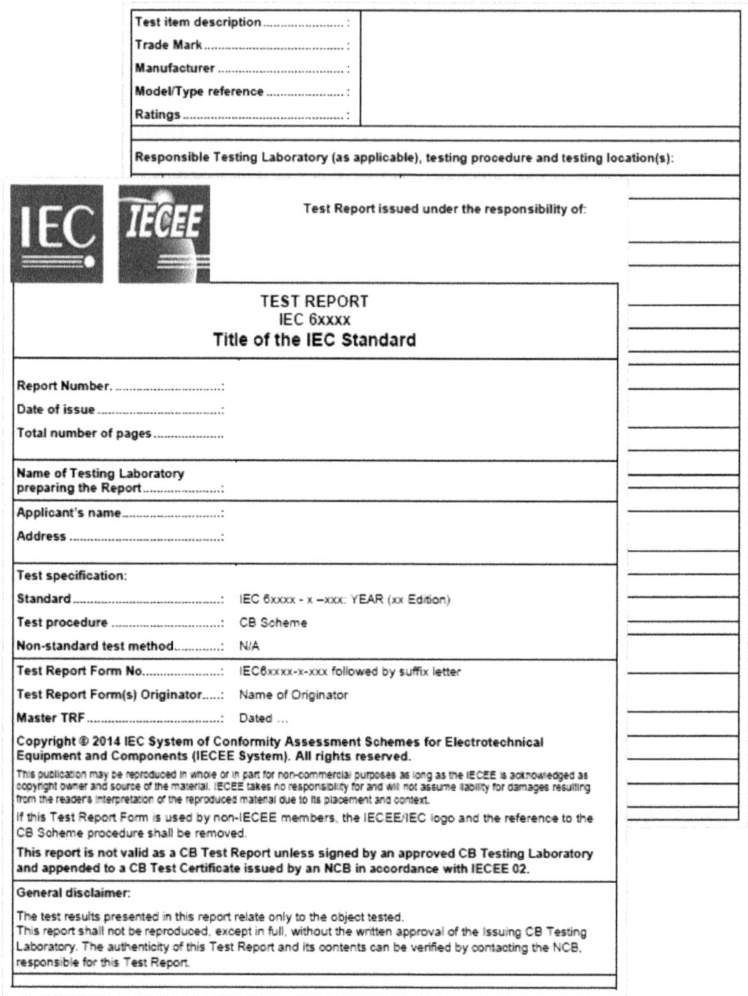

Test item description .... :
Trade Mark .... :
Manufacturer .... :
Model/Type reference .... :
Ratings .... :

Responsible Testing Laboratory (as applicable), testing procedure and testing location(s):

Test Report issued under the responsibility of:

TEST REPORT
IEC 6xxxx
Title of the IEC Standard

Report Number. ....:
Date of issue ....:
Total number of pages ....

Name of Testing Laboratory
preparing the Report........................:

Applicant's name..............................:
Address ....:

Test specification:
Standard ....: IEC 6xxxx - x –xxx: YEAR (xx Edition)
Test procedure ....: CB Scheme
Non-standard test method.............: N/A

Test Report Form No.......................: IEC6xxxx-x-xxx followed by suffix letter
Test Report Form(s) Originator.....: Name of Originator
Master TRF ....: Dated ...

Copyright © 2014 IEC System of Conformity Assessment Schemes for Electrotechnical Equipment and Components (IECEE System). All rights reserved.

This publication may be reproduced in whole or in part for non-commercial purposes as long as the IECEE is acknowledged as copyright owner and source of the material. IECEE takes no responsibility for and will not assume liability for damages resulting from the readers interpretation of the reproduced material due to its placement and context.

If this Test Report Form is used by non-IECEE members, the IECEE/IEC logo and the reference to the CB Scheme procedure shall be removed.

This report is not valid as a CB Test Report unless signed by an approved CB Testing Laboratory and appended to a CB Test Certificate issued by an NCB in accordance with IECEE 02.

General disclaimer:

The test results presented in this report relate only to the object tested.
This report shall not be reproduced, except in full, without the written approval of the Issuing CB Testing Laboratory. The authenticity of this Test Report and its contents can be verified by contacting the NCB, responsible for this Test Report.

Figure 4.6 IECEE Test Report form (TRF) template – pages 1 and 2 [34].

- Are there appropriate mitigations of potential risks?
- Are the enrollment criteria appropriate?
- Are patients adequately informed (e.g., via the Patient Informed Consent)?
- Is the sample size appropriate? [33]

A final and comprehensive verification, a considerable portion of which is done by third-party laboratories, is usually performed when there is enough confidence that it can be completed with positive results and if no major re-design is expected should some tests not meet pass/fail criteria in the first round. The aim is to avoid as much as possible having to repeat testing again and again. Final verification needs to be documented in V&V reports in accordance with the company's document control procedures.

When using third-party laboratories, it is recommendable to select independent test labs that are officially accredited for the scope required. This will ensure that their test results are obtained in accordance with Good Laboratory Practices (GLPs) and/or the ISO/IEC standard 17025:2005, *General requirements for the competence of testing and calibration laboratories*.

Manufacturing process validation activities cover equipment installation qualification (IQ) and operational qualification (OQ), sterilization process validation and sterile packaging validation. Long-term validation activities such as process qualification (PQ), ageing, stability and reliability typically run over many months and years and as such are not required to be completed at this stage, but there should be plans, protocols and interim reports in place, as applicable.

Almost always, the design and manufacturing processes need to be tweaked, adjusted or significantly changed before all V&V is completed with positive results. Good configuration management and traceability of design versions used during specific tests, also referred to as *build standards*, is extremely important during this time.

Test reports and associated test data sheets containing original measurements, inspection and test results must comply with document control requirements, that is, be uniquely identified by a document number and a version number. They also need to include information of what was tested (model designation and build standard identifier), how it was tested (inspection and test method, including equipment identification, if applicable), who tested it (name and job title), date and location (e.g., internal or external laboratory).

Test Report forms (TRFs) prepared by members of the IECEE (IEC System of Conformity Assessment Schemes for Electrotechnical Equipment and Components) are excellent examples of professional templates that comply with document controls requirements as well as GLPs. The examples shown in Fig. 4.7 (report first two pages) and Fig. 4.8 (examples of test data sheets) are pages from the IECEE Master template for IEC TRFs [34].

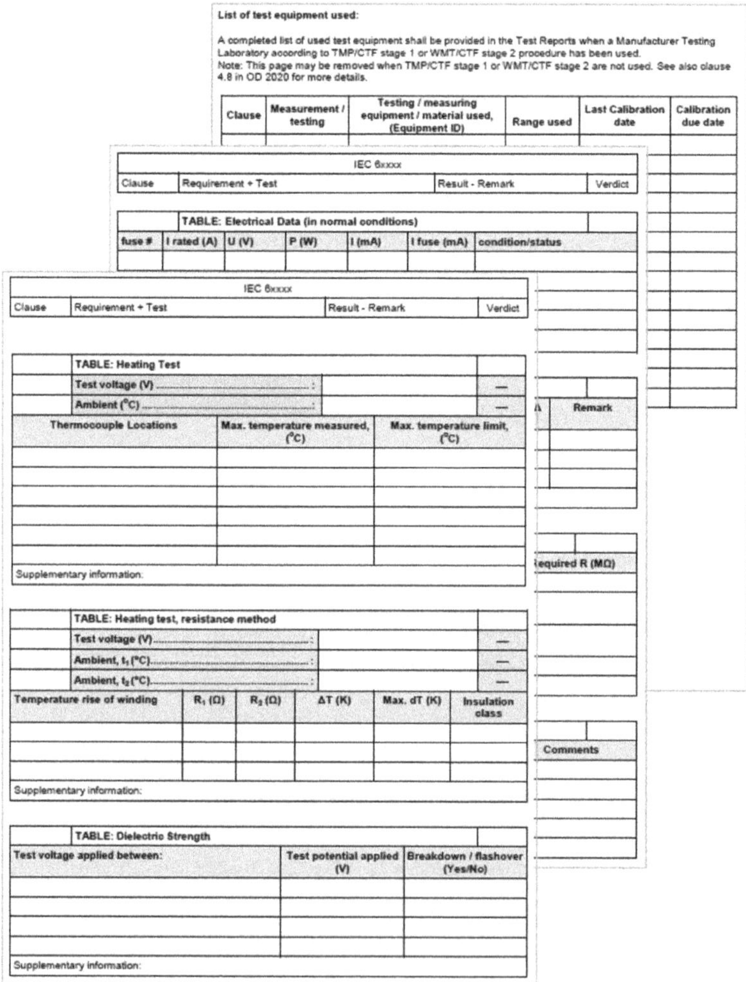

Figure 4.7 IECEE Test Report form (TRF) template – test data sheets [34].

Design validation activities include clinical evaluation, usability and consumer preference testing. They are usually performed once the design is stable enough and no significant changes are expected. Significant changes include changes in the indications for use and intended use, principle of operation and basic design and performance characteristics related to device safety and effectiveness. For high-risk medical devices and some moderate-risk medical devices clinical evaluation would typically need to include data collected from pivotal clinical trials. A pivotal study:

- Is generally intended as the primary clinical support for a marketing application;
- Is designed to demonstrate a "reasonable assurance of safety and effectiveness";
- Has endpoints and sample size that are statistically driven; and
- Is designed to assess both safety and effectiveness.

The regulatory review of a pivotal study is much more complex than that of a feasibility study, as it focuses on safety and the plan for collecting and evaluating study data and additional critical issues such as:

- Primary and secondary trial endpoints, including appropriateness of endpoint parameters, hypotheses and success criteria; generally endpoints are divided into *safety* endpoints and *effectiveness* endpoints.
- Study design – control, randomization, blinding, follow-up, etc., including a rationale for the chosen study design.
- Study conduct and monitoring – data collection, handling and adjudication process by independent committees (e.g., Clinical Trial Data Monitoring Committee).
- Statistical analysis plan – clearly defined safety and effectiveness hypotheses, type 1 error and multiplicity, missing data handling, sample size calculations and assumptions, assessment of critical covariates, adaptive design plans, interim analyses and early stopping rules and data handling.

Clinical trials for medical devices are designed to support a reasonable assurance of safety and effectiveness for the marketing application. Some clinical investigations involve novel devices, but many are run with "me too" devices. Typically, a single pivotal study follows feasibility stage(s): early feasibility study, first-in-human and traditional feasibility study. Device trials are unique, in that they tend to be smaller than drug trials and:

- Many are difficult to blind, randomize and control;
- Many depend on physician technique (e.g., implants);
- Device modifications occur during the trial; and
- The endpoints are highly diverse [33].

Clinical trials require careful planning. An appropriate and scientifically robust clinical trial design is essential. Poorly designed investigations can result in data that fails to sufficiently support safety and/or performance claims. Typical flaws and errors in a Clinical Investigation Plan that impede the regulatory approval process and delay market access include, but are not limited to:

- The plan fails to identify rules and procedures for data collection, management and adjudication.
- The sample size identified in the Clinical Investigation Plan is not based on scientific and statistical principles but solely on a manufacturer's experience.
- The plan fails to select a study protocol that minimizes sample bias.

An aspect often forgotten or ignored during the V&V stage is reimbursement. To have a successful business, a manufacturer must be able to demonstrate the clinical and economic benefits of its medical devices compared to standard medical practice or competitor devices. Collecting appropriate and relevant clinical and economic data is crucial for winning tenders and obtaining reimbursement approvals.

Clinical trials can be very expensive to run; therefore they should be panned carefully. Clinical Investigation Plans should make provisions for gathering the economic data required for reimbursement applications. The selection of the clinical study design should take into consideration the expected level of rigour required for regulatory and reimbursement approvals (see also Section 2.6.2.1, "Study Designs").

For example, in the United States, the Centers for Medicare & Medicaid Services (CMS) ranks clinical study designs from most to least methodologically rigorous as follows:

- Randomized controlled trials
- Non-randomized controlled trials
- Prospective cohort studies
- Retrospective case control studies
- Cross-sectional studies
- Surveillance studies (e.g., using registries or surveys)
- Consecutive case series
- Single case reports [35]

HTA refers to the systematic evaluation of properties, effects and/or impacts of health technology. It is a multi-disciplinary process to evaluate the social, economic, organizational and ethical issues of a health intervention or health technology. The main purpose of conducting an assessment is to inform a policy decision making [36].

HTA uses scientific evidence to assess the quality, safety, efficacy, effectiveness and cost-effectiveness of health services. The key questions that HTA typically aims to answer for each new health technology, in comparison to alternative interventions, are:

- Is it safe?
- Does it improve health outcomes?
- Is it cost effective? [37]

HTA should compare the cost and benefit of *the care using the product* with *the care that is actually being delivered to the target population in healthcare facilities*, also taking into consideration staff training or changes to the current systems that may be required to adopt the new technology.

Economic evaluations should use appropriate methodologies for measuring the costs and consequences of using the devices, therapies or methods of diagnosis being compared, such as cost analysis, cost-effectiveness analysis, cost–utility analysis or cost–benefit analysis (see also Table 4.8).

It is important to ensure that all requirements are addressed by the design and that they are traceable to V&V results but also

Table 4.8 Measurement of costs and consequences in economic evaluation

Type of study	Measurement/valuation of costs in two alternative therapies	Identification of consequences	Measurements/valuation of consequences
Cost analysis	Monetary units	None	None
Cost-effectiveness analysis	Monetary units	Single effect of interest, common to both alternatives, but achieved to different degrees	Natural units (e.g., life-years gained, disability-days saved, points of blood pressure reduction, etc.)
Cost–utility analysis	Monetary units	Single or multiple effects, not necessarily common to both alternatives	Healthy years (typically measured as quality-adjusted life-years)
Cost–benefit analysis	Monetary units	Single effect of interest, common to both alternatives, but achieved to different degrees	Monetary units

Source: *Methods for the Economic Evaluation of Health Care Programmes, Third Edition* [38]

that no unnecessary testing is performed (tests that are not called by any particular requirements). There must be full traceability between high-level system requirements and detailed sub-system and assembly requirements (vertical traceability, see also Fig. 4.5 and Fig. 4.2) and between user needs, including statutory ERs/EPs and final V&V results (horizontal traceability, see also Fig. 4.1).

Requirements management is the systematic process of defining, organizing and tracking the requirements of a product or system, and it is usually the responsibility of the company's Systems Engineering function. Traceability is achieved by establishing the source and dependencies between requirements. Relationships between parent and child requirements can be one-to-many and many-to-one (see Fig. 4.8). Complex products require specialist software tools for requirements management.

A fourth D&D milestone review needs to check that all relevant V&V has been completed with positive results as per the Master V&V Plan and V&V protocols.

The fourth D&D project milestone review (V&V completed with positive results) – typical deliverables:

- *Overall V&V Summary Report*;
- *Requirements Traceability Report*;
- Risk management file (finalized);
- ER/EP checklists;
- Design verification reports – performance, electrical safety, EMC, mechanical safety and environmental conditions, chemical and biological safety, software validation;
- Manufacturing validation reports – manufacturing processes IQ and OQ, sterilization validation;
- Usability studies and consumer preference testing; and
- *Clinical Evaluation Report*, Post-Market Surveillance Plan, Clinical Investigation Plan, protocol and report and other essential study documentation, if applicable.

The regulatory professional should check that all documents required for regulatory submissions have been generated and are in a submission-ready state (see also Chapter 3, "Technical Documentation"). Design outputs and V&V reports must address all applicable ERs/EPs and performance requirements. Depending on

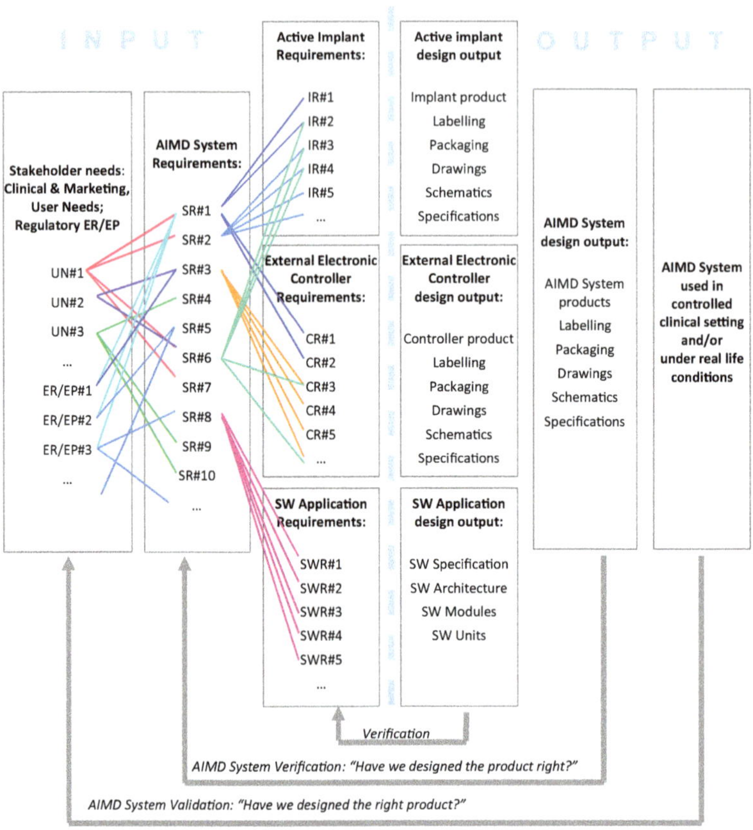

Figure 4.8 Example illustrating requirements traceability, verification and validation for an AIMD system (indicative only).

their individual knowledge and experience, regulatory professionals may advise the project teams on the application of international, EN Harmonised and any other relevant national standards.

Authorities in some emerging markets require a Certificate of Analysis (CoA) similar with what is required for pharmaceutical products. For medical devices this requirement can be addressed by providing a declaration that summarizes the critical quality control (QC) inspection steps performed during manufacturing (e.g., visual inspection, electrical, functional, sterility assurance tests). The results can be presented in tabular form and should cover three

Table 4.9 Example of Certificate of Analysis summary table

[Product model designation], [Batch No/ Serial No.]/ [Sterilization Batch No.] Date:			
#	Test/Visual inspection	Test/inspection method	Results
1	[*Short description/purpose*]	[*Short description – inspection/test method and equipment*]	Pass
2	[*Short description/purpose*]	[*Short description – inspection/test method and equipment*]	Pass
...	...	...	...

batches of the manufactured product, with short descriptions of what was tested, using what method and equipment, and what were the final results (must be pass to be acceptable) – see Table 4.9. The CoA must be signed by the qualified person responsible for product release.

4.4.4 *Design Transfer*

After completion of the V&V stage, the project team can proceed with transferring the design to production. During the design transfer stage the D&D project team needs to carefully assess the design specifications, selection of components and production methods and *how they all fit together*. Once a medical device enters the production phase it is placed under strict change control. An effective design transfer is therefore important in order to avoid changes that might be required to fix problems not picked up earlier, especially if the production or parts of it are subcontracted to other companies.

According to the FDA regulation 21 CFR 820.30(h), *Design Transfer*, "Each manufacturer shall establish and maintain procedures to ensure that the device design is correctly translated into production specifications". Although the ISO 13485:2009 standard does not use the term "design transfer" it contains equivalent requirements in Sections 5.4.2, "Quality management system planning", and 7.1, "Planning of product realization" [3].

Procedures for design transfer should address at least the following basic elements:

- Include a qualitative assessment of the completeness and adequacy of the production specifications – this can be addressed during design transfer.
- Ensure that all documents and articles that constitute the production specifications are reviewed and approved – this is addressed by implementing document controls and configuration management best practices.
- Ensure that only approved specifications are used to manufacture production devices – this is addressed by implementing document controls and configuration management best practices.

Records containing the specifications and manufacturing procedures for a finished device need to be compiled in a set of documentation that the FDA defines as the Device Master Record, or DMR. The DMR includes "engineering drawings and documents used to procure components, fabricate, test, inspect, install, maintain, and service the device" [30].

While a Design History File (DHF) can typically cover entire product families (products that have the same indications for use and intended use, same basic design and performance characteristics related to device safety and effectiveness and same risk-based classification), a DMR is required for each product type and should be traceable to the product model designation and part number (or bill of materials [BOM] identifier) – refer also to Section 4.5.1, "Product Identifiers".

Failure to transfer a design effectively can lead to gaps or contradictions in the DMR documentation, which in turn could result in unnecessary design changes, re-work, or low-quality products. A design transfer plan should be put in place, with checklists of required items, including:

- Updated and approved specifications for off-the shelf and custom made components and materials;
- Incoming inspections procedures;
- A BOM and a bill of operations (BOO);

- Work instructions;
- Equipment and process settings;
- In-process inspection and testing procedures;
- Final testing and inspection procedures; and
- Product release procedures.

Design transfer is a good opportunity to correct errors, resolve any outstanding issues and finalize design and manufacturing specifications. It is therefore recommendable to start submitting regulatory applications only after design transfer has been completed successfully.

4.5 Product Identification and Traceability

Identification and traceability of medical devices are essential for ensuring patient safety. They enable the retrieval of information on how a particular product was designed and manufactured, when it was manufactured and under what conditions. The required level of traceability often depends on the device risk classification. High-risk implanted devices must be traceable to individual patients, whereas traceability of lower-risk devices can be done to the manufactured batch or lot.

More importantly, in the case of a serious adverse event, sponsors and manufacturers must be able to identify a device quickly and precisely, and track it through the distribution chain, so that all products that have been placed on the market can be promptly located and recalled, if needed. Tracking information is also used to facilitate communication and notifications of product recalls between various stakeholders – manufacturers, regulatory agencies, distributors and healthcare providers.

Medical device identification and traceability require a holistic approach. Manufacturers must understand what product identifiers are needed for what purpose and when each of those identifiers should change if there are changes in the product design or manufacturing process. Quality system procedures should define a process for assigning product identifiers and for managing changes in sync with identification and traceability rules. Typical product identifiers that a manufacturer might be using during the life cycle of a medical device are described hereafter.

4.5.1 *Product Identifiers*

Model designation (also referred to as *model number* or *product name*) identifies a finished medical device with specific indications for use, intended use, design and performance characteristics. It includes any information necessary for the user to identify the device and to distinguish it from similar devices. A model designation should be assigned as early as possible in the D&D process, ideally during the D&D planning stage, once the user needs are defined and before the design input requirements are specified (see also Section 4.4.1, "Design Inputs"), so the design dossier documents can be correctly identified as belonging to the relevant product or product family. Usually, the model designation remains unchanged as long as the indications for use, intended use, design and performance characteristics and the manufacturer or sponsor remain the same.

The model designation appears on the product label, user manual and in the technical documentation supporting claims of safety and effectiveness, such as design descriptions, V&V protocols and reports.

The model designation is also used for regulatory and reimbursement purposes to identify the medical device on certificates, registrations, listings, etc.

The *catalogue number* identifies a saleable item (an item, separately packed and shipped, that can be ordered by a customer), which can be a finished medical device, an accessory, spare parts packed and shipped separately or combinations thereof. Catalogue numbers are also used to distinguish regional variants of the same medical device (e.g., US version, EU version, Japanese version) or design variants of the same medical device (e.g., range of colours or dimensions). There can be one or more catalogue numbers associated with the same model designation.

Differences between regional versions are typically related to labelling, for example, with or without the Conformité Européenne (CE) marking or other approval marks, use of symbols and translations, use of medical terminology specific to the country or variations in the approved indications for use and intended use.

Catalogue numbers distinguishing between design variants of the same medical device are often required to be listed in regulatory and reimbursement documents (application forms, product lists, certificates, registrations, listings, etc.), along with the model designation.

The *part number* identifies the production build or BOM of a product. Part numbers allow manufacturers to differentiate between iterations or variations of the same design, including those that do not require a change in the model designation or catalogue number, for instance, different manufacturing methods for the same design requirements – hence different BOOs, optimization of a design without significantly changing the design or performance characteristics, using alternative parts, materials or manufacturing sub-contractors that meet the design input requirements. In other words, the same model designation or catalogue number can have one or more part numbers associated with it.

Part numbers should not be used as product identifiers in regulatory documents or on product labelling, because they need to change relatively often. They can and should be included in dispatch records (invoice, delivery note, shipping list, bill of lading, etc.) to have a record of the design build that was actually delivered to the customer.

Changing a product identifier listed in a regulatory or reimbursement approval invalidates the approval for that product. Therefore the model designation and catalogue numbers are the more appropriate product identifiers that should be used for regulatory and reimbursement documents (application forms, product lists, certificates, registrations, listings, etc.).

Changing a product identifier that is affixed on a product label or included in the instructions for use (IFUs) would require revising all relevant labels, packaging and manuals for that product. Scrapping or re-working existing stock, re-printing new labels and packaging can be laborious and expensive. Therefore the model designation and serial or batch numbers are the more appropriate product identifiers that should be used for labeling purposes (device labels, sales packaging and IFUs).

The *serial number or batch/lot number* identifies a unit (serial number) or a group of units (batch or lot number) of a product manufactured at a certain time under specified conditions. All units belonging to the same batch or lot are manufactured under uniform conditions using the same specifications, production methods and equipment. The serial and batch numbers allow a manufacturer to trace a product back to the manufacturing date and production records, including the design build identified by the part number.

There must be full traceability between the model number, catalogue number, (production) part number and serial or batch/ lot number of the same product.

4.5.2 *Software Identifiers*

In addition to a model designation (commercial branding), software should be identified following international best practices, for instance, as defined in IEEE 828:2012, *Standard for Configuration Management in Systems and Software Engineering*, and IEEE 1042:1987, *Guide to Software Configuration Management*.

Typically, a naming convention scheme for software includes the model designation and a 3-digit identifier according to IEEE 828. For example, "3.5.8" is a 3-digit identifier, where "3" is the *Release* (to the customer), "5" is the *Version* (internal release by the developer) and "8" is the *Revision* (by the developer).

Version identifies an initial release or re-release of a configuration item associated with a complete compilation or recompilation of the item. Different versions have *different functionalities*.

Revision identifies a change to a version that corrects only errors in the design/code but does *not* affect the documented functionality.

Release identifies the formal distribution of an approved version.

If this method is chosen to identify medical device software products, the release and the version would be the only identifiers that would need to be included on physical, hardware items such as CD/DVD labels and printed IFUs. The software application itself should always be identified by the release, version *and* revision.

Regulatory and reimbursement approvals (certificates, registrations, listings, etc.) should only include the model designation so that they are not invalidated every time the release and version change. However, changes in software functionality are almost always considered significant and require notification or approval by regulators. Therefore regulatory agencies may require that software is identified by release and version in the initial application forms and/or product lists so that they can keep track of all subsequent significant changes.

4.5.3 *Product Grouping*

Most regulatory agencies allow manufacturers to group similar products and register them together as a product family, instead of submitting and registering them individually. This helps streamline the review and approval process and save costs in regulatory fees and charges. To take advantage of this, early planning and good organization of product information are needed.

The design input requirements and development process should utilize a modular structure as much as possible to allow scalability from a single product to a product family comprised of similar devices. DHFs should be set up for product families rather than separately for each individual product in order to take advantage of the fact that a significant portion of the technical documentation or design dossier can be shared among the products within the same family.

In reality, many medical device companies start by developing one system comprised of a few main components, for instance, an active implantable, and an external electronic controller and a software application. Subsequently, as the main components of the system evolve to the next generations, a system is put together by mixing and matching various versions of the main components that are compatible with each other (see example in Fig. 4.9).

In the example given earlier, grouping the main components of a system into product families enables flexibility in how system components are combined together into systems. It is not necessary to identify all these possible combinations by a system name or model designation, because combinations or systems are put together according to compatibility between the main components.

Also, the development and maintenance of the main system components become much easier if products are grouped into

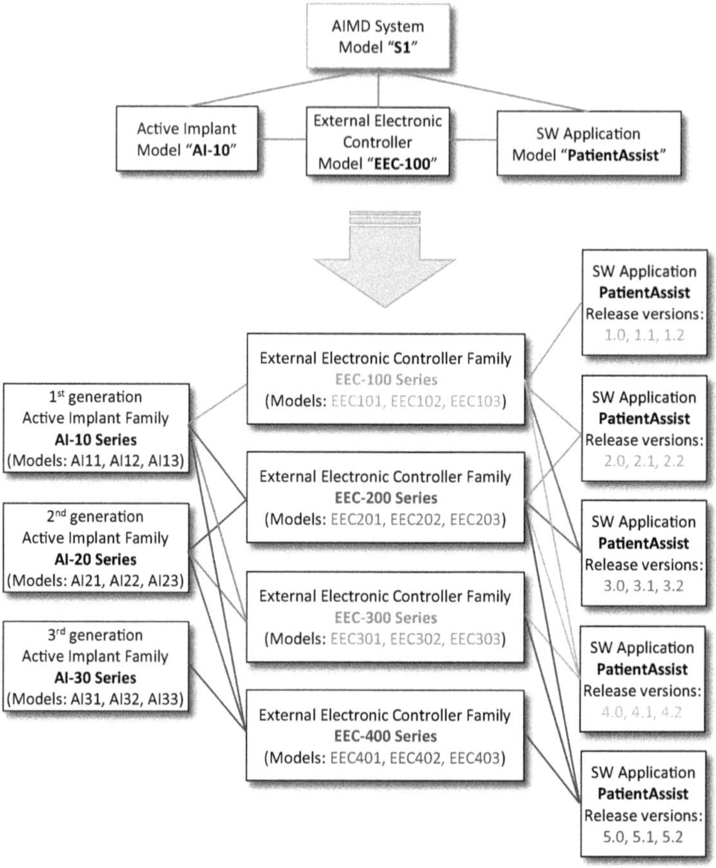

Figure 4.9 Example of evolution from one system to product families (subsequent generations of main system components) that are combined into flexible systems; connecting lines represent interface compatibility/interoperability.

families, especially when the life cycles of the main components vary greatly, for instance, a few years for an active implantable to a few months for a software application.

Where available, definitions from regulations and regulatory guidelines for the terms "kind of product", "product type", "product family", "product category or range", "group of products", "systems" and "procedure packs or kits" are reproduced in the next sub-sections and should be considered when grouping own products and formulating the regulatory strategy.

4.5.3.1 European terminology

Although there is no specific definition for *device family* in the EU regulations, Article 1 of the MDD defines *device subcategory* as "a set of devices having common areas of intended use or common technology", which is similar in intent with other definitions for *device family*. Grouping products that share the same intended use, technology and performance characteristics into device families is a widely accepted practice with EU Notified Bodies.

The NB-MED guidance 2.1/Rec2, *Explanation of Terms*, provides definitions for individual product or device, product category and product range [39]; they are reproduced hereafter.

A *product* or *device* (medical device and/or medical device accessory) is an article or articles manufactured to a defined specification and labelled for a specific intended use. In MDD the term "product" is also used to indicate individual items instead of "type" (as this term is used in MDD).

A *product category* (medical device group) designates products or product and any accessories needed for their proper use that have common attributes of technology and application. This term must be regarded as being the best equivalence to the terms "medical device group" used in ENV 12611:1997, *Medical informatics – Categorial structure of systems of concepts – Medical devices*, and "generic device group" used in EN ISO 15225:2010, *Medical devices – Quality management – Medical device nomenclature data structure*, and defined as a "set of devices having the same or similar intended use, common technology, or both".

Product range refers to different products or product categories marketed by the same manufacturer under the directives. This term is not equivalent with the term "device category" used in EN ISO 15225 and defined as the "broadest grouping within the nomenclature". The term "product range" is not used in EN ISO 15225.

Kits, systems and *procedure packs* are covered in Article 12 of the MDD. Although no specific definition is provided, the terms "kit", "system" and "procedure pack" are synonymous and are understood to be a combination of products including at least one medical device packaged together and placed on the market for use in medical treatment or surgical procedures.

4.5.3.2 US terminology

A *device family* is a group of one or more devices that:

- Are manufactured by or for the same manufacturer;
- Have the same basic design and performance characteristics related to device safety and effectiveness;
- Have the same intended use and function; and
- Have the same device classification and product code [40].

Devices that differ only in minor ways not related to safety or effectiveness can be considered in the same device family. Factors such as brand name and common name of the device and whether the devices were introduced into commercial distribution under the same 510(k) or pre-market approval (PMA) application may be considered in grouping products into device families.

Convenience kits are defined as being comprised of legally marketed devices that are simply being assembled in kit form strictly for the convenience of the user. According to the FDA's terminology, the terms "kit", "set" and "tray" are considered synonymous.

4.5.3.3 Australian terminology

A medical device is considered to be of the *same kind* as another medical device if they both:

- Have the same sponsor;
- Have the same manufacturer;
- Have the same device nomenclature system code (GMDN code);
- Have the same medical device classification; and
- Are the same in relation to such other characteristics as the regulations prescribe, either generally or in relation to medical devices of the kind in question.

In the case of Class I, Class I sterile, Class I measuring, Class IIa and Class IIb medical devices, one medical device is considered to be of the *same kind* as another medical device if both devices:

- Have the same manufacturer;
- Have the same sponsor;
- Are the same classification; and
- Have the same GMDN code.

For Class III and Class AIMD medical devices a further requirement is added to the definition of the *same kind* of medical device – they must have the same Unique Product Identifier (UPI) (41 p. 169). In other words, Class III and Class AIMD devices are considered to be of the same kind if they are identical.

Systems are comprised of components, including at least a medical device, that are intended by the manufacturer to be used in combination as a unit. One or more components of a system may be supplied in a number of sizes in order to accommodate differences in patient anatomy (41 p. 241). Examples include:

- Orthopaedic drill system, incorporating a drill, drill bits, burs, cables, a foot pedal;
- Knee joint- replacement system, incorporating a femoral component, an articulating surface, a stemmed tibial plate, wedges, pins, screws; and
- Patient monitoring system, incorporating a monitor, ECG leads, a blood pressure cuff with a cable, an infusion pump with a tubing set.

Procedure packs are comprised of components that are packaged together, including at least one medical device, and intended by the manufacturer to be used in a medical, surgical or diagnostic procedure (41 p. 241). Examples include:

- Appendectomy surgical procedure pack, incorporating clamps, drapes, sutures, needles, forceps, scalpels, gauze, swabs, kidney dishes; and
- First-aid kit, incorporating bandages, antiseptic ointment, tweezers, pain relief tablets, adhesive strips, cotton buds, swabs.

Composite packs contain only medicines and their containers and are used for a single treatment or for a single course of treatment. They are classified as medicines or "Other Therapeutic Goods". Composite packs cannot contain any medical devices as, by definition, a collection of goods that includes at least one medical device is defined as a system or procedure pack (41 pp. 242–243).

Therapeutic kits comprise a collection of medicines, other therapeutic goods and non-therapeutic goods (e.g., a multi-vitamin pack supplied with fish oil capsules and iron tablets). Therapeutic kits are regulated as medicines or as "Other Therapeutic Goods". If the combination of products contains at least a medical device, it is regulated as a system or procedure pack under the medical device regulations. The term "kit" has a specific meaning in the Australian legislation. Although some products use the word "kit" in their name, they may not meet the definition of kit according to the Therapeutic Goods Act. For example, first-aid kits meet the definition of procedure pack under the legislation but do not meet the definition of therapeutic kit (41 p. 243).

4.5.3.4 Canadian terminology

A *single medical device* is identified with a unique name by its manufacturer and is sold as a distinct package entity.

A *medical device family* means a group of medical devices that are made by the same manufacturer, that differ only in shape, colour, flavour or size, that have the same design and manufacturing process and that have the same intended use.

A *medical device group* means a medical device comprising a collection of medical devices, such as a procedure pack or tray that is sold under a single name.

A *medical device group family* means a collection of medical device groups that are made by the same manufacturer, that have the same generic name specifying their intended use and that differ only in the number and combination of products that comprise each group.

A *system* means a medical device comprising a number of components or parts intended to be used together to fulfil some or all of the device's intended functions and that is sold under a single name.

A *test kit* means an in vitro diagnostics (IVD) device that consists of reagents or articles, or any combination of these, and that is intended to be used to conduct a specific test [42].

4.5.3.5 Singapore terminology

A *single medical device* is a medical device from a product owner identified by a medical device proprietary name with a specific intended purpose. It is sold as a distinct packaged entity and does not meet the criteria for a family, IVD test kit, system, IVD cluster or group [43].

A *medical device family* is a collection of medical devices and each medical device *family* member:

- Is from the same product owner;
- Is of the same risk classification class;
- Has the same medical device proprietary name;
- Has a common intended purpose;
- Has the same design and manufacturing process; and
- Has variations that are within the scope of the permissible variants.

A characteristic of a medical device may be considered a permissible variant if:

- The physical design and construction of the medical device(s) are the same or very similar;
- The manufacturing processes, including the sterilization method, for the medical devices are same or very similar;
- The intended purpose of the medical devices is the same; and
- The risk profile of the medical devices, taking into account the above factors, is the same.

An *IVD test kit* is an IVD device that consists of reagents or articles that are:

- From the same product owner;

- Intended to be used in combination to complete a specific intended purpose;
- Sold under a single test kit name or the labelling, IFUs, brochures or catalogues for each reagents or article states that the component is intended for use with the IVD test kit; and
- Compatible when used as a test kit.

A *medical device system* comprises a number of constituent-components that are:

- From the same product owner;
- Intended to be used in combination to complete a common intended purpose;
- Compatible when used as a system; and
- Sold under a single system name or the labelling, IFUs, brochures or catalogues for each component states that the constituent component is intended for use with the system.

If several *systems* fulfil the following conditions to be grouped as a *family*, they may be registered as a *family*:

- The systems are from the same product owner;
- The systems are of the same risk classification class;
- The systems have a common intended purpose;
- The systems have the same design and manufacturing process; and
- Key constituent-components of the system have variations that are within the scope of the permissible variants.

An *IVD cluster* comprises a number of IVD reagents or articles that are:

- From the same product owner;
- Within risk classification A or B;
- Of a common methodology (e.g., clinical chemistry, immuno-chemistry, haematology/histology/cytology, microbiology culture, molecular biology); and

- Of the same IVD cluster category (e.g., enzymes, electrolytes reagents, allergy, cancer markers, haemoglobin testing, immunological culture identification, oncogenes).

A *medical device group* is a collection of two or more medical devices, supplied in a single package by a product owner (e.g., first-aid kits, dressing trays, promotional packs). The medical device group has the following:

- A single proprietary *group* name; and
- A common intended purpose.

4.5.4 *Unique Device Identifier*

In an increasingly interconnected world, information about medical devices travels from manufacturers to health authorities, from sponsors to distributors and healthcare providers worldwide and between regulatory agencies from different countries.

Without a consistent, harmonized method of identifying medical devices, it is very difficult to know what device is actually being discussed or talked about. When regulatory agencies receive adverse event reports they must be able to quickly determine what specific device is being reported on and what patients have which devices. Regulators also need to be able to aggregate post-market surveillance data to identify trends and react in a timely fashion.

In 2013 the FDA released a final rule establishing a unique device identification system designed to adequately identify medical devices throughout their distribution chain and use. The final rule requires device labelers to include a Unique Device Identifier (UDI) on device labels and packages, unless exceptions or alternatives are allowed [44].

The FDA rule defines a UDI as a unique numeric or alphanumeric code that consists of two parts:

- A Device Identifier (DI), a mandatory, fixed portion of a UDI that identifies the labeler and the specific version or model of a device; and

- A Production Identifier (PI), a conditional, variable portion of a UDI that identifies one or more of the following when included on the label of a device:
  - The lot or batch number within which a device was manufactured;
  - The serial number of a specific device;
  - The expiration date of a specific device;
  - The date a specific device was manufactured; and
  - The distinct identification code required by regulation 21 CFR Part 1271.290(c) for a human cell, tissue, or cellular and tissue-based product (HCT/P) regulated as a device.

All DIs must be issued under a system operated by an FDA-accredited issuing agency. At the time of going to print there were three FDA-accredited organizations authorized to assign UDIs: GS1, Health Industry Business Communications Council (HIBCC) and the International Council for Commonality in Blood Banking Automation (ICCBBA) [45].

Each UDI must be provided in a plain-text version allowing human-readable interpretation (HRI) and in a form that uses automatic identification and data capture (AIDC) technology such as 1D/linear bar code, 2D/matrix bar code, smart cards and radio frequency identification (RFID). The UDI will also be required to be directly marked on a device that is intended for more than one use and intended to be reprocessed before each use.

Dates on device labels and packages are to be presented in a standard format that is consistent with international standards and international practice – for example, "January 2, 2014" must be presented as "2014-01-02" [46].

As part of the US UDI system, device labelers are required to submit information to the Global Unique Device Identification Database (GUDID), a publicly searchable database administered by the FDA that will serve as a reference catalogue for every device with an identifier. Details on setting up a GUDID account and submitting device identification information are available on the FDA's website [47].

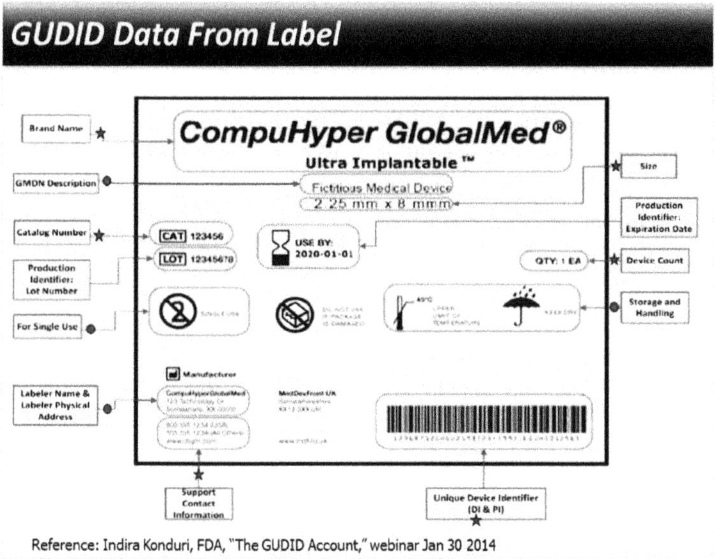

Figure 4.10 Example of a label containing information required for the GUDID; Device Identifier (DI) record = Device Identifier (DI) + GUDID attributes. *Source*: FDA.

The GUDID contains *only* the DI, which serves as the primary key to obtain device information in the database. PIs are not submitted to or stored in the GUDID, but the GUDID will contain PI flags to indicate which PI attribute(s) are on the device label (see example in Fig. 4.10).

The UDI system will be phased in the United States in over several years, as shown in Table 4.10.

Shortly after the FDA's final rule came out, the International Medical Device Regulatory Forum (IMDRF) published a guidance document that provides a framework for those Regulatory Authorities that intend to develop their UDI systems, with the aim of achieving a globally harmonized approach to the UDI. It states that:

> The UDI System is intended to provide a single, globally harmonized system for positive identification of medical devices. Healthcare professionals and patients will no longer have to access multiple, inconsistent, and incomplete sources in an attempt to identify a medical device and, its key attributes [49].

Table 4.10 Compliance dates for UDI requirements in the United States

Compliance date	Requirement
1 year after publication of the final rule (September 24, 2014)	The labels and packages of Class III medical devices and devices licensed under the Public Health Service Act (PHS Act) must bear a UDI. §801.20. Dates on the labels of these devices must be formatted, as required by §801.18. Data for these devices must be submitted to the GUDID. §830.300. A 1-year extension of this compliance date may be requested under §801.55; such a request must be submitted no later than June 23, 2014. Class III stand-alone software must provide its UDI, as required by §801.50(b).
2 years after publication of the final rule (September 24, 2015)	The labels and packages of implantable, life-supporting, and life-sustaining devices must bear a UDI. §801.20. Dates on the labels of these devices must be formatted, as required by §801.18. A device that is a life-supporting or life-sustaining device that is required to be labelled with a UDI must bear a UDI as a permanent marking on the device itself if the device is intended to be used more than once and intended to be reprocessed before each use. §801.45. Stand-alone software that is a life-supporting or life-sustaining device must provide its UDI, as required by §801.50(b). Data for implantable, life-supporting and life-sustaining devices that are required to be labelled with a UDI must be submitted to the GUDID. §830.300.
3 years after publication of the final rule (September 24, 2016)	Class III devices required to be labelled with a UDI must bear a UDI as a permanent marking on the device itself if the device is a device intended to be used more than once and intended to be reprocessed before each use. §801.45. The labels and packages of Class II medical devices must bear a UDI. §801.20. Dates on the labels of these devices must be formatted, as required by §801.18. Class II stand-alone software must provide its UDI as required by §801.50(b). Data for Class II devices that are required to be labelled with a UDI must be submitted to the GUDID. §830.300.

(*Contd.*)

Table 4.10 (*Contd.*)

Compliance date	Requirement
5 years after publication of the final rule (September 24, 2018)	A Class II device that is required to be labelled with a UDI must bear a UDI as a permanent marking on the device itself if the device is a device intended to be used more than once and intended to be reprocessed before each use. §801.45. The labels and packages of Class I medical devices and devices that have not been classified into Class I, Class II or Class III must bear a UDI. §801.20. Dates on the labels of all devices, including devices that have been exempted from UDI labelling requirements, must be formatted, as required by §801.18. Data for Class I devices and devices that have not been classified into Class I, Class II or Class III that are required to be labelled with a UDI must be submitted to the GUDID. §830.300. Class I stand-alone software must provide its UDI, as required by §801.50(b).
7 years after publication of the final rule (September 24, 2020)	A Class I device and a device that has not been classified into Class I, Class II or Class III that is required to be labelled with a UDI must a bear UDI as a permanent marking on the device itself if the device is a device intended to be used more than once and intended to be reprocessed before each use. §801.45.

Source: FDA [48]

The IMDRF UDI guidance lays down the fundamental concepts of a globally harmonized UDI system; they include:

- The UDI and UDI Carrier – the means to convey the UDI by using AIDC (bar codes, smart cards, RFID, etc.) and, if applicable, its HRI – are based on standards.
- A UDI applied to a medical device anywhere in the world should be able to be used globally and to meet the UDI requirements of its Regulatory Authority.
- National or local identification numbers should NOT be a substitute for UDIs.
- Regulatory Authorities should not specify the procedure for modifying these UDI standards.

- The UDI Database (UDID) core elements should not be modified.
- The UDID should use the Health Level Seven International (HL7) Structured Product Label (SPL) and web-based interface for data submission (SPL is a HL7 standard for the exchange of product information using extensible markup language [XML]).
- Every medical device needs to be identified by a UDI, unless it is exempted.

A UDI system, once implemented, will offer a range of benefits to industry, regulatory agencies, consumers, healthcare providers and healthcare systems by:

- Allowing more accurate reporting, reviewing and analyzing of adverse event reports so that problem devices can be identified and corrected more quickly.
- Reducing medical errors by enabling healthcare professionals and others to more rapidly and precisely identify a device and obtain important information concerning the characteristics of the device.
- Enhancing analysis of devices on the market by providing a standard and clear way to document device use in electronic health records, clinical information systems, claim data sources and registries. A more robust post-market surveillance system can also be leveraged to support premarket approval or clearance of new devices and new uses of currently marketed devices.
- Providing a standardized identifier that will allow manufacturers, distributors and healthcare facilities to more effectively manage medical device recalls.
- Providing a foundation for a global, secure distribution chain, helping to address counterfeiting and diversion and prepare for medical emergencies.
- Leading to the development of a medical device identification system that is recognized around the world [50].

4.6 Case Study: Why Is It Always Taking So Long?

Despite putting a lot of effort during the pre-market phase and generating an impressive amount of engineering documents, a medical device company was struggling with lengthy approval timelines and multiple rounds of questions and answers with its EU Notified Body and the FDA in the United States. Delayed time to market was hurting the company's bottom line. To find out the root cause of this ongoing situation senior management decided to engage an external consultancy specializing in regulatory and quality for medical devices.

The consultant performed a thorough audit of the D&D processes. He looked into the records of D&D projects and regulatory submissions from the previous three years, including questions and deficiencies raised by agency reviewers.

After completing the audit, the consultant presented his findings. They included a number of recurring issues leading directly or indirectly to multiple rounds of questions and answers with regulatory agencies, product re-tests and documentation re-work:

- Lack of appropriate rationale or justification for the selection of V&V test items as representative of a whole product family.
- Tested items not sufficiently identified; instead of using build standard identification (part numbers), V&V reports make reference to drops (1, 2, 3), releases (first, second) or builds (A, B, C); no QMS procedure describes how these references were assigned or controlled.
- Use of build standard identifiers (part numbers) instead of catalogue numbers on sales packaging and in regulatory registration documents results in uncontrolled, poorly defined references to build standards in V&V documentation (previous finding) because there is a reluctance to change part numbers – the production department does not want to scrap sales packaging already printed with the part numbers on them, and the regulatory department does not want to have registrations including references to part numbers invalidated.

- Breakdown in the document version tree; assigning a new document number instead of a new version number for the same V&V protocols and reports causes a breakdown in traceability for critical V&V documents.
- Software application release 2.2 mislabeled and shipped as 2.0 in a major market because the company wanted to avoid another regulatory submission for the change from the previously approved 2.0 release to the latest 2.2 release; this was a misbranding of the medical device software and represented a high non-compliance risk; additionally, it raised additional issues for any future submissions where the technical documentation would have to be customized for that market alone.
- Responses to regulatory agency questions are often rushed, resulting in mistakes, they do not respond to the actual questions asked or information contained is contradictory.
- Outcomes of clinical evaluations often do not support the indications for use and intended use of the medical device under evaluation.

4.7 Concluding Summary

Chapter 4 covers some of the basic regulatory controls applicable to D&D in the pre-market phase, also referred to as design controls. Takeaway points:

- Some of the most common D&D methodologies are the waterfall model, the V-model and the Agile model for software.
- Managing high volumes of documentation will be easier if the information is organized into QMS procedures, project documentation and product-specific documentation.
- The D&D planning stage is important to ensure that the main tasks, key deliverables and resources are identified upfront. The example of a market strategy template includes sections for regulatory, clinical and reimbursement strategies.

- D&D process stages are explained – design inputs, design outputs and V&V – and the typical deliverables that would be required for each of the four milestones before transferring the design to manufacturing.
- The use of product identifiers – model designation, catalogue numbers, part numbers and product identifiers (serial numbers and batch or lot numbers) – needs to be well understood and applied consistently. For software, release, version and revision numbers may be used in addition to model designation.
- Various jurisdictions allow for products to be grouped and submitted in one application, which streamlines the review and approval process for similar products or products belonging to a kit or a system.
- The UDI is a unique number pertaining to a medical device that enables the identification of different types of devices and the access to useful and relevant information stored in a UDI database. Due to the UDI's specificity, it can make traceability of devices more efficient, allow easier recall of devices, fight against counterfeiting and improve patient safety.

References

1. Food and Drug Administration. 21 CFR Parts 808, 812 and 820 cGMP Final Rule – Federal Register Vol. 61, No. 195. *www.gpo.gov.* [Online] October 7, 1996. [Cited: May 10, 2014.] http://www.gpo.gov/fdsys/pkg/FR-1996-10-07/html/96-25720.htm.
2. Food and Drug Administration. Medical Device Recall Report FY2003 to FY2012. *www.fda.gov.* [Online] [Cited: May 10, 2014.] http://www.fda.gov/downloads/AboutFDA/CentersOffices/OfficeofMedicalProductsandTobacco/CDRH/CDRHTransparency/UCM388442.pdf.
3. Food and Drug Administration. Design Control Guidance for Medical Device Manufacturers. *www.fda.gov.* [Online] March 11, 1997. [Cited: May 10, 2014.] http://www.fda.gov/medicaldevices/deviceregulationandguidance/guidancedocuments/ucm070627.htm#_Toc382720784.

4. IEC. IEC 62304:2006 Medical device software – Software life cycle processes. s.l. : IEC. 2006-05. 62304.
5. Food and Drug Administration. General Principles of Software Validation; Final Guidance for Industry and FDA Staff. *www.fda.com.* [Online] January 11, 2002. [Cited: May 10, 2014.] http://www.fda.gov/medicaldevices/deviceregulationandguidance/guidancedocuments/ucm085281.htm.
6. AAMI. AAMI TIR45 – Guidance on the use of AGILE practices in the development of medical device software. *www.ibm.com.* [Online] August 20, 2012. [Cited: May 10, 2014.] http://www.ibm.com/developer works/rational/library/compliant-agile-medical-device/index.html?ca=dat.
7. Food and Drug Administration. PMA Application Content. *www.fda.gov.* [Online] [Cited: May 10, 2014.] http://www.fda.gov/MedicalDevices/DeviceRegulationandGuidance/HowtoMarketYourDevice/Premarket Submissions/PremarketApprovalPMA/ucm050289.htm.
8. Health Canada. Guidance Document: Preparation of Summary Technical Documentation (STED)-based Class III and Class IV Premarket Medical Device Licence Applications, not including In Vitro Diagnostic Devices (IVDDs). *www.hc-sc.gc.ca.* [Online] November 2, 2011. [Cited: May 10, 2014.] http://www.hc-sc.gc.ca/dhp-mps/md-im/applic-demande/guide-ld/md_gd_im_ld_sted-eng.php#a347.
9. Pharmaceuticals and Medical Devices Agency. Yakushokuhatsu No. 0216003 Applications for Marketing Approval for Medical Devices. *www.pmda.go.jp.* [Online] February 16, 2005. [Cited: August 10, 2014.] http://www.pmda.go.jp/english/service/pdf/notifications/PFSB-0216002.pdf.
10. Pharmaceuticals and Medical Devices Agency. Yakushokuki No. 0216003 – Handbook for Preparation of Summary Technical Documentation Submitted in Applications for Marketing Approval for Medical Devices. *www.pmda.go.jp.* [Online] February 16, 2005. [Cited: August 10, 2014.] http://www.pmda.go.jp/english/service/pdf/notifications/PFSB-ELD-OMDE-0216003.pdf.
11. ASEAN. Common Submission Dossier Template. *www.asean.org.* [Online] October 21, 2010. [Cited: May 10, 2014.] http://www.asean.org/archive/SnC/ASEAN%20MDPWG%20CSDT_ Final_ 21%20Oct%202010.pdf.
12. Global Harmonization Taskforce. Summary Technical Documentation (STED) for Demonstrating Conformity to the Essential Princi-

ples of Safety and Performance of Medical devices. *www.imdrf.org.* [Online] February 21, 2008. [Cited: May 10, 2014.] http://www.imdrf.org/docs/ghtf/final/sg1/technical-docs/ghtf-sg1-n063-2011-summary-technical-documentation-ivd-safety-conformity-110317.pdf.

13. Independent Hospital Pricing Authority (IHPA). Australian refined diagnosis-related groups (AR-DRG) data cubes. *www.ihpa.gov.au.* [Online] October 11, 2013. [Cited: October 3, 2014.] http://www.ihpa.gov.au/internet/ihpa/publishing.nsf/Content/Classifications.
14. Australian Department of Health. Prostheses List. *www.health. gov.au.* [Online] August 15, 2014. [Cited: October 3, 2014.] http://www.health.gov.au/internet/main/publishing.nsf/content/prostheses-list-pdf.htm.
15. International Society for Pharmaeconomics and Outcomes Research (ISPOR). ISPOR Global Health Care Systems Road Map; Canada – Medical devices and diagnostics. *www.ispor.org.* [Online] February 2014. [Cited: October 3, 2014.] http://www.ispor.org/HTA RoadMaps/CanadaMDD.asp#4.
16. International Society for Pharmacoeconomics and Outcomes research (ISPOR). ISPOR GLobal Health Care Systems Road Map; China Mainland – Medical devices. *www.ISPOR.org.* [Online] January 2011. [Cited: October 3, 2014.] http://www.ispor.org/HTARoadMaps/ChinaMD.asp.
17. International Society for Pharmaeconomics and Outcomes Research (ISPOR). ISPOR Global Health Care Systems Road Map; France – Medical devices. *www.ispor.org.* [Online] October 2011. [Cited: October 3, 2014.] http://www.ispor.org/HTARoadMaps/FranceMD.asp#4.
18. l'Assurance Maladie. Liste des produits et prestations (LPP). *www.ameli.fr.* [Online] October 10, 2014. [Cited: October 26, 2014.] http://www.ameli.fr/professionnels-de-sante/directeurs-d-etablissements-de-sante/codage/liste-des-produits-et-prestations-lpp/liste-des-produits-et-prestations-lpp/consultation-et-telechargement-de-la-lpp.php.
19. Federal Joint Committee (Gemeinsamer Bundesausschuss). The Federal Joint Committee. *www.english.g-ba.de.* [Online] [Cited: October 3, 2014.] http://www.english.g-ba.de/structure/.
20. International Society for Pharmacoeconomics and Outcomes Research (ISPOR). ISPOR Global Health Care Systems Road Map; Germany – Medical devices. *www.ispor.org.* [Online] April 2011. [Cited: October 3, 2014.] http://www.ispor.org/HTARoadMaps/GermanyMD.asp#4.

21. GKV-Spitzenverband. Hilfsmittelverzeichniss. *www.gkv-spitzenverband.de.* [Online] March 14, 2013. [Cited: October 3, 2014.] http://www.gkv-spitzenverband.de/krankenversicherung/hilfsmittel/hilfsmittelverzeichnis/hilfsmittelverzeichnis.jsp.
22. International Society for Pharmacoeconomics and Outcomes Research (ISPOR). ISPOR Global Health Care Systems Road Map; Italy – Medical devices & Diagnostics. *www.ispor.org.* [Online] February 2012. [Cited: October 3, 2014.] http://www.ispor.org/HTARoadMaps/Italy/Italy_MDD.asp#4.
23. Junikon, K.K. Japan Medical Technology Market Overview. *www.junicon.net.* [Online] 2010. [Cited: May 10, 2014.] http://www.junicon.net/JapanMedicalTechnologyOverview.pdf.
24. International Society for Pharmacoeconomics and Outcomes Research (ISPOR). ISPOR Global Health Care Systems Road Map; Suoth Korea – Medical devices & Diagnostics. *www.ispor.org.* [Online] September 2014. [Cited: October 3, 2014.] http://www.ispor.org/HTARoadMaps/S-KoreaMD.asp#4.
25. International Society for Pharmacoeconomics and Outcomes research (ISPOR). ISPOR Global Health Care Systems Road Map. *www.ispor.org.* [Online] November 2009. [Cited: October 3, 2014.] http://www.ispor.org/HTARoadMaps/Spain.asp#4.
26. International Society for Pharmacoeconomics and Outcomes Research (ISPOR). ISPOR Global Health Care Systems Road Map; USA – In-Vitro Diagnostics. *www.ispor.org.* [Online] May 2010. [Cited: October 3, 2014.] http://www.ispor.org/HTARoadMaps/USMD.asp.
27. Centers for Medicare & Medicaid Services (CMS). ICD-10 MS-DRG Conversion Project. *www.cms.gov.* [Online] August 25, 2014. [Cited: October 3, 2014.] http://www.cms.gov/Medicare/Coding/ICD10/ICD-10-MS-DRG-Conversion-Project.html.
28. Centers for Medicare & Medicaid Services (CMS). Indexes – Lists of National and Local Coverage. *www.cms.gov.* [Online] [Cited: October 3, 2014.] http://www.cms.gov/medicare-coverage-database/indexes/national-and-local-indexes.aspx.
29. International Society for Pharmacoeconomics and Outcomes Research (ISPOR). ISPOR Global Health Care Systems Road Map; United Kingdom – Diagnostics. *www.ispor.org.* [Online] May 2010. [Cited: October 3, 2014.] http://www.ispor.org/HTARoadMaps/UKDiagnostics.asp#4.
30. Food and Drug Administration. 21 CFR Part 820.3 Definitions. *www.accessdata.fda.gov.* [Online] [Cited: May 10, 2014.] http://www.accessdata.fda.gov/scripts/cdrh/cfdocs/cfcfr/CFRSearch.cfm?fr=820.3.

31. Food and Drug Administration. 21 CFR Part 820 Quality System Regulation, subpart C – Design Controls. *www.accessdata.fda.gov.* [Online] [Cited: May 10, 2014.] http://www.accessdata.fda.gov/scripts/cdrh/cfdocs/cfcfr/CFRSearch.cfm?CFRPart=820&showFR=1&subpartNode=21:8.0.1.1.12.3.
32. Hu, C., Shorrock, S., Hu, Y., Goldbenberg. S.J. *Strategies for Registering and Testing Medical Devices under China's New Rules.* April 2014, s.l. : Informa UK, 2014.
33. Faris, O., Food and Drug Administration. Clinical trials for medical devices: FDA and the IDE process. *www.fda.gov.* [Online] November 12, 2013. [Cited: October 3, 2014.] http://www.fda.gov/downloads/Training/ClinicalInvestigatorTrainingCourse/UCM378265.pdf.
34. IECEE. IECEE Test Report Forms (TRFs). *www.iecee.org.* [Online] 2013. [Cited: May 31, 2014.] http://www.iecee.org/cbscheme/html/cbtrep.htm.
35. Centers for Medicare & Medicaid Cervices (CMS). Decision Memo for Implantable Cardioverter Defibrillators (ICDs) (CAG-00157N), Chapter VI General Methodological Principles, Section 1. Assessing Individual Studies. *www.cms.gov.* [Online] June 6, 2003. [Cited: May 10, 2014.] http://www.cms.gov/medicare-coverage-database/details/nca-decision-memo.aspx?NCAId=39&fromdb=true.
36. WHO. Health technology assessment. *www.who.int.* [Online] 2014. [Cited: November 18, 2014.] http://www.who.int/medical_devices/assessment/en/.
37. About Health Technology Assessment. *www.health.gov.au.* [Online] September 16, 2010. [Cited: October 3, 2014.] http://www.health.gov.au/internet/hta/publishing.nsf/Content/about-1.
38. Drummond, M.F., Sculpher, M.J., Torrance, G.W., O'Brien, B.J., Stoddard. G.L. *Methods for the Economic Evaluation of Health Care Programmes.* Oxford University Press, Oxford, 2005. ISBN-13:978-0198529453.
39. NB-MED. NB-MED 2.1/Rec2 Explanation of Terms. *www.team-nb.org.* [Online] February 9, 1998. [Cited: October 3, 2014.] http://www.team-nb.org/documents/2010/Recommendation-NB-MED-2_ 1-2_ rev5_ Explanation_ of_ Terms.pdf.
40. Food and Drug Administration. Medical Device Reporting for Manufacturers. *www.fda.gov.* [Online] March 1997. [Cited: October 3, 2014.] http://www.fda.gov/MedicalDevices/DeviceRegulationandGuidance/GuidanceDocuments/ucm094529.htm.
41. Therapeutic Goods Administration. Australian Regulatory Guidelines for Medical Devices (ARGMD). *www.tga.gov.au.* [Online] May 2011.

[Cited: May 31, 2014.] http://www.tga.gov.au/pdf/devices-argmd-p2.pdf.

42. Health Canada. Medical devices Regulations SOR/98-282. *laws-lois.justice.gc.ca.* [Online] December 16, 2011. [Cited: October 3, 2014.] http://laws-lois.justice.gc.ca/PDF/SOR-98-282.pdf.
43. Singapore HSA. GN-12: Guidance on Grouping of Medical Devices for Product Registration. *www.hsa.gov.sg.* [Online] January 2011. [Cited: October 3, 2014.] http://www.hsa.gov.sg/content/dam/HSA/HPRG/Medical_Devices/Overview_Framework_Policies/Guidances_for_Medical_Device_ Registration/GN-12-R1_Guidance%20on%20 Grouping%20of%20Medical%20Devices%20for%20Product%20Registration.pdf.
44. Food and Drug Administration. Unique identification System. *www.federalregister.gov.* [Online] September 24, 2013. [Cited: October 3, 2014.] https://www.federalregister.gov/articles/2013/09/24/2013-23059/unique-device-identification-system.
45. Food and Drug Administration. UDI Issuing Agencies. *www.fda.gov.* [Online] September 30, 2014. [Cited: October 3, 2014.] http://www.fda.gov/MedicalDevices/DeviceRegulationandGuidance/UniqueDeviceIdentification/UDIIssuingAgencies/default.htm.
46. US Government Printing Office. e-CFR Title 21: Food and Drugs, Part 801 Labeling, Subpart A – General Labeling Provisions; §801.18 Format of Dates Provided on a Medical Device Label. *www.ecfr.gov.* [Online] September 24, 2013. [Cited: October 3, 2014.] http://www.ecfr.gov/cgi-bin/text-idx?SID=b3889284e807a2e8e7c446b6e9e7dea7&node=21:8.0.1.1.2.1.1.8&rgn=div8.
47. Food and Drug Administration. Global UDI Database (GUDID). *www.fda.gov.* [Online] September 30, 2014. [Cited: October 3, 2014.] http://www.fda.gov/MedicalDevices/DeviceRegulationandGuidance/UniqueDeviceIdentification/GlobalUDIDatabaseGUDID/ucm20038750.htm.
48. Food and Drug Administration. Compliance Dates for UDI Requirements. *www.fda.gov.* [Online] September 30, 2014. [Cited: October 3, 2014.] http://www.fda.gov/MedicalDevices/DeviceRegulationandGuidance/UniqueDeviceIdentification/CompliancedatesforUDIRequirements/default.htm.
49. IMDRF. IMDRF WG/N7Final:2013 Unique Device Identification (UDI) of Medical devices. *www.imdrf.org.* [Online] December 9, 2013. [Cited: October 3, 2014.] http://www.imdrf.org/docs/imdrf/final/technical/imdrf-tech-131209-udi-guidance-140901.pdf.

50. Food and Drug Administration. Benefits of a UDI System. *www.fda.gov.* [Online] September 30, 2014. [Cited: October 3, 2014.] http://www.fda.gov/MedicalDevices/DeviceRegulationandGuidance/UniqueDeviceIdentification/BenefitsofaUDIsystem/default.htm.

Chapter 5

Regulatory Submissions, Approvals and Registrations

This chapter explains basic terminology related to regulatory submissions, such as entities responsible for placing medical devices on the market, administrative provisions for establishment registration and product listing and applications for marketing authorizations. Processes of submitting applications for regulatory approvals, as well as procedures for making available unapproved devices, are explained for each of the established jurisdictions. The chapter concludes with recent developments in key emerging markets.

5.1 Administrative Provisions

5.1.1 *Manufacturer, Sponsor, Authorised Representative, Agent*

Regulators need to be able to identify the entity legally responsible for the manufacturing and distribution of medical devices, also known as the (legal) manufacturer or sponsor. This can be the actual manufacturer of the product or a different natural or legal entity.

Medical Device Regulatory Practices: An International Perspective
Val Theisz

ISBN 978-981-4669-10-8 (Hardcover), 978-981-4669-11-5 (eBook)
www.panstanford.com

European Union (EU) medical devices directives define a *manufacturer* as being "the natural or legal person with responsibility for the design, manufacture, packaging and labelling of a device before it is placed on the market under his own name, regardless of whether these operations are carried out by that person himself or on his behalf by a third party". The *manufacturer obligations* also apply to "the natural or legal person who assembles, packages, processes, fully refurbishes and/or labels one or more ready-made products and/or assigns to them their intended purpose as a device with a view to their being placed on the market under his own name". This definition does not apply to persons who "assemble or adapt devices already on the market to their intended purpose for an individual patient". Foreign manufacturers without a registered place of business within the EU must appoint an EU Authorised Representative. Legal manufacturers located within the EU and EU Authorised Representatives appointed by manufacturers outside the EU are legally liable for medical devices and in vitro diagnostics (IVDs) they place on the EU market.

The Food and Drug Administration (FDA) regulations define a *manufacturer* as "any legal person or entity engaged in the manufacture of a product subject to license under the act; 'Manufacturer' also includes any legal person or entity who is an applicant for a license where the applicant assumes responsibility for compliance with the applicable product and establishment standards". Foreign manufacturers without a US subsidiary must designate a US Agent. Manufacturers are legally liable for devices marketed in the United States; however, US Agents designated by foreign manufacturers are not.

Although wording for the *manufacturer* definition varies slightly in other jurisdictions, the meaning is the same. In Australia, a sponsor is the equivalent of a legal manufacturer, responsible for the importation of medical devices into Australia, the supply of medical devices in Australia and the export of medical devices from Australia, as well as making application to the Therapeutic Goods Administration (TGA) to have the device included in the Australian Register of Therapeutic Goods, or ARTG. A manufacturer may also be the Australian Sponsor if it has a registered place of business in Australia. Foreign manufacturers without a local subsidiary need to appoint a local sponsor. Australian manufacturers and Australian Sponsors of foreign manufacturers are legally liable for devices marketed in Australia.

Canadian regulations require that a person importing or selling a medical device hold an establishment licence. Exempt from this requirement are retailers, healthcare facilities and, in the case of Class II, III or IV medical devices, manufacturers of such devices. Manufacturers of Class I devices are exempt only if they distribute their products through a person who holds an establishment licence [1].

In Japan, a Marketing Authorization Holder (MAH) is the equivalent of a legal manufacturer, responsible for the development, manufacture and distribution of drugs, quasi-drugs, cosmetics and medical devices. Only entities with a registered place of business in Japan holding an MAH licence are permitted to place the above-mentioned products on the Japanese market. The MAH has legal liability for devices placed on the Japanese market.

Under the previous J-PAL regulations foreign manufacturers were required to obtain a Foreign Manufacturer Accreditation (FMA), but under the new Pharmaceutical and Medical Device (PMD) Act this is no longer required. Foreign manufacturers that do not have a local subsidiary have to either appoint their Japanese distributor as the MAH for their products or designate an independent local agent – a so-called Designated Marketing Authorization Holder (DMAH) – to deal with the Pharmaceuticals and Medical Devices Agency (PMDA) and apply for an MAH on their behalf. Allowing a local distributor to be the MAH poses business risks, for instance, if the foreign manufacturer wants to change to a different distributor or give the distributor access to confidential product information. Using an independent DMAH enables foreign manufacturers to retain ownership of the MAH licence for their products [2].

Local agents or representatives must be notified to the relevant authorities. The contract between the legal manufacturer and the local agent needs to define clearly the obligations of each party to ensure compliance with regulatory requirements. The key responsibilities of local agents in established markets are summarized in the next paragraphs.

5.1.1.1 EU Authorised Representative

An EU Authorised Representative must:

- Have a registered place of business within the European Economic Area (EEA), in Switzerland or in Turkey. The EEA encompasses all EU countries, plus Iceland, Lichtenstein and Norway.
- Be the single Authorised Representative within the EU for at least all devices of the same type.
- Register with the Competent Authority of the member state in which he or she is located; provide the manufacturer's registered place of business and a description of the devices being placed on the market, if designated for devices covered by the obligation to notify the Competent Authorities (MDD Class I, procedure packs and custom-made devices and Active Implantable Medical Device Directive [AIMDD] custom-made devices).
- Unless this obligation is undertaken by the manufacturer, notify of the intention to carry out a clinical investigation to the Competent Authorities of the member states in which the investigations are to be conducted and when the investigation ends.
- Provide to the Competent Authority of the member state in which he or she is located information on the manufacturer's registered place of business and a declaration required for IVD devices for performance evaluation.
- Unless this obligation is undertaken by the manufacturer, initiate the procedures for conformity assessment according to MDD Annexes II, IV, VII and VIII; AIMDD Annexes 3, 4 and 6; or IVDD Annexes II, V, VI and VIII.
- Provide upon request Declarations of Conformity (DoCs), technical documentation and any other information that a market surveillance authority may require for the purpose of market surveillance; the manufacturer is obliged to keep this information up to date at all times.
- Keep the manufacturer informed of matters relating to the devices placed on the EU market, especially decisions to withdraw devices from the market and the reporting of

serious adverse events (SAEs) during clinical investigations [3].

5.1.1.2 US Agent

A US Agent must:

- Have a registered place of business in the United States;
- Be the single US Agent designated by a foreign manufacturer;
- Register with the FDA using the FDA Unified Registration and Listing Systems (FURLS);
- Assist the FDA in communicating with the foreign manufacturer;
- Respond to questions concerning the foreign manufacturer's devices that are imported or offered for import into the United States;
- Assist the FDA in scheduling inspections of the foreign establishment; and
- If the FDA is unable to contact the foreign establishment directly or expeditiously, be the contact person for and receive information or documents from the FDA [4].

5.1.1.3 Australian Sponsor

An Australian Sponsor must:

- Be a resident of Australia or be an incorporated body in Australia and be conducting business in Australia where the representative of the company is residing in Australia;
- Have procedures in place, including a written agreement with the manufacturer, to obtain information from the manufacturer when requested by the TGA;
- Ensure that:
  - He or she has available sufficient information to substantiate compliance with the Essential Principles (EPs) or have procedures in place to ensure that such information can be provided from the manufacturer to the TGA within 20 working days;

  - An appropriate conformity assessment procedure has been applied to the medical devices;
  - The manufacturer has appropriate conformity assessment evidence for the medical device; and
  - The conformity assessment evidence remains valid while the device is supplied in Australia.

- For devices other than Class I not supplied sterile or with a measuring function, submit the conformity assessment evidence to the TGA;
- Apply to include the medical devices in the ARTG, including certifying that the information provided is complete and correct;
- Pay the fee for applying to include the medical device in the ARTG and, where applicable, pay the fee for an application audit to be conducted;
- Upon request:
  - Provide documentation relating to the medical device to the TGA;
  - Deliver samples of the medical device to the TGA; and
  - Allow a person authorized by the TGA to enter and inspect any premises, including outside Australia, where the devices are manufactured or located.
- Notify the TGA of certain incidents and performance issues;
- Ensure the information about the device complies with the regulatory requirements; and
- Pay the annual charges for ongoing inclusion of the medical device in the ARTG [5].

5.1.1.4 Canadian importer or distributor

A Canadian importer or distributor must:

- Maintain distribution records for devices placed on Canadian market;
- Maintain records related to complaint handling;
- Report incidents related to the device safety and performance according to medical device vigilance requirements; and

- Notify the authorities of any recalls involving medical devices marketed in Canada [6].

5.1.1.5 Japanese Designated Marketing Authorization Holder

A Japanese DMAH must:

- Have a registered place of business in Japan;
- Meet the personnel and organizational requirements for an MAH, including the appointment of following controller roles as full-time employees:
  - General Manager overseeing operations, with overall responsibility for the safety and quality of marketed products;
  - Quality Manager responsible for ensuring the quality system in compliance with the Ministerial Ordinance for Good Quality Practices (GQPs); and
  - Safety Manager responsible for the post-market surveillance activities according to the Ministerial Ordinance on Good Vigilance Practices (GVPs).
- Obtain the appropriate type of MAH licence for the products intended to be marketed – a medical device or an IVD DMAH licence; and
- Implement a quality management system (QMS) compliant with MHLW Ordinance No. 169 and GVPs [7, 8, 9].

5.1.2 *Establishment Registration, Device Listing, Notification to Local Authorities*

5.1.2.1 EU: registration of legal manufacturer and Authorised Representative

In the EU, natural or legal persons engaging in the activities listed hereafter must inform the Competent Authority of the member state in which they have their registered place of business of the address of the registered place of business and the generic description of the devices concerned (e.g., using definitions provided in the GMDN database), in accordance with Article 14 of the MDD, Article 10a of the AIMDD or Article 10 of the In Vitro Diagnostics Directive

(IVDD). A list of EU Competent Authorities is available from the official website of the European Commission [10].

Activities requiring registration with local Competent Authorities:

- Manufacture of Class I or custom-made devices with a view to placing them on the market under own name or trading name(s);
- Full refurbishment of Class I devices, or labelling of one or more ready-made devices, with a view to placing them on the market under own name;
- Placing devices bearing the Conformité Européenne (CE) marking on the market, under own name, in a system or a procedure pack within their intended purposes and within the limits of uses specified by their original manufacturers;
- Sterilization, for the purpose of placing on the market under own name, of systems or procedure packs or other CE-marked medical devices designed by the manufacturer to be sterilized before use;
- Acting as the EU Authorised Representative of a manufacturer who does not have a registered place of business in the EU or, if importing and placing on the EU market for a manufacturer, who has no Authorised Representative in the EU, devices within the above-listed categories;
- Manufacture of IVD medical devices and placing them on the market under own name or trading name(s);
- Manufacture of IVDs for performance evaluation and making them available under own name or trading name(s); and
- Acting as the EU Authorised Representative of a manufacturer who does not have a registered place of business in the EEA countries, Switzerland or Turkey [11].

Manufacturers of medical devices, including IVDs, need to register when first applying the CE marking to their products. Manufacturers of custom-made devices, systems or procedure packs and sterilization companies, who do not need to affix a CE marking, should register no later than the first time they claim compliance with the EU directives. More details about the CE marking are provided in Section 5.2.1 in this chapter.

Individual EU member states such as France, Italy, the Netherlands, Portugal and Spain have additional registration or notification requirements. Others such as Germany and Ireland have additional requirements for marketing, sales and distribution personnel. Regulatory professionals should always check with the relevant Competent Authorities about what additional national requirements apply before placing medical devices on their territories [12].

5.1.2.2 United States: establishment registration

Owners or operators of places of business (also called establishments or facilities) that are involved in the production and distribution of medical devices intended for use in the United States are required to register annually with the FDA. This process is known as establishment registration.

The purpose of registering the name and place of business of medical device companies is to provide regulatory agencies with the physical location of establishments involved in the development, production and commercial distribution of medical devices. Authorities must be able, particularly in emergencies, to contact the person responsible for placing the products on the market.

Most establishments that are required to register with the FDA are also required to list the devices that are made there and the activities that are performed on those devices. The FDA identifies 11 types of activities that an establishment may be engaged in, reproduced below [13].

Definitions of establishment activities:

- Contract Manufacturer – Manufactures a finished device to another establishment's specifications.
- Contract Sterilizer – Provides a sterilization service for another establishment's devices.
- Foreign Exporter – Exports or offers for export to the United States a device manufactured, prepared, propagated, compounded or processed in a foreign country, including

devices originally manufactured in the United States. A foreign exporter must have an establishment address outside the United States.

- Initial Importer – Takes first title to devices imported into the United States. An Initial Importer must have a US address.
- Manufacturer – Makes by chemical, physical, biological or other procedures any article that meets the definition of *device* in Section 201(h) of the federal Food, Drug, and Cosmetic (FD&C) Act.
- Repackager – Packages finished devices from bulk or repackages devices made by a manufacturer into different containers (excluding shipping containers).
- Relabeler – Changes the content of the labelling from that supplied from the original manufacturer for distribution under the establishment's own name. A relabeler does not include establishments that do not change the original labelling but merely add their own name.
- Remanufacturer – Processes, conditions, renovates, repackages, restores or does any other act to a finished device that significantly changes the finished device's performance or safety specifications or intended use.
- Reprocessor of Single-Use Device – Performs re-manufacturing operations on a single-use device.
- Specification Developer – Develops specifications for a device that is distributed under the establishment's own name but performs no manufacturing. This includes establishments that, in addition to developing specifications, also arrange for the manufacturing of devices labeled with another establishment's name by a contract manufacturer.
- US Manufacturer of Export-Only Devices – Manufactures medical devices that are not sold in the United States and are manufactured solely for export to foreign countries.

Once a manufacturer has paid the registration fee and submitted the registration and listing information, the FDA will send a notification confirming that the establishment has been registered. The information is then included in the Establishment Registration & Device Listing database (see screenshot in Fig. 5.1).

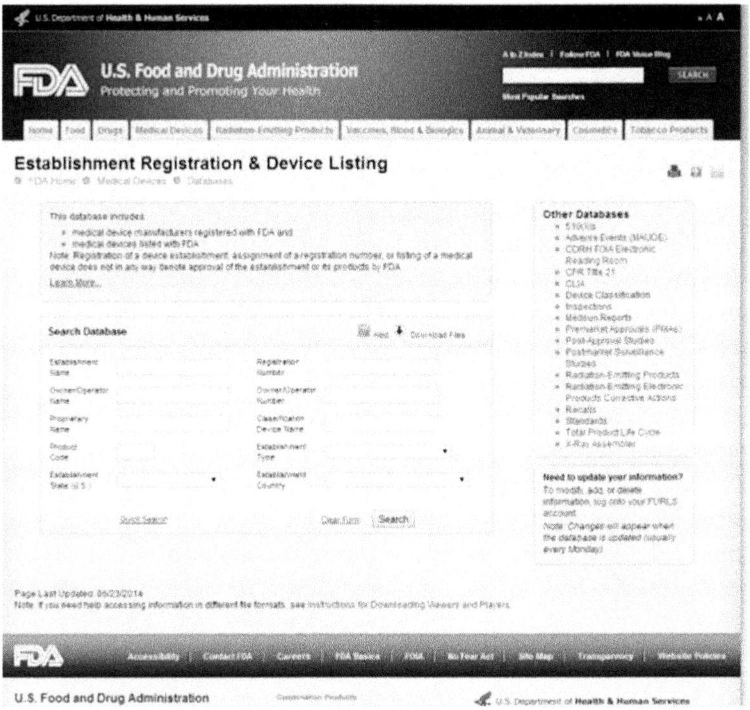

Figure 5.1 The FDA Establishment Registration & Device Listing database available online.

Since 2007, establishment registration and listing information must be submitted electronically, unless a waiver has been granted. Step-by-step instructions on how to create an account with the FDA and how to register a facility using the FDA's Unified Registration and Listing System (FURLS) are available on the FDA's website [14].

Overseas manufacturers should watch out for unscrupulous agents selling "certificates" of establishment registration with wording that imply the company's products or QMSs are approved by the FDA. Some of these "certificates" even have official-looking seals, the US eagle logo and the "FDA" acronym on them, but they have no FDA endorsement. Establishment registration is an administrative obligation that requires no certificate. On its own, the establishment registration does not confer any rights to a manufacturer or importer to claim that the FDA has approved the manufacturer's devices or quality system.

5.1.2.3 Australia: registration of sponsor and manufacturer

In Australia, manufacturers, sponsors or their local agents involved with the supply of therapeutic goods must register their details with the TGA by submitting a client details form [15]. This information is then recorded in the ARTG, an electronic database with information on all therapeutic goods that can be lawfully supplied in Australia. As applications are submitted electronically, applicants must also establish an account with TGA eBusiness Services, or eBS [16].

Manufacturers or sponsors of Class I non-sterile and non-measuring devices only need to lodge an application for inclusion of the product category onto the ARTG via TGA eBS. For all other classes of devices manufacturers must obtain marketing approval according to one of the applicable conformity assessment procedures before lodging the application for inclusion onto the ARTG.

5.1.2.4 Canada: establishment licence for manufacturers, importers and distributors

In Canada, information about manufacturers of Class II, II or IV devices is captured in medical device licences issued by Health Canada. Manufacturers, importers and distributors of Class I devices for which a medical device licence is not required must obtain an establishment licence from the Canada Health Products and Food Branch Inspectorate (HPFBI), unless the manufacturer imports or distributes solely through a person who holds an establishment licence. The establishment licence is valid for one year and must be reviewed by Health Canada every year before being renewed. All current medical device licences are listed on the Health Canada MDALL website [17].

5.1.2.5 Japan: registration of place of business

In Japan, companies placing medical devices on the market must have a registered place of business in Japan and hold a marketing authorization licence. Typically, local distributors are MAHs. If a foreign manufacturer doesn't have a local subsidiary, he or she needs to either appoint his or her Japanese distributor as the MAH or appoint an independent local agent as the DMAH.

Under the previous J-PAL, domestic manufacturers had to obtain a Manufacturer License (*Kyoka*). Foreign manufacturers had to obtain an FMA (*Nintei*) containing their name, address and other required details [18].

The recently enacted PMD Act has introduced a new registration system for manufacturing facilities (*Toroku*), whereby domestic manufacturers must register their manufacturing facilities with authorities at their local prefectures and foreign manufacturers must register their manufacturing facilities with the PMDA [9].

An overview of the Japanese supply chain licensing requirements for medical devices is provided in Table 5.1. Under the revised regulations, listing is required for establishments undertaking the following activities: design and development (D&D), manufacturing, sterilization and final inspection and product release. Listing is not required for (subcontracted) sub-assembly, incoming inspection, packing and supply of critical components and materials.

5.1.3 *Fees and Charges*

Unlike EU Notified Bodies, which are for-profit organizations competing with each other, Regulatory Authorities in the other developed markets operate on a cost recovery basis. Cost recovery is the practice of charging fees for services provided by regulatory agencies.

Fees are charged for establishment registrations, applications for product approvals, QMS audits and assessments of certain changes in the post-market phase. Some agencies provide a reduction in fees to eligible small businesses. EU Notified Bodies, Health Canada and the TGA in Australia charge annual certification or licence fees, in addition to the one-off application fees. From time to time Regulatory Authorities revise their fees upwards.

Medical device approvals issued by the EU Notified Bodies and the TGA have limited validity of five years and must be renewed if the manufacturer wishes to continue to market the products. The

Table 5.1 Overview of supply chain licensing requirements in Japan

Legal entity	Supply chain licensing and registration requirements	
	Marketing Authorization Holder (MAH)	Manufacturing Facility Registration (*Toroku*)
Local Manufacturer	Marketing Authorization Holder (MAH)	Registration with local prefectures (replaces previous Manufacturer License, or *Kyoka*)
Foreign Manufacturer	Through local MAH (Japanese distributor) who is also the approval holder OR Through local DMAH (independent Japanese local agent); Foreign Manufacturer is the MAH	Registration with PMDA (replaces previous Foreign Manufacturer Accreditation, or *Nintei*)
Wholesaler/Seller/Leaser	High-risk devices: Seller/Leaser License; Moderate-risk devices: Notification; Low-risk devices: Self-declaration	
Repairer	Repairer License	

FDA, Health Canada and product approvals in Japan, on the other hand, do not have an expiry period.

Considering that the total cost of a regulatory approval in a developed market can go over 200,000 dollars for a high-risk device, manufacturers need to adequately budget for regulatory expenditures. Some agencies publish information about applicable fees and charges on their websites – see examples below:

- FDA Medical Device User Fee and Modernization Act (MDUFMA) [19]
- Health Canada Establishment Licences [20]; Guidance Document – Fees for the Review of Medical Device Licence Applications [21]
- TGA Schedule of fees and charges [22]; *Australian Regulatory Guidelines for Medical Devices* (ARGMD) Section 2. Fees and charges for medical devices (23 pp. 34–38)
- PMDA List of user fees for reviews, etc., of medical devices under the Pharmaceutical Affairs Law (Law No. 145, 1960) (24 pp. 181–184)

EU Notified Bodies fees vary greatly. Quotes for a CE marking certification can range between a few thousand euros and tens of thousands of euros, with equally variable levels of competency [25].

5.2 Regulatory Submissions and Approvals

5.2.1 *Europe*

Firstly, a manufacturer must determine whether his or her products fall under one of the EU medical devices directives and, if so, determine their risk classification (see also Sections 1.4, "Medical Devices", and 1.5. "Risk-Based Classification").

5.2.1.1 Declaration of conformity and CE marking

For Class I non-sterile, non-measuring medical devices and for general IVDs the manufacturer can self-declare compliance; hence he or she only needs to affix the CE marking on the device labelling and packaging, draw up an EC DoC and register with the relevant

Competent Authorities, as mentioned in Section 5.1.2.2 in this chapter. The technical documentation has to be maintained and made available upon request.

For all other medical devices and IVDs a Notified Body needs to be involved; hence the manufacturer must select a Notified Body that is accredited to perform conformity assessments for the categories of devices in question. The accreditation scope of every Notified Body is listed in the New Approach Notified and Designated Organizations (Nando) Information System [26].

Manufacturers need to choose carefully and take into consideration competence, expertise and reputation, not just price, when selecting a Notified Body. In the wake of recent scandals involving faulty breast implants, metal-on-metal hip implants and vaginal meshes, EU member states had re-assessed designations of Notified Bodies, and by the end of 2012, almost half of designations for high-risk devices were withdrawn. When a Notified Body loses its accreditation for certain product categories all certificates issued for products in those categories become invalid. The impact on manufacturers can be critical. Products certified by a Notified Body that had its designation canceled can only be sold up to the batches released to market when the certificate was still valid. After that, they cannot market the products impacted by the designation withdrawal [27].

A reputable Notified Body can better weather such situations. Take, for instance, the notorious case of the French company Poly Implant Prothèse (PIP). For many years PIP had fraudulently used industrial silicone instead of the approved medical-grade silicone in many of its breast implants that were marketed worldwide, and it concealed this fact during the pre-announced audits of its Notified Body. The Notified Body had a good track record and argued that its role in the conformity assessment of the manufacturer is to avoid inadvertent errors by the manufacturer, not to protect against intentional fraud, and managed thus to keep its designation for non-active implants. Nevertheless this case was the catalyst that galvanized the European Commission to recently tighten the regulatory controls on medical devices [28].

The application for CE marking approval must include the products for which certification is sought, their risk classification and the selected conformity assessment procedure. Notified Bodies may assist inexperienced manufacturers to correctly classify their devices and select the appropriate conformity assessment procedure. Once the manufacturer obtains approval, he or she can affix the CE marking on the device labelling and packaging and draw up a DoC.

The DoC is a legally binding document signed by an authorized person whereby the manufacturer declares compliance of the device with the applicable EC directive(s) (see example in Fig. 5.2). The CE mark is a symbol with a design prescribed by the EC directives (see Fig. 5.3).

"CE" stands for *Conformité Européenne*, the French term for *European Conformity*. By affixing the CE mark on a product, the manufacturer takes full responsibility for its conformity with EU law.

For medical devices where a Notified Body must be involved, that is, for medical devices classified as Class I sterile or with measuring function, Class IIa, Class IIb, Class III, active implantable medical devices (AIMDs), self-testing IVDs, and Annex II IVDs devices, the CE symbol must be accompanied by the identification number of the Notified Body responsible for implementation of the conformity procedures involving the audit of the QMS set out in the relevant directives, that is:

- MDD Annexes II, IV, V and VI;
- AIMDD Annexes 2, 3, 4 and 5; or
- IVDD Annexes III, IV, VI and VII.

The Notified Body identification number is a four-digit number assigned to the Notified Body and listed in the Nando Information System.

5.2.1.2 Conformity assessment procedures

The risk classification determines which conformity assessment procedures can be applied. Conformity assessment modules applicable to the various risk classes are shown in the next figures: Fig. 5.4 for MDD, Fig. 5.5 for AIMDD and Fig. 5.6 for IVDD, where modules are identified by the Annex (and section, if relevant) of the directive. For instance, the "Annex II.4 Design Examination" module in Fig. 5.4

[Manufacturer's letterhead]

EC Declaration of Conformity

Manufacturer:	*[Name and Address]*
EU Authorised Representative:	*[Name and Address]*
Products:	*[Name and Model designation]*
Classification:	*[MDD risk class and classification rule according to Annex IX; or AIMD; or IVD]*

We herewith declare that the above mentioned products meet the provisions of Council Directive [93/42/EEC *for Medical devices*] / [90/385/EEC *for Active implantable medical devices*] / [98/79/EC *for In vitro diagnostic medical devices*] and the conformity assessment route [*Annex applied*] and [*other EC directives if applicable*] and the conformity assessment route of [*Annex applied*].

All supporting documentation is retained at the premises of the [Manufacturer/ EU Authorised Representative].

Notified Body:	*[Name, Address and Identification Number]*
EC Certificates:	*[EC Certificates Numbers, as applicable]*
Start of CE marking:	*[Date, Lot Number or Serial Number of first CE-marked products]*
Place and Date of Issue:	*[City, Date]*
Authorised Signature:	______________________
Name, Position:	

Figure 5.2 Example of an EC Declaration of Conformity template.

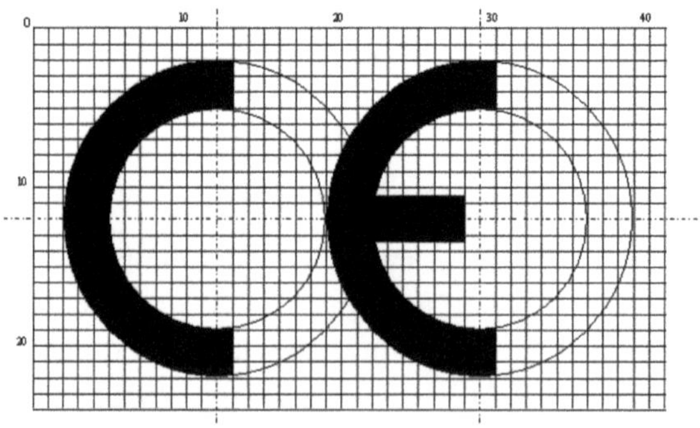

Figure 5.3 CE marking design according to Council Decision 93/465/EC) [29].

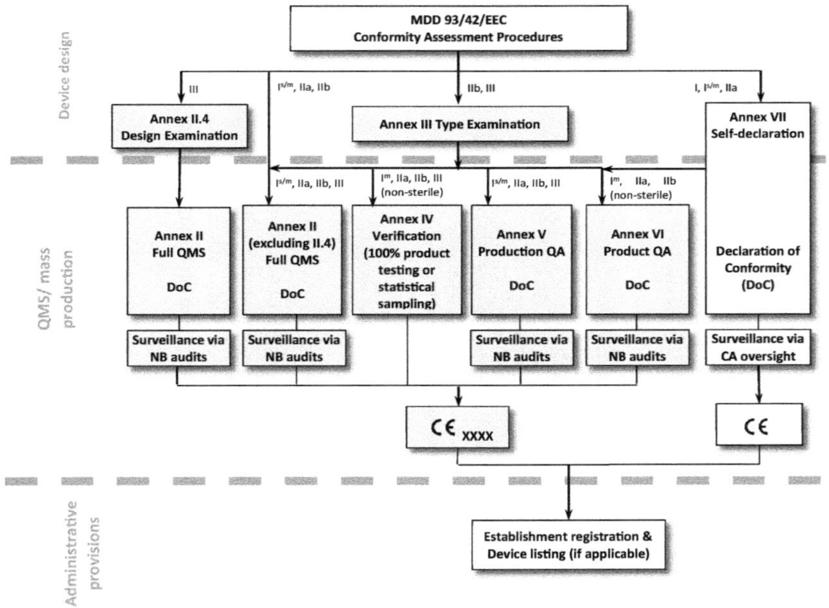

Figure 5.4 MDD 93/42/EEC, *Conformity assessment procedures.*
Notes: Shaded boxes indicate the procedures for which a Notified Body must be involved. The four-digit number "XXXX" represents the Notified Body identification number accompanying the CE marking. Letters "s" and "m" in superscript indicate Class I devices supplied sterile and with a measuring function, respectively.

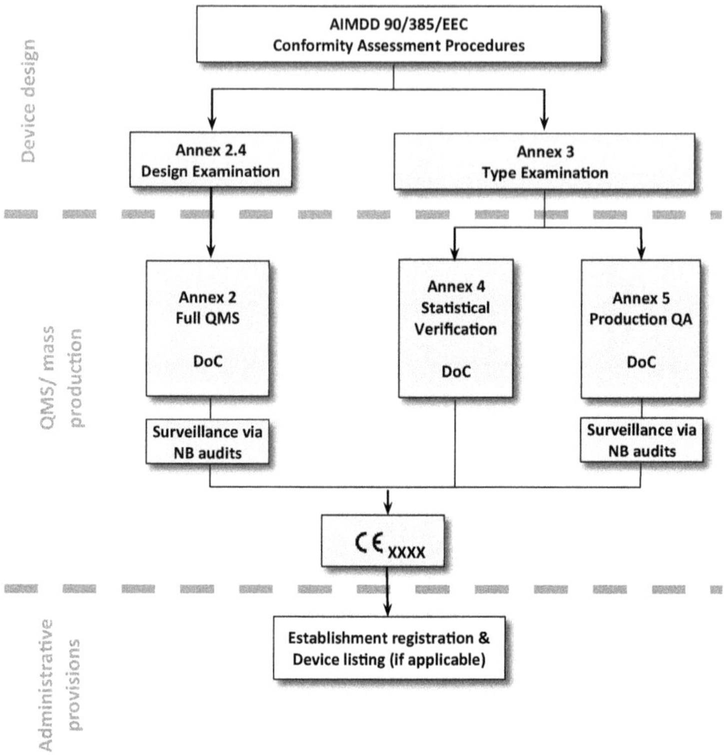

Figure 5.5 AIMDD 90/385/EEC, *Conformity assessment procedures.*
Notes: Shaded boxes indicate the procedures for which a Notified Body must be involved; for AIMDs a Notified Body must always be involved. The four-digit number "XXXX" represents the Notified Body identification number accompanying the CE marking.

refers to Section 4, "Examination of the Design of the Product", of MDD Annex II.

Conformity assessment for high-risk devices such as Class III medical devices, AIMDs and IVDs in List A and List B requires both a design examination or a type examination and a quality system assessment. Usually, the design or type examination is done first, followed by the QMS audit or statistical verification of manufactured product, as applicable.

The manufacturer must generate and maintain product-specific documentation in accordance with regulations and guidelines

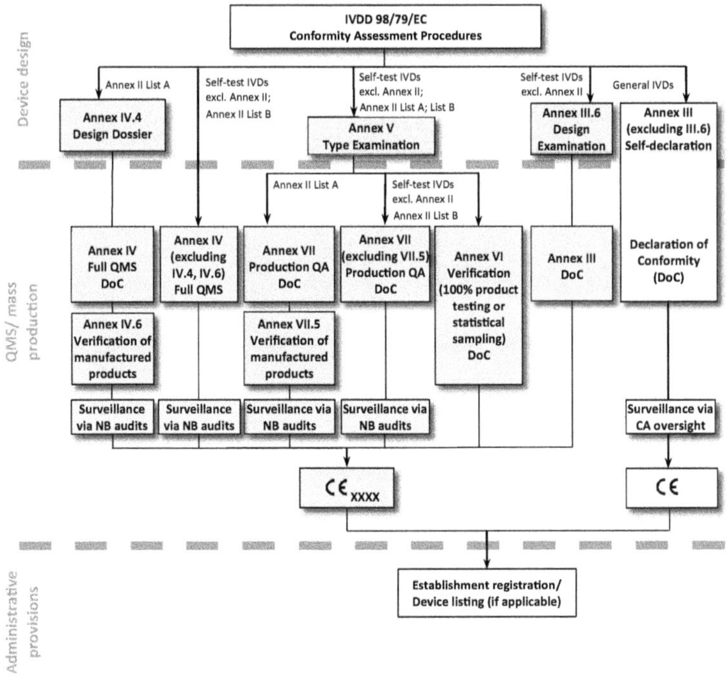

Figure 5.6 IVDD 98/79/EEC, *Conformity assessment procedures.*
Notes: Shaded boxes indicate the procedures for which a Notified Body must be involved. The four-digit number "XXXX" represents the Notified Body identification number accompanying the CE marking.

as detailed in Section 3.1.1, "Documentation Mandated by EU Regulations".

Furthermore, if clinical trials are required, the clinical data can be submitted as a self-contained module. It is well known that clinical trials can take many months to run, and in these situations the manufacturer may negotiate with the Notified Body to first submit the design dossier without the clinical data, so that the Notified Body can commence the assessment, and then submit the clinical data after completion of the trial.

The unwritten rule is that in the event that the submission is managed in modules (design dossier without clinical trial data, clinical trial data and QMS audit), the individual modules should not be submitted by more than six months apart from each other

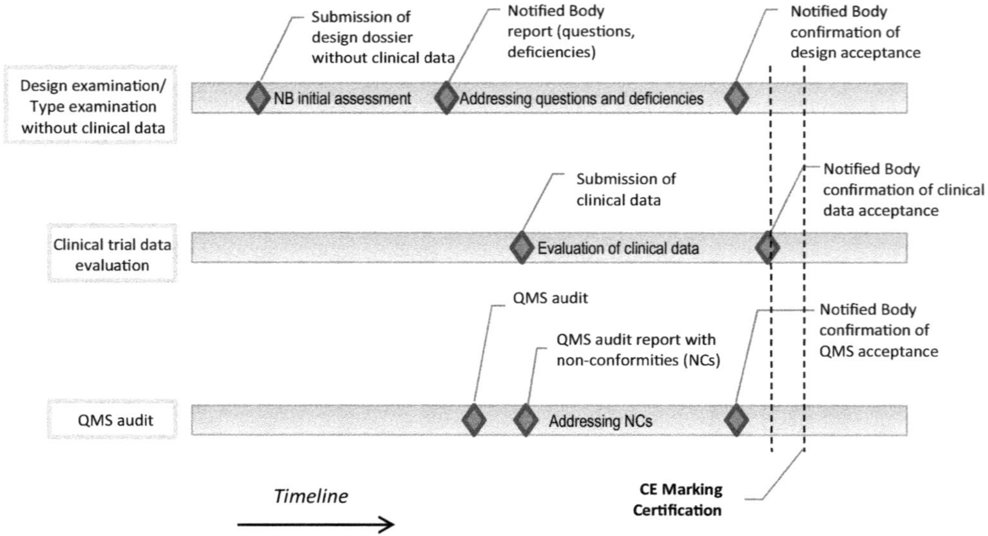

Figure 5.7 Example of timelines for a modular CE marking submission, including clinical trial data for a high-risk medical device.

so that the information remains in sync across the modules during the assessment process. An example of how timelines for a modular submission of a high-risk medical device might look like is shown in Fig. 5.7. Depending on the complexity of the high-risk device, how well the design control process is implemented and how good the technical documentation is, approval for a high-risk device can take six months or a few years.

5.2.1.3 EC Certificates of Conformity

Certificates issued by EU Notified Bodies represent the proof that a medical device (other than Class I non-sterile and non-measuring) and/or an IVD medical device (other than general IVD) is compliant with relevant regulations and can be legally placed on the EU market. There are product certificates (see Table 5.2) and quality system certificates (Table 5.3) that can be issued under the EU medical devices directives [30].

High-risk devices such as Class III medical devices, AIMDs and IVDs in List A and List B require both a product certificate and a quality system certificate according to the applicable conformity assessment procedures.

The same product or product category cannot be certified by more than one Notified Body. Medical devices directives require that each application to a Notified Body include a written declaration that no application has been lodged with any other Notified Body for the same product-related quality system or for the same product type, depending on the conformity assessment procedure applied. This means that only one CE mark is allowed on the product, namely the one accompanied by the identification number of the Notified Body responsible for implementation of the conformity procedures set out in MDD Annexes II, IV, V and VI; AIMDD Annexes 2, 3, 4 and 5; or IVDD Annexes III, IV, VI and VII.

There may be situations, however, where a manufacturer obtains, for the same medical device, an EC Type Examination Certificate according to MDD Annex III from Notified Body A and an EC Certificate for Production Quality Assurance according to MDD Annex V from Notified Body B. In this case the manufacturer must

Table 5.2 Product certificates that can be issued under the EU medical devices directives

Type of certificate	Annex of EC directive	Device risk classification
EC Type Examination Certificate	MDD Annex III	MDD Class IIb, III
	AIMDD Annex 3	AIMDs
	IVDD Annex V	IVDs List A, List B, self-testing
EC Design Examination Certificate	MDD Annex II.4	MDD Class III
	AIMDD Annex 2.4	AIMDs
	IVDD Annex III.6	IVDs self-testing
	IVDD Annex IV.4, IV.6	IVDs List A
EC Certificate of Conformity	MDD Annex IV	MDD Class I sterile and/or measuring, Class IIa, Class IIb, Class III
	AIMDD Annex 4	AIMD
	IVDD Annex VI	IVDs List B, self-testing

affix the identification number of Notified Body B (i.e., the Notified Body that has certified the QMS) on its products.

QMS certification for the full quality system, production quality assurance and product quality assurance requires surveillance audits "to ensure that the manufacturer duly fulfills the obligations imposed by the approved quality system". Surveillance is mandated by:

- MDD Annex II.5, Annex V.4 and Annex VI.4;
- AIMDD Annex 2.5 and Annex 5.4; and
- IVDD Annex IV. and Annex VII.4.

Typically, the EU Notified Body would perform annual surveillance audits for the next four years after initial certification (see Fig. 5.8). Surveillance of Class I medical devices non-sterile, non-measuring and general IVDs is the responsibility of national Competent Authorities.

In the wake of the PIP scandal mentioned earlier (in Section 5.2.1.1 in this chapter) the European Commission published a

Table 5.3 Quality system certificates that can be issued under the EU medical devices directives

Type of certificate	Annex of EC directive	Device risk classification
EC Certificate for Full Quality Assurance System	MDD Annex II (excluding II.4)	MDD Class I sterile and/or measuring, IIa, IIb, III, sterilized systems or procedure packs
	AIMDD Annex 2 (excluding II.4)	AIMDs
	IVDD Annex IV (excluding IV.4, IV.6)	IVDs List B, self-testing
	IVDD Annex IV	IVDs List A
EC Certificate for Production Quality Assurance	MDD Annex V	MDD Class I sterile and/or measuring, IIa, IIb, III, sterilized systems or procedure packs
	AIMDD Annex V	AIMDs
	IVDD Annex VII (excluding VII.5)	IVDs List B, self-testing
	IVDD Annex VII	IVDs List A
EC Certificate for Product Quality Assurance	MDD Annex VI	MDD Class I sterile and/or measuring, IIa, IIb

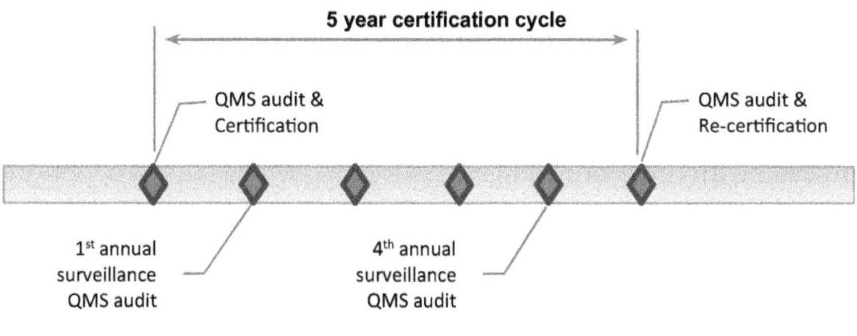

Figure 5.8 Diagram representing the five-year certification cycle during which the EU Notified Body performs an initial certification QMS audit and four annual surveillance QMS audits.

Joint Action Plan for Immediate Actions under the existing medical devices legislation. The plan, put forward in February 2012, proposed to the member states joint actions aimed at tightening controls on medical devices in the framework of the current legislation. It covers actions by the Commission (e.g., adoption of clearer rules on designation of Notified Bodies), member states (e.g., re-assessment of Notified Bodies) and Notified Bodies (e.g., undertaking unannounced audits).

According to the Joint Action Plan, "Even though Notified Bodies were entitled to carry out unannounced audits, at the time of the PIP-scandal, in most cases, those audits did not take place". The plan goes on saying that "a majority of member states have requested their Notified Bodies to carry out unannounced audits and have asked Notified Bodies to ensure they are informed about incident reports". Hence starting with 2014 manufacturers need to be prepared for unannounced audits as well [31].

Although the basic requirement is one unannounced audit per certification every three years, the frequency of unannounced audits can be increased in these situations:

- If the devices bear a high risk;
- If the devices of the type in question are frequently non-compliant; or
- If specific information provides reasons to suspect non-conformities of the devices or of their manufacturer [32].

Before the end of the five-year certification period, the manufacturer needs to decide whether to renew the certification and, if so, proceed with re-certification.

5.2.1.4 Re-certification

EC certificates have a validity period of five years, during which time the manufacturer must ensure that the product and the QMS maintain compliance with all relevant requirements. An application for re-certification should be submitted at latest six months before the certificate expiry date.

The application for re-certification must include the following documentation:

- A report of all the changes to the approved design or type made since the previous submission to the Notified Body;
- A reference document of the key data submitted for the renewal process, including any cross-references to any previously submitted data held by the Notified Body;
- A report demonstrating the compliance with the requirements of the directives for the devices involved, taking into consideration the current state of the art, including:

  - Experience gained from the devices in the post-production phase, including comparable products in the market (manufacturer's post-market surveillance);
  - Change of suppliers, subcontractors;
  - Modifications of production or test methods;
  - New experience regarding materials, components, etc., used, including biocompatibility;
  - Results of the risk management process (updated risk analysis);
  - Risk assessment in relation to new medical treatments and medical technology (risk–benefit ratio for the patient);
  - Experience from changes of the updating of the Essential Requirements;
  - Results of new clinical investigations and/or the post-marketing clinical follow-up, including results of comparable products in the market (updated clinical evaluation); and
  - Modifications according to regulatory changes.

- If the device contains a medicinal product or it is a device utilizing materials of animal origin or a device assisted by human blood derivatives the manufacturer shall provide an updated statement on the rationale and justification for the use of the medicinal product, the material of animal origin or the human blood derivatives for each of their product types [33].

5.2.1.5 Switching to another Notified Body

Sometimes a manufacturer may choose or may be forced to transfer from one Notified Body to another. If the change is voluntary, the transition plan must take into account the expiry date of existing certificates, placing on the market of devices covered by existing certificates, changing labelling to the CE mark with the new Notified Body's identification number, providing technical documentation to the new Notified Body for review and planning for an audit by the new Notified Body, if necessary.

If the change is forced, for instance, due to a withdrawal of designation, the Competent Authority responsible for the Notified Body's designation would typically need to review the impact on existing certifications and in some cases may require affected manufacturers to switch to a new Notified Body. More detailed guidance is provided in the Notified Body Operations Group (NBOG) Best Practice Guide (BPG) 2006-1 *Change of Notified Body* [34].

5.2.1.6 Custom-made devices

Custom-made devices are "devices for special purposes" specifically made in accordance with a duly qualified medical practitioner's written prescription for the sole use of a particular patient, for example, patient-specific orthopaedic footwear, hearing aid moulds, artificial eyes, prosthetics and orthotics. Mass-produced devices, which need to be adapted to meet the specific requirements of a healthcare professional (and which are supplied for the sole use of a particular patient), such as contact lenses and stock footwear, are not considered to be custom-made devices [35].

Custom-made devices must meet the relevant provisions of the directives set out in MDD Annex VIII and AIMDD Annex 6 that apply to them, including drawing up a DoC and maintaining a technical documentation file.

Custom-made devices neither require nor are allowed to be CE marked. They must, however, be labeled with the wording "custom-made device" according to MDD Annex I, Paragraph 13.3(g), and AIMDD Annex 1, Paragraph 14.1.

5.2.1.7 Devices intended for clinical investigations

Devices intended for clinical investigations are "devices for special purposes" intended for use by a duly qualified medical practitioner when conducting clinical investigations in an adequate human clinical environment. A clinical investigation is a systematic investigation or study in human subjects for the purpose of assessing the safety and/or performance of a medical device (for more details refer to Section 2.6.2, "Clinical Trials").

The conformity assessment procedures for active implantables and for Class III and implantable medical devices require that a clinical investigation be undertaken unless it is duly justified to rely on existing data (AIMDD Annex 7, Section 1.2, and MDD Annex X, Section I.1a). Justifications for not performing clinical investigations would have to be well documented and supported by the risk management file. Devices in a lower-risk classification may also require clinical investigations, depending on indications for use and intended use, clinical claims and risk management outcomes.

Annex 7 Clinical Evaluation of the Active Implantable Medical Devices Directive (AIMDD) 90/385/EEC states the following:

> 1.2. Clinical investigations shall be performed unless it is duly justified to rely on existing clinical data.
>
> 1.5. Where demonstration of conformity with essential requirements based on clinical data is not deemed appropriate, adequate justification for any such exclusion has to be given based on risk management output and under consideration of the specifics of the device/body interaction, the clinical performances intended and the claims of the manufacturer. Adequacy of demonstration of conformity with the essential requirements by performance evaluation, bench testing and pre-clinical evaluation alone has to be duly substantiated.

Annex X Clinical Evaluation of the Medical Devices Directive (MDD) 93/42/EEC states the following:

> 1.1a In the case of implantable devices and devices in Class III clinical investigations shall be performed unless it is duly justified to rely on existing clinical data.

1.1d Where demonstration of conformity with essential requirements based on clinical data is not deemed appropriate, adequate justification for any such exclusion has to be given based on risk management output and under consideration of the specifics of the device/body interaction, the clinical performances intended and the claims of the manufacturer. Adequacy of demonstration of conformity with the essential requirements by performance evaluation, bench testing and pre-clinical evaluation alone has to be duly substantiated.

In Europe, clinical trials for medical devices should be conducted in line with the following guidelines:

- MEDDEV 2.7/4:2010, *Guidelines on clinical investigations* [36] – they are based on the GHTF guidance SG5/N3:2010 Clinical investigations.
- MEDDEV 2.7.2:2008, guide for Competent Authorities in making an assessment of clinical investigation notification [37].

If the aim of the clinical investigation is to establish the safety and effectiveness for a novel device or for new indications of an existing device, the investigational devices are neither required nor allowed to bear the CE marking. They must, however, be labeled with the wording "exclusively for clinical investigations" according to MDD Annex I §13.3(h) and AIMDD Annex 1 §14.1 fifth dash and §14.2 fourth dash.

If the purpose of the clinical investigation is to test the usability or customer preference (other than safety or effectiveness) it should only be carried out on a CE-marked (i.e., approved) device, unless they form part of a study to investigate safety and performance for CE marking purposes.

According to Article 15 of the MDD and Article 10 of the AIMDD the manufacturer or sponsor must notify the relevant Competent Authorities in the member states in which the clinical trials are to be conducted, at least 60 days before commencement of the trials. At the end of the 60-day waiting period the trials may commence unless the Competent Authorities inform the manufacturer of a decision to the contrary. A member state may, however, authorize manufacturers to start the clinical investigations before the expiry of the 60-day period, provided that an Ethics Committee with jurisdiction in that area has issued a favourable opinion.

Roles of Competent Authorities may vary between member states in relation to assessment of clinical investigation notifications therefore it is important to check directly with each Competent Authority. A list of EU Competent Authorities is available from the official website of the European Commission [10].

Changes to the clinical investigation plan or other amendments and updates to the original clinical trial notification must be submitted in a timely manner to the relevant authorities.

If a clinician uses a CE-marked device for a new, off-label purpose that is not supported by the manufacturer's indications for use or intended uses, the clinician and the relevant healthcare establishment effectively take on the responsibilities of "the manufacturer," as defined by the regulations and are liable for the off-label use of the device [38].

5.2.1.8 IVDs for performance evaluation

IVDs for performance evaluation are special-purpose IVDs intended by the manufacturer to be subject to one or more performance evaluation studies in laboratories for medical analyses or in other appropriate environments outside his or her own premises.

IVDs for performance evaluation must meet the relevant provisions of the IVDD set out in Annex VIII that apply to them, including drawing up a DoC and maintaining a technical documentation file.

IVDs for performance evaluation neither require nor are allowed to be CE marked. They must, however, be labeled with the wording "for performance evaluation only" according to IVDD Annex I §8.4(f).

5.2.1.9 Humanitarian-use devices

Competent Authorities may authorize the use of non-CE-marked medical devices or IVDs on humanitarian grounds, provided that the manufacturer can demonstrate it is in the interests of the patient and the protection of health and if the following conditions are met:

- There are no alternative CE-marked devices available for this treatment.
- It has been demonstrated that the morbidity and/or mortality are significantly reduced with the use of the device in question compared to those using alternative available treatment.

For instance, in the U.K. a humanitarian-use device may not be used until an application requesting such use has been made by the manufacturer and due authorization has been given by the Medicines & Healthcare products Regulatory Agency (MHRA), the UK Competent Authority. The authorization applies only to the use of the individual device for a named individual within that member state. Failure to comply with these requirements constitutes a criminal offence [39].

5.2.2 *The United States*

Before marketing a medical device in the United States, a manufacturer needs to go through the following steps:

(1) Classify the device.
(2) Choose the correct pre-market submission.
(3) Prepare the appropriate information for the pre-market submission to the FDA.
(4) Send the pre-market submission to the FDA and interact with FDA staff during the review.
(5) Complete the establishment registration and device listing.

Unless exempt (see also Section 1.7.1, "Regulatory Controls in the United States"), medical devices require one of the following types of pre-market submissions:

- 510(k) Premarket Notification – applicable to some Class I and most Class II devices;
- Premarket Approval (PMA) – applicable to most Class III devices;

- De Novo Evaluation of Automatic Class III designation – applicable to novel devices with low to moderate risk for which there is no predicate device; or
- Humanitarian Device Exemption (HDE) – applicable to Class III devices intended to benefit patients with rare diseases or conditions, that is, affecting less than 4,000 individuals in the United States per year.

The third Medical Devices User Fee Act (MDUFA III) enacted on October 1, 2012, re-authorizes the FDA to collect fees for its regulatory activities over the period between financial years FY13 and FY17. MDUFA III also introduced process improvements and new or updated policies to enhance predictability, consistency, transparency, efficiency and timeliness of FDA review and approval procedures. Areas of improvement are listed below along with explanations of terminology [40].

Presubmission Process – A Presubmission is a formal written request from an applicant for FDA feedback, which is provided in the form of a formal written response or, if the manufacturer chooses, a meeting or tele-conference in which the feedback is documented in meeting minutes. A Presubmission meeting is a meeting or tele-conference in which the FDA provides its substantive feedback on the Presubmission. It represents an opportunity for applicants to obtain FDA feedback prior to intended submission of a marketing application or an investigational-device exemption (IDE) (application for approval to conduct a clinical trial in the United States). Presubmissions and meeting requests will be assigned a "Q" number.

Submission acceptance criteria – Submission acceptance criteria are checklists with objective criteria for "refuse to accept/refuse to file" applications. Their purpose is to screen out submissions that lack basic requirements, allowing thus FDA reviewers to concentrate resources on complete applications. If a submission is not accepted for in-depth review, the review clock does not start until the FDA receives a revised submission that meets required elements.

Interactive Review – The purpose of the Interactive Review process is to provide for, and encourage, informal communication between the FDA and applicants to ensure that the FDA's concerns are clearly communicated to the applicant during the review process and thus minimize the number of review cycles. Increased informal interaction will facilitate timely completion of the review process on the basis of accurate and complete information.

Substantive Interaction – Substantive Interaction is an email, letter, tele-conference, video conference, fax or other form of communication by the FDA notifying the applicant of substantive deficiencies identified in the initial submission review or a communication stating that the FDA has not identified any deficiencies in the initial submission review and any further minor deficiencies will be communicated through Interactive Review. An approval or clearance letter issued prior to the Substantive Interaction goal date will qualify as a Substantive Interaction.

Guidance development – An updated FDA guidance for guidance development includes publication of a priority list of topics for development and a more structured approach to gathering stakeholder input.

Third-party review – The third-party review program is aimed at providing manufacturers of eligible devices with an alternative 510(k) review process by private third parties accredited by the FDA (Accredited Persons). This program enables the FDA to use its scientific review resources for higher-risk devices, while maintaining confidence in the review by third parties of low- to moderate-risk devices and yielding a more rapid marketing clearance decisions for manufacturers. Currently, under the program all Class I devices that were not exempt from 510(k) in 1996 and 30 Class II devices are eligible for third-party review. Lists with Accredited Persons and eligible devices are available from the FDA website [41]. The FDA will establish new procedures to improve transparency, including the publishing of criteria for third parties' re-accreditation.

Patient safety and risk tolerance – Patient safety and risk tolerance refer to factors to consider when making benefit risk determinations, including patient tolerance for risk, magnitude of the benefit and the availability of other treatments or diagnostic tests. A final FDA guidance on factors to consider when making benefit–risk determinations in medical device PMA and de novo classifications has been published and will be fully implemented.

Low-risk medical device exemptions - On August 1, 2014, the FDA published a draft guidance proposing to exempt additional 107 Class II and Class I Reserved medical devices from 510(k) Premarket Notification requirements [42]. The FDA intends to issue a final rule exempting additional low-risk medical devices from Premarket Notification within two years of this proposal, that is, by 2016.

Emerging diagnostics - The FDA will work with industry to develop a transitional IVD approach for the regulation of emerging diagnostics.

In addition, MDUFA III introduced a statutory requirement for applicants to provide an electronic copy (eCopy) with any pre-submission or submissions for devices. The eCopy must meet the technical standards outlined in the FDA guidance document *eCopy Program for Medical Device Submissions* [43].

New and revised guidance documents explaining the key provisions of MDUFA III are available on the FDA website [44] – they include:

- *Requests for Feedback on Medical Device Submissions: The Presubmission Program and Meetings with FDA Staff* [45];
- *Types of Communications During the Review of Medical Device Submissions* [46];
- *Refuse to Accept (RTA) Policy for 510(k)s* [47];
- *FDA and Industry Actions on Premarket Notifications (510(k)) Submissions* [48];
- *Acceptance and Filing Reviews for Premarket Approval Applications (PMAs)* [49];
- *FDA and Industry Actions on Premarket Approval Applications (PMAs)* [50]; and
- *Factors to Consider When Making Benefit-Risk Determinations in Medical Device Premarket Approvals and De Novo Classifications* [51].

5.2.2.1 510(k) Premarket Notification

A 510(k) is a pre-market submission made to the FDA to demonstrate that a device that is not subject to PMA is at least as safe and effective, that is, substantially equivalent, to a legally marketed or predicate device. A legally marketed or predicate device is a device that:

- Was legally marketed in the United States prior to the 1976 Amendments of the FD&C Act, for which a PMA is not required; or
- Has been re-classified from Class III to Class II or I; or
- Has been found substantially equivalent through the 510(k) process; and
- Is not in violation of the FD&C Act.

Any legally marketed device may be used as a predicate. However, because medical technology has changed greatly since 1976, almost all 510(k) submissions claim substantial equivalence to a post-amendment device that has been recently cleared under the 510(k) process. Predicate devices can be found searching the FDA 510(k) database for devices with the same indications for use and intended use as the new device [52].

A claim of substantial equivalence does not mean the new and predicate devices must be identical. A medical device is substantially equivalent to a predicate if it:

- Has the same indications for use and intended use as the predicate; and
- Has the same technological characteristics as the predicate;

or

- Has the same indications for use and intended use as the predicate; and
- Has different technological characteristics, and the information submitted to the FDA:
  - Does not raise new questions of safety and effectiveness; and

- Demonstrates that the device is at least as safe and effective as the legally marketed device.

Substantial equivalence is established by comparing the new device with the predicate device with regard to indications for use and intended use, principle of operation, design, labelling, performance, energy used or delivered, materials, manufacturing process and other characteristics, as applicable.

A 510(k) submission must comply with the requirements described in 21 CFR 807 Subpart E, *Premarket Notification Procedures* [53]. In addition to demonstrating substantial equivalence to a predicate device, the manufacturer must provide evidence of compliance with applicable FDA guidance documents or FDA Recognized Consensus Standards. A side-by-side comparison table together with a discussion of similarities and differences, for instance, like the one in Table 5.4, needs to be included in the 510(k) submission [54].

The 510(k) content and structure should follow the requirements in the relevant FDA regulations and guidance documents listed in Section 3.1.2, "Documentation Mandated by US Regulations". The FDA requires two copies of the 510(k), one of which must be an eCopy.

A simplified overview of the 510(k) submission process is provided in Fig. 5.9.

The 510(k) submission process consists of four steps:

Step 1 – Log-in and Acknowledgement Procedure

The FDA's Document Control Center (DCC) receives the 510(k) submission and checks whether the applicant submitted the correct user fee and a valid eCopy. Within seven days from receiving the 510(k) submission the FDA sends either an Acknowledgment Letter to confirm that the 510(k) submission and the user fee payment were received or a Hold Letter in the case of unresolved issues with the user fee or the eCopy. The FDA Acknowledgment Letter will include the 510(k) unique reference number, also known as the "K number".

Table 5.4 Example of substantial equivalence comparison table

Substantial equivalence	*[New device model designation]*	*[Predicate device model designation]*	Comparison/conclusion
Indications for use	*[indications for use statement]*	*[indications for use statement]*	Same
Intended use	*[intended use statement]*	*[intended use statement]*	Same
Principle of operation	*[short description]*	*[short description]*	Same
Design	*[short description]*	*[short description]*	*[similarities, differences]*
Energy used/delivered	*[short description]*	*[short description]*	*[similarities, differences]*
Materials	*[include or reference material list]*	*[include or reference material list]*	*[similarities, differences]*
Human factors	*[short description]*	*[short description]*	*[similarities, differences; references to V&V reports]*
Performance	*[short description]*	*[short description]*	*[similarities, differences; references to V&V reports]*
Safety Electrical Mechanical Chemical Thermal Radiation Biocompatibility	*[short summary]*	*[short summary]*	*[references to V&V reports]*
Compliance with guidance documents/standards	*[short summary]*	*[short summary]*	*[references to V&V reports]*
Other characteristics	...	...	...

If the applicant receives a Hold Letter, he or she has 180 calendar days to fully address issues with the user fee or eCopy submission, otherwise the 510(k) is considered withdrawn.

Step 2 – Acceptance Review

After the Acknowledgment Letter is sent, the 510(k) is assigned to the FDA branch that performs the review. The lead reviewer checks whether the 510(k) submission can

Step 1 ▪ What happens during this stage: ▪ How long does it take: ▪ Possible outcomes:	**Log-in & Acknowledgment (Day 1)** ▪ Document Control Center (DCC) checks whether applicant submitted correct user fee & valid eCopy ▪ 7 days from submission receipt ▪ FDA sends either: ☑ **Acknowledgement Letter**; or ☒ **Hold Letter** (applicant has 180 days to fully address issues with the user fee or eCopy submission)
Step 2 ▪ What happens during this stage: ▪ Reference: ▪ How long does it take: ▪ Possible outcomes:	**Acceptance Review** ▪ Screening by Lead Reviewer to check whether 510(k) submission meets the minimum threshold of acceptability for substantive review ▪ Acceptance Checklist for 510(k) guidance ▪ 15 days from submission receipt ▪ FDA notifies applicant of: ☑ **Acceptance for Substantive Review**; or ☒ **Refuse to Accept - (RTA) Hold** (applicant has 180 days to fully address cited deficiencies)
Step 3 ▪ What happens during this stage: ▪ How long does it take: ▪ Possible outcomes:	**Substantive Review** ▪ Comprehensive review of 510(k) submission and **Substantive Interaction** with applicant ▪ 60 days from submission receipt ▪ FDA proceeds with: ☑ **Interactive Review** (review clock does not stop); or ☒ **Additional Information (AI) request** (review clock stops; applicant has 180 days to fully address cited deficiencies)
Step 4 ▪ What happens during this stage: ▪ How long does it take: ▪ Possible outcomes:	**FDA Decision** ▪ Notification of FDA decision ▪ 90 days from submission receipt, excluding the days the submission was on hold for an AI request ▪ FDA notifies applicant that: ☑ Device found substantially equivalent (SE) - 510(k) has been cleared; ☒ Device found not substantially equivalent (NSE)

Figure 5.9 Simplified overview of the 510(k) process. *Source*: FDA [55].

be accepted for review according to the FDA's guidance *Refuse to Accept Policy for 510(k)s* [47]. The purpose of a rigorous acceptance review screening is to allow FDA reviewers to concentrate resources on complete applications. The Refuse to Accept (RTA) criteria for 510(k) is a checklist of objective criteria for screening out submissions that lack basic requirements.

Within 15 days of the 510(k) receipt, depending on the outcome of this initial screening, the applicant receives an electronic notification either that the 510(k) was accepted for review (i.e., Acceptance Review) or that the 510(k) was not accepted for review (i.e., considered RTA).

A 510(k) that has been accepted for review proceeds to the Substantive Review. If the 510(k) is placed on RTA Hold, the applicant has 180 calendar days to fully address the deficiencies cited in the RTA Hold, otherwise the 510(k) is considered withdrawn. If the submission is refused for acceptance the review clock does not start until the FDA receives a revised submission that meets the acceptance criteria.

Step 3 – Substantive Review, including Substantive Interaction and Interactive Review

During a Substantive Review the lead reviewer performs a comprehensive assessment of the 510(k) submission.

Within 60 days of the 510(k) receipt the FDA lead reviewer informs the applicant through a Substantive Interaction whether outstanding deficiencies may be resolved via an Interactive Review or whether an Additional Information (AI) Request will be issued placing the file on hold.

If the applicant receives an AI Request, he or she has 180 calendar days from the date of the AI Request to submit a complete response to all deficiencies raised, otherwise the 510(k) is considered withdrawn. Any additional information submitted to the FDA lead reviewer during the Interactive Review or to address an AI Request must include a valid eCopy.

Step 4 – 510(k) Decision

Within 90 days of the 510(k) receipt, excluding the days the submission was on hold for an AI Request, the FDA notifies the applicant of its decision, that is, whether the device was found to be substantially equivalent or "not substantially equivalent" (NSE) to the predicate device(s).

If the FDA determines that the device is substantially equivalent, the applicant receives an order, in the form of a letter, that states that the device can be marketed

in the United States. This order "clears" the device for commercial distribution; therefore the FDA uses the term "clearance", not "approval", in the context of a 510(k). Until the applicant receives clearance declaring the device substantially equivalent, the applicant may not proceed to market the device in the United States.
If the FDA determines that the device is NSE, the applicant may either:

- Re-submit another 510(k) with new data;
- Request a Class I or II designation through the de novo process;
- File a re-classification petition; or
- Submit a PMA.

There is no requirement for the FDA to perform facility inspections (audits) prior to issue a 510(k) clearance. The applicant may market the device immediately after 510(k) clearance is granted; however, the manufacturer should be prepared for an FDA inspection of its quality system, including design controls, at any time after 510(k) clearance.

The 510(k) process described so far represents the Traditional 510(k). In 1998 the FDA has introduced two optional approaches for obtaining 510(k) marketing clearance if certain conditions are met:

Special 510(k) Device Modification applies to modifications to a manufacturer's own devices that rely on results from design control process.

Abbreviated 510(k) applies to devices for which there are guidance documents, special controls and FDA Recognized Consensus Standards.

The decision tree for determining which type of 510(k) can be used is shown in Fig. 5.10 [56].

5.2.2.2 Premarket Approval

PMA, required for Class III devices, is the most stringent type of premarket submission for medical devices in the United States. It involves an in-depth assessment and a determination by FDA that

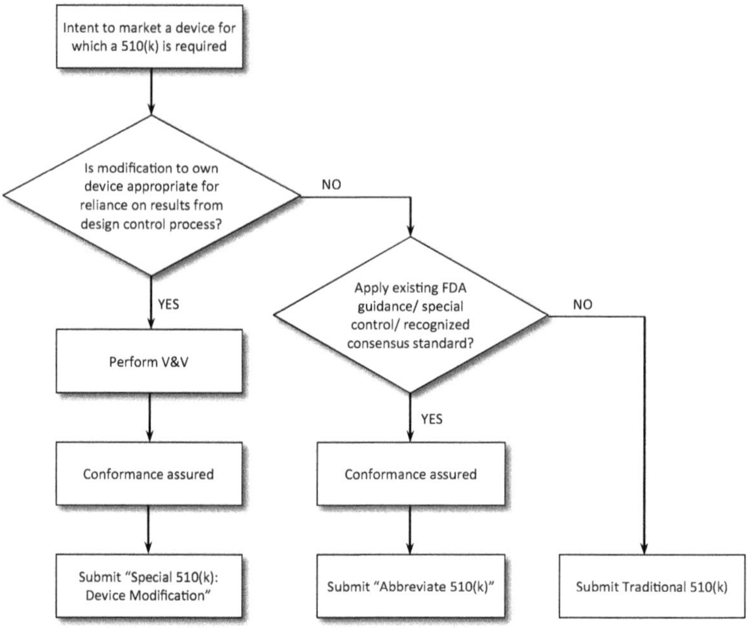

Figure 5.10 Decision tree for determining which type of 510(k) can be used. *Source*: FDA, 510(k) submission methods.

there is sufficient valid scientific evidence to assure that the device is safe and effective for its indications for use and intended use(s).

A PMA application must comply with the requirements described in 21 CFR Part 814, *Premarket Approval of Medical Devices* [57]. A Class III device that fails to meet PMA requirements is considered to be adulterated under Section 501(f) of the FD&C Act and cannot be marketed [58].

The PMA application content and structure should follow the requirements in the relevant FDA regulations and guidance documents listed in Section 3.1.2, "Documentation Mandated by US Regulations". The FDA requires six copies of the PMA application, one of which must be an eCopy.

A simplified overview of the PMA application submission process is provided in Fig. 5.11.

The PMA application submission process consists of four steps:

Step 1 ▪ What happens during this stage: ▪ Reference: ▪ How long does it take: ▪ Possible outcomes:	**Filing Review** ▪ Administrative and limited scientific review to determine whether the PMA meets minimum threshold of acceptability ▪ Acceptance and Filing Reviews for PMAs guidance ▪ 45 days from submission receipt ▪ FDA notifies applicant that either: ☑ **PMA has been filed**; or ☒ **PMA has been rejected** (applicant may either resubmit PMA with additional information, or request a meeting with ODE Division);
Step 2 ▪ What happens during this stage: ▪ Reference: ▪ How long does it take: ▪ Possible outcomes:	**Substantive/ In-depth Review** ▪ Comprehensive review of PMA submission and interaction (Day-100 meetings) ▪ Guidance on PMA Interactive Procedures for Day-100 Meetings and Subsequent Deficiencies; ▪ 180 days from submission filing ▪ FDA notifies applicant: ☑ **PMA review complete** and whether a **Panel Review** is required; or ☒ **Major/ minor deficiencies** (applicant may submit PMA amendment; review period may be extended by 180 days);
Step 3 ▪ What happens during this stage: ▪ When is it required: ▪ Reference: ▪ Possible outcomes:	**Panel Review** ▪ Review and recommendation by an outside panel of experts (advisory committee) ▪ PMAs for first-of-a-kind device ▪ Panel Review of PMAs - Blue Book memo ▪ Public meeting & advisory committee vote to: ☑ **Recommend approval**; or ☒ **Recommend rejection;**
Step 4 ▪ What happens during this stage: ▪ Possible outcomes:	**FDA Decision** ▪ Final deliberations, documentation and notification of the FDA decision: ▪ ☑ Approval Order - §814.44(d); ☑ Approvable Letter - §814.44(e) – FDA inspection of facilities; ☒ Not Approvable Letter - §814.44(f) ☒ Order Denying Approval - §814.45

Figure 5.11 Simplified overview of the PMA process. *Source*: FDA [59].

Step 1 – Filing Review

The Filing Review is an administrative and limited scientific review by FDA staff to determine whether the PMA application submission can be accepted for review according to FDA's guidance *PMA Acceptance and Filing Review Policy* [49]. The purpose of the Filing Review is to allow FDA reviewers to concentrate resources on complete applications. The PMA Acceptance and Filing

Review is a checklist of objective criteria for screening out submissions that lack basic requirements. Filing of a PMA application means that the FDA has made a threshold determination that the application is sufficiently complete to begin an in-depth review.

Within 45 days from application receipt, the agency notifies the applicant whether the PMA application has been filed, that is, if the PMA application has been accepted for in-depth review. If the application is accepted for filing, the FDA letter will include the PMA reference number and the date of filing. The date of filing is the date that the PMA application accepted for filing was received by the agency.

If the application is rejected during this initial screening, for instance, due to incomplete information or a lack of clarity, the FDA will notify the applicant of the reasons for the refusal. The letter will identify the deficiencies in the application that prevent filing and will include the PMA reference number. The FDA will advise the manufacturer of what information must be provided, or steps to be taken, to accept the application for filing.

Step 2 – Substantive/ In-Depth Review

This step begins after the PMA application has been accepted for filing and it consists of an in-depth scientific, regulatory and quality system review by FDA personnel with relevant expertise. During this phase the FDA examines submitted documentation containing data from nonclinical studies (microbiological, toxicological, immunological, biocompatibility, shelf life, analytical [for IVDs], animal studies and engineering tests such as stress, wear and fatigue) and clinical studies and prepares the Summary of Safety and Effectiveness Data (SSED). FDA field personnel perform quality system inspection(s) of the manufacturer's establishment(s) against the FDA's Quality System Regulation 21 CFR Part 820.

During the in-depth review process, the FDA will notify the PMA applicant via major/minor deficiency letters of any information needed by the FDA to complete the review of the application. The applicant may request to meet with the FDA within 100 days of the filing of the PMA to discuss the review status of the application. If he or she chooses to do so, he or she must follow the FDA guidance *PMA Interactive Procedures for Day-100 Meetings and Subsequent Deficiencies* [60].

FDA regulations stipulate a time frame of 180 days to review the PMA application and make a determination, starting from the date of filing [61]. In reality, the review time is normally longer.

An applicant may amend a pending PMA application to revise existing information or to provide additional information, which may result in the FDA extending the time required for its review of the PMA application for up to another 180 days. An applicant may also voluntarily withdraw a PMA application or resubmit a PMA application that was withdrawn, not accepted for filing or not approved.

If the FDA requests an applicant to submit a PMA amendment, and a written response to the FDA's request is not received within 180 days, the FDA will consider the pending PMA application or PMA supplement to be withdrawn voluntarily by the applicant (abandoned) [62].

Step 3 - Panel Review

Before approving or denying a PMA application, the FDA may refer the PMA application to an advisory committee comprised of external experts. A panel review would typically be required for all novel devices. The panel must review the PMA application at a public meeting (according to 21 CFR Part 14) and provide the FDA with the committee's recommendation on whether the FDA should approve the application or not and the basis for such recommendation. More detailed guidance for panel review is found in the FDA's memo *Panel Review of Premarket Approval Applications #P91-2* [63].

Step 4 - FDA Decision

This step involves final deliberations, documentation and notification of the FDA decision.

After completion of the in-depth review and of the advisory committee's report and recommendation, the FDA will issue one of the following:

- An approval order under 21 CFR Part 814.44(d) – An approval order is issued to the applicant informing him or her of the PMA application's approval. The PMA application approval is then notified to the public via a notice published on the FDA's website [64].
- An approvable letter under 21 CFR Part 814.44(e) – An approvable letter is sent to the applicant if the PMA application substantially meets the regulatory requirements, and the FDA believes it can be approved, provided specified additional information is submitted or specific conditions are agreed to by the applicant. The applicant may either amend the PMA application, as requested; if he or she disagrees with the FDA's findings, file a petition under 21 CFR Part 10.33; or withdraw the PMA application.

An FDA inspection (audit) to establish that manufacturing facilities, methods and controls are in compliance with the quality system regulations (QSRs) defined in 21 CFR 820 is typically required prior to granting a PMA application approval.

- A not-approvable letter under 21 CFR Part 814.44(f) – A not-approvable letter is sent to the applicant if the PMA application has significant deficiencies. The not-approvable letter will describe the deficiencies in the application, including each applicable ground for denial under Section 515(d)(2)(A)-(E) of the FD&C Act and, where practical, will identify what is necessary to make the PMA application approvable. The applicant may amend the PMA application, as requested; file a petition under 21 CFR Part 10.33, if he or she disagrees with the FDA's findings; or withdraw the PMA application.
- An order denying approval under 21 CFR Part 814.45 – A denial of approval order is issued to the applicant if, for

instance, the PMA application contains a false statement of material fact, if the labelling is not compliant with relevant regulations, if the FDA inspector is denied access to manufacturer's facilities in which the device is made; if an essential nonclinical study was not conducted in accordance with Good Laboratory Practice (GLP) regulations in 21 CFR Part 58 or if any clinical investigation involving human subjects was not conducted in accordance with the institutional review board (IRB) regulations in 21 CFR Part 56 or the Informed Consent Regulations in 21 CFR Part 50. The denial of approval order will list the deficiencies in the PMA application, including each applicable ground for denial under Section 515(d)(2) of the FD&C Act and the regulations under Part 814 and, where practical, will identify measures required to place the PMA application in approvable form.

The FDA may impose post-approval requirements in a PMA application approval order by regulation at the time of approval of the PMA application or by regulation subsequent to approval. Post-approval requirements may include as a condition of approval of the device:

- Restriction of the sale, distribution or use of the device;
- Ongoing evaluation and periodic reporting on the safety, effectiveness and reliability of the device for its intended use;
- Any warnings and precautions to be displayed prominently in the device labelling, including any advertising;
- Inclusion of identification codes on the device or its labelling where required, for example, for implants;
- Traceability to individual patients, where required;
- Submission, at specified intervals, of periodic reports ("Annual Reports") containing the information required by §814.84(b);
- Batch testing of the device;
- Any other requirements determined by the FDA to be necessary to provide reasonable assurance, or continued

reasonable assurance, of the safety and effectiveness of the device; and
- Device tracking requirements under §821.

The PMA process described so far represents the traditional PMA method, whereby a complete PMA application is submitted to the FDA at once. This method is generally used if the device has already undergone clinical testing and has been approved in a country with established medical device regulations.

The FDA has put in place alternative methods that encourage early collaboration with the sponsor, allowing devices to be brought to market as early as possible. These alternative methods include:

- **Modular PMA** – The content of a PMA application is organized into well-delineated modules (pre-clinical, clinical, manufacturing), and each module is submitted to the FDA as soon as it is completed. The FDA reviews each module separately as soon as it is received, allowing manufacturers to receive timely feedback during the review process. This may allow more rapid closure when the last components are submitted, because much of the review work will have already been done. This method is recommended for products that are in early stages of clinical study. This method is not appropriate when the applicant is very close to being ready to submit a PMA application or when the device design is in a state of flux or likely to change [65].
- **Streamlined PMA** – A complete PMA application is submitted as in a traditional PMA application, but the sponsor must be available for an interactive review process during the protocol and PMA review. Ideally, prior to beginning studies to determine the safety and effectiveness of the product to be included in this pilot program, the sponsor would submit its protocol for FDA review. Familiarity with the product and protocol as part of this upfront evaluation should streamline the review of the PMA application once filed. This method is suitable for a device in which the technology and use are well known to the FDA. A streamlined PMA review may be appropriate

for PMA applications when there is either an FDA guidance document or other published methods for review, which have been evaluated by the FDA, or an FDA review history dealing with like products (two or more of a kind).

- **Product Development Protocol (PDP)** – The PDP is essentially a contract that describes the agreed-upon details of design and development (D&D) activities, the outputs of these activities and the acceptance criteria for these outputs. It establishes reporting milestones that convey important information to the FDA as it is generated, where they can be reviewed and responded to in a timely manner. The sponsor would be able to execute their PDP at their own pace, keeping the FDA informed of its progress with these milestone reports. A PDP that has been declared completed by the FDA is considered to have an approved PMA application.
- **Expedited Access PMA (EAP)** – In April 2014 the FDA published the draft guidance *Expedited Access for Premarket Approval Medical Devices Intended for Unmet Medical Need for Life Threatening or Irreversibly Debilitating Diseases or Conditions*. The intent of this guidance is to propose a new, voluntary program to help patients have more timely access to medical devices that demonstrate the potential to address unmet medical needs for life-threatening or irreversibly debilitating diseases or conditions by expediting their development, assessment and review, while preserving the statutory standard of reasonable assurance of safety and effectiveness for PMA, consistent with the FDA's statutory mission to protect and promote public health [66].

To qualify for the EAP program a device must meet at least one the following criteria:

(a) The device represents a breakthrough technology that provides a clinically meaningful advantage over existing technology.
(b) No approved alternative treatment or means of diagnosis exists.
(c) The device offers significant, critically meaningful advantages over existing approved alternatives.

(d) The availability of the device is in the best interest of patients (e.g., addresses an unmet clinical need).

Elements of the EAP process include:

- Interactive PMA review based on a prior agreement for a Data Development Plan;
- Involvement of the FDA office- and centre-level senior management and experienced review staff in a proactive, collaborative, cross-disciplinary review;
- Appointment of a cross-disciplinary case manager to facilitate efficient review of the Data Development Plan; and
- Assigning of priority review status to PMA applications for EAP devices under Section 515(d)(5) of the FD&C Act.

PMA application approvals of EAP devices may be supported by:

- Clinical evidence from intermediate and surrogate endpoints; that are reasonably likely to predict clinical benefit (on the condition that remaining uncertainty about the predictive relationship between a surrogate and clinical benefit is minimized through confirmatory post-approval studies or on the condition that clinical benefit is verified through confirmatory post-approval studies).
- Two-phase studies – a smaller pre-market study and a post-market study specified in the PMA conditions of approval; the design of the pre-market study would have to ensure that the probability of statistical type I error at the pre-market phase is controlled at a level agreed upon by the FDA and the sponsor at the design stage (refer also to Section 2.6.2.1, "Clinical Study Designs").

  For example, if the FDA would normally require a study with 200 subjects followed for 2 years, the FDA may approve the device after receiving promising results from 100 subjects who use the device for 6 months, and condition the approval of the device on the sponsor providing the remaining data on the completion of the study – that is, the data from 200 subjects using the device for 2 years.

- Alternative experimental designs (specific to diagnostics) to generate evidence demonstrating the analytical and clinical validity of an IVD for PMA.
- Less manufacturing information, provided the sponsor has a good track record for quality systems and there are not new, unique manufacturing issues that could adversely impact product quality or performance.

5.2.2.3 De novo classification process (evaluation of automatic Class III designation)

Novel devices that the FDA has not previously classified are "automatically" or "statutorily" classified as Class III according to Section 513(f)(1) of the FD&C Act regardless of the level of risk they pose. This is because, by definition, a new type of device would not be within a type that was on the market before the 1976 Amendments to the FD&C Act or that has since been classified into Class I or Class II.

The evaluation of automatic Class III designation of novel devices with low to moderate risk for which there is no predicate device is referred to as the de novo process because it requires the FDA to evaluate novel devices anew, from an independent, risk-based standpoint under the criteria at Section 513(a)(1) of the FD&C Act.

A novel medical device may be eligible for the de novo classification after the FDA has made an NSE determination in response to a 510(k) submission. In this case, the applicant may, within 30 days of receipt of an NSE determination for that 510(k), submit a de novo petition requesting the FDA to make a risk-based classification determination for the device under Section 513(a)(1) of the FD&C Act. The FDA must make a classification determination by written order within 60 days of the request, placing the device into one of the three statutory device classes.

If the agency re-classifies the device from Class III into Class I or Class II, the device may be commercially distributed, subject to other applicable regulatory requirements. Low- to medium-risk devices that are classified through the de novo process may be marketed and used as predicates for future 510(k) submissions.

If the device is classified as Class III it may not be marketed based on the classification order and will require an approved PMA application or completed PDP before commercial distribution can commence.

Section 513(f)(2) of the FD&C Act was amended on July 9, 2012, to allow a sponsor to submit a de novo classification request to the FDA for novel low- to moderate-risk devices without first being required to submit a 510(k) [67].

5.2.2.4 Humanitarian-device exemptions

Manufacturers are unlikely to spend resources on developing and obtaining regulatory approvals for medical devices for rare diseases or conditions because of limited commercial potential. A device manufacturer's R&D and regulatory costs could exceed its market returns for diseases or conditions affecting small patient populations. Hence, the FD&C Act includes provisions with reduced regulatory burden for "humanitarian" devices in order to provide an incentive for the development of devices for use in the treatment or diagnosis of diseases affecting these populations.

A humanitarian-use device (HUD) is defined in 21 CFR Part 814.3(n) as a "medical device that is intended to benefit patients by treating or diagnosing a disease or condition that affects or is manifested in fewer than 4,000 individuals in the United States per year". To obtain HUD designation, the applicant must provide documentation, with appended authoritative references, to demonstrate that the device meets the definition of 21 CFR 814.3(n). If the FDA determines that the device is indeed an HUD, the applicant can then submit an application for humanitarian-device exemption (HDE) to obtain marketing approval for the HUD. The HDE application must include the FDA's HUD designation letter [68].

The format and content of an HDE application is similar to a PMA application, except that an HDE application is not required to contain clinical data demonstrating that the device is effective for its intended purpose. It must, however, contain sufficient information for the FDA to determine that the device does not pose an unreasonable or significant risk of illness or injury and that the probable benefit to health outweighs the risk of injury or illness from its use, taking into account the probable risks and benefits of currently available devices or alternative forms of treatment. Additionally, the applicant must demonstrate that no comparable devices are available to treat or diagnose the disease or condition and that he or she could not otherwise bring the device to market.

An approved HDE authorizes marketing of the HUD. However, an HUD may only be used in facilities that have established a local IRB to supervise clinical testing of devices and after an IRB has approved the use of the device to treat or diagnose the specific disease. The labelling for an HUD must include the following wording: "Humanitarian device. Authorized by Federal law for use in the [treatment or diagnosis] of [disease or condition]. The effectiveness of this device for this use has not been demonstrated" [69].

A difficult grey area is an HUD indication that represents a sub-set of a common disease or condition, a so-called orphan sub-set. The applicant must demonstrate that the sub-set is medically plausible, not just readily identifiable. A medically plausible sub-set is one in which use of the device is limited to that sub-set because of some inherent property of the device and/or the disease. That is, the applicant must explain why the device couldn't also be used in all patients with the disease or condition.

5.2.2.5 Investigational-device exemption

An investigational-device exemption (IDE) allows a device without marketing approval to be used for clinical research or to collect safety and effectiveness data required to support a PMA application, an HDE, or a 510(k) submission to the FDA. IDEs or clinical investigations are regulated under 21 CFR Part 812. An investigational device is defined in §812.3(g) as a "device, including a transitional device, that is the object of an investigation".

Most PMAs and about 10%–15% of 510(k)s – especially those for devices that are significantly different from existing predicate devices, for instance, with a new indication for use or new technology – require data collected from clinical studies to support claims of safety and effectiveness (70 p. 4). Certain modifications or new intended uses of legally marketed devices may also require clinical evaluation via an IDE.

An excerpt from the 21 CFR 814.20 regulation on PMA regarding clinical data is reproduced below:

> (B) A summary of the clinical investigations involving human subjects submitted in the application including a discussion of subject selection and exclusion criteria, study population, study period, safety and effectiveness data, adverse reactions and complications, patient discontinuation, patient complaints, device failures and replacements, results of statistical analyses of the clinical investigations, contraindications and precautions for use of the device, and other information from the clinical investigations as appropriate (any investigation conducted under an IDE shall be identified as such).
>
> (ii) A section containing results of the clinical investigations involving human subjects with the device including clinical protocols, number of investigators and subjects per investigator, subject selection and exclusion criteria, study population, study period, safety and effectiveness data, adverse reactions and complications, patient discontinuation, patient complaints, device failures and replacements, tabulations of data from all individual subject report forms and copies of such forms for each subject who died during a clinical investigation or who did not complete the investigation, results of statistical analyses of the clinical investigations, device failures and replacements, contraindications and precautions for use of the device, and any other appropriate information from the clinical investigations.

If required for a 510(k), clinical data needs to address the requirements of 21 CFR 807.92 on content and format of a 510(k), which are reproduced below:

> (2) A brief discussion of the clinical tests submitted, referenced, or relied on in the premarket notification submission for a determination of substantial equivalence. This discussion shall include, where applicable, a description of the subjects upon whom the device was tested, a discussion of the safety or effectiveness data obtained from the testing, with specific reference to adverse effects and complications, and any other information from the clinical testing relevant to a determination of substantial equivalence; and [3] The conclusions drawn from the nonclinical

and clinical tests that demonstrate that the device is as safe, as effective, and performs as well as or better than the legally marketed device.

All clinical investigations, unless exempt, must obtain approval of an IDE by the FDA before the study is initiated. An IDE allows the investigational device to be used in a clinical study in order to collect safety and effectiveness data. The decision whether a clinical trial is exempt from obtaining approval from the FDA before the start of the investigation depends on the level of risk to human subjects.

Clinical trials or investigations covered under the IDE regulations are subject to different levels of regulatory control, depending on the level of risk. There are three levels of regulatory controls for IDEs, reproduced hereafter:

- **Significant-risk device** investigations – involve significant-risk devices such as implants, life-supporting devices and devices that are substantially important for diagnosing, curing, mitigating or treating disease or in preventing impairment to human health.
- **Non-significant-risk device** investigations – do not pose a significant risk to the human subjects, for example, daily-wear contact lenses and lens solutions and ultrasonic dental scalers.
- **IDE-exempt** investigations – these include:

(a) A legally marketed device when used in accordance with its labelling;
(b) A diagnostic device if it complies with the labelling requirements in 21 CFR 809.109c) and if the testing is non-invasive; does not require an invasive sampling procedure that presents a significant risk; does not by design or by intention introduce energy into a subject; and is not used as a diagnostic procedure without confirmation by another medically established diagnostic product or procedure;
(c) Consumer preference testing, testing of a modification or testing of a combination of devices if the device(s) are legally marketed device(s) – that is, if the devices are exempt from 510(k) or have a cleared 510(k) or an

approved PMA application – *and* if the testing is not for the purpose of determining safety or effectiveness and does not put subjects at risk;

(d) A device intended solely for veterinary use; and

(e) A device shipped solely for research with laboratory animals and contains the labelling "CAUTION – Device for investigational use in laboratory animals or other tests that do not involve human subjects".

Clinical investigations involving significant-risk devices require both FDA and Ethics Committee (referred to in the United States as "IRB") approval *prior* to initiation of the study. Clinical investigations involving non-significant-risk devices only require an IRB approval *prior* to initiation of the study. IDE-exempt investigations do not need FDA approval, but sponsors should consult with the relevant IRBs to confirm whether they are required to obtain an IRB approval and informed consent from study participants.

Clinical investigations must comply with all applicable IDE regulations and Good Clinical Practices (GCPs) – an overview is provided in Table 5.5.

Foreign companies wanting to conduct a clinical trial in the United States must have a US sponsor, who is then responsible for submitting the IDE application to the FDA. IDE sponsors do not need to submit a PMA application or 510(k), register their establishment or list the device while the device is under investigation. Sponsors of IDEs are also exempt from the QSR except for the requirements for design controls in 21 CFR 820.30.

Details on how to prepare and submit an IDE application are available on the FDA's website [71]. Important elements required for an IDE application include:

- Scientific literature review;
- Investigational plan;
- Description of the methods, facilities and controls used for the manufacture, processing, packing, storage and installation of the device;
- Participating investigators and investigating sites; and
- Approving IRBs.

Table 5.5 Overview of regulatory requirements for clinical investigations in the United States

Applicable regulations and requirements	Significant-risk devices	Non-significant-risk devices	IDE-exempt investigations
FDA approval of IDE application – 21 CFR 812.20, 812.25, 812.27	√	N/A	N/A
Institutional review board (IRB) approval – 21 CFR 812.56			Case by case
Labelling to include statement: "CAUTION - Investigational Device. Limited by Federal (or United States) law to investigational use." – 21 CFR 812.5	√	√	N/A
Distribution of investigational devices to qualified investigators only – 21 CFR 812.43(b)	√	√	N/A
Informed consent to be signed by each subject prior to study commencement – 21 CFR 50	√	√	Case by case
Monitoring to ensure ongoing compliance with approved protocols – 21 CFR 812.46	√	√	N/A
Prohibition of commercialization, promotion and misrepresentation of an investigational device and prolongation of the study – 21 CFR 812.7	√	√	N/A
Records and reports to investigators, IRBs and the FDA – 21 CFR 812.140, 812.150	√	√	N/A

There are three possible outcomes following an IDE application and they are explained in the recent FDA guidance, *FDA Decisions for Investigational Device Exemption Clinical Investigations* [72]:

- **Approval** – the sponsor may begin subject enrollment upon receipt of IRB approval and in accordance with the limits described in FDA's decision letter.
- **Approval with Conditions** – the sponsor may begin subject enrollment upon receipt of IRB approval and in accordance with the limits described in the FDA's decision letter and

must submit information addressing the issues identified as conditions of approval in the FDA's letter within 45 days.

- **Disapproval** – the sponsor may not initiate enrollment in the clinical investigation until the sponsor submits an amendment to the IDE to respond to the deficiencies identified in the FDA's letter and subsequently receives a new letter from the FDA granting approval or approval with conditions.

Sponsors are encouraged to use the pre-submission process mentioned earlier, especially for new and novel devices, to avoid delays in the IDE review and approval process.

The FDA has published on its website common problems with original IDE applications – useful to know in order to avoid in own IDE applications. They include:

- Premature IDE submission with inadequate report of prior investigations, inadequate investigational plan and inadequate or incomplete design and manufacture information;
- Laboratory studies with inadequate description of methods, inadequate or no summary or conclusion or conclusions not supported by data;
- Reports of animal studies with no rationale for animal selection, no scientific justification for the number of animals selected, inappropriate duration or follow-up, failure to address compliance with *Good Laboratory Practices for Nonclinical Studies* in 21 CFR Part 58;
- Reports of prior publications with incomplete searches, copies of relevant publications not included, omission of adverse information and failure to identify relevant parts or information and to summarize;
- Investigational plan that does not clearly define study objectives, inadequate description of the protocol, failure to identify all risks, investigational plan includes elements that would expose study subjects to unacceptable probable risks, failure to develop proper monitoring procedures and inadequate informed consent documents;
- Inadequate characterization or description of the device and its operation due to inadequate or omitted: design/

engineering drawing of device, rationale for device design, device and performance specifications, description of materials (including biocompatibility information), description of function – how does device and/or components/subsystems work together to achieve desired function, validation testing for subsystems and main system; and
- Inadequate or missing description of the controls used to ensure that the devices are produced consistently and as designed [73].

5.2.2.6 IDE early/expanded access

There are circumstances under which a healthcare professional may wish to use an unapproved device to save the life of a patient or to help a patient suffering from a serious disease or condition for which no other alternative therapy exists. Patients and physicians faced with these circumstances may have access to investigational devices under one of five main mechanisms by which the FDA may make an unapproved device available [74]:

- **Emergency Research** – The human subject is in a life-threatening situation and it is not feasible to obtain informed consent. To allow such research to go ahead, special provisions for exception from informed consent requirements must be met. In addition, the IRB and a physician not participating in the investigation must review and approve the investigation. The sponsor must also submit a separate original IDE application to the FDA.
- **Emergency Use** – The human subject has a life-threatening or serious disease or serious condition requiring *immediate* use, for which there is no generally accepted alternative and there is no time to obtain FDA approval. The sponsor must notify the FDA of the emergency use within five days through a submission of an IDE report describing the details of the case and the patient protection measures that were followed. (Emergency use is not research!)
- **Compassionate Use** – The human subject has a serious disease or condition and there is no alternative treatment

or diagnose. It allows access for patients who do not meet the requirements for inclusion in the clinical investigation but for whom the treating physician believes the device may provide a benefit in treating and/or diagnosing their disease or condition. This provision is typically approved for individual patients but may be approved to treat a small group. (Compassionate use is not research!)

- **Treatment Use** – An approved IDE specifies the maximum number of clinical sites and the maximum number of human subjects that may be enrolled in the study. During the course of the clinical trial, if the data suggests that the device is effective, then the trial may be expanded to include additional patients with life-threatening or serious diseases, for whom there is no alternative.
- **Continued Access** – The FDA may allow continued enrollment of subjects after the controlled clinical trial under an IDE has been completed in order to allow access to the investigational medical device, while the marketing application is being prepared by the sponsor or reviewed by the FDA, provided this is in the interest of public health or if preliminary evidence indicates that the device will be effective and there are no significant safety concerns.

5.2.2.7 Custom-device exemption

Custom devices are those developed or modified in order to comply with the order of an individual physician or dentist. To qualify for a custom-device exemption, no more than 5 units per year must be produced.

The custom-device exemption provision allows for development of two different categories of custom devices, patient-centric and physician-centric. A custom device made to treat a patient's sufficiently rare condition leaves a medical practice with the patient, while a custom device made to satisfy a physician's unique special need remains with that physician for use in his or her practice.

Custom devices are exempt from PMA requirements and conformance to mandatory performance standards, but they are not exempt from any other requirements, including, but not limited to:

- *Quality System Regulation, including Design Controls* (21 CFR Part 820);
- *Medical Device Reporting* (21 CFR Part 803);
- *Labelling* (21 CFR Part 801); in addition, the labelling accompanying a custom device should include the following information: (1) a statement that the device is a custom device, (2) the name of the ordering physician, (3) identifying information for the patient (if applicable) whom the device is intended to treat, (4) indications for use, (5) sterilization status, (6) relevant composition information (materials, components, etc.) and (7) storage conditions;
- *Corrections and Removals* (21 CFR Part 806); and
- *Registration and Listing* (21 CFR Part 807).

More details are available in the FDA guidance document *Custom Device Exemption* [75].

5.2.2.8 Research-use-only and investigational-use only IVDs

The distribution of IVD products without approval or clearance labeled "Research Use Only" (RUO) or "Investigational Use Only" (IUO), but intended for purposes other than research or investigation (e.g., for clinical diagnostic use), has led, in some cases, to the clinical diagnostic use of products with unproven performance characteristics and with manufacturing controls that are inadequate to ensure consistent manufacturing of the finished product. Use of such tests for clinical diagnostic purposes may mislead healthcare providers and cause serious adverse health consequences to patients, who are not aware that they are being diagnosed with or treated on the basis of the results of tests with research or investigational products. The FDA guidance *Distribution of In Vitro Diagnostic Products Labeled for Research Use Only or Investigational Use Only* clarifies the requirements applicable to RUO and IUO IVD products, including that RUO and IUO labelling must be consistent with the manufacturer's intended use of the device [76].

An RUO product is an IVD product that is in the laboratory research phase of development and is being shipped or delivered for an investigation that is not subject to IDE regulations under 21

CFR Part 812. During the research phase of development, the focus of manufacturer-initiated studies is typically to evaluate design, limited-scale performance and issues such as usability of the test. Some examples of products in this research phase include:

- Tests that are in development to identify test kit methodology, necessary components and analytes to be measured;
- Instrumentation, software or other electrical/mechanical components under development to determine correct settings, subcomponents, subassemblies, basic operational characteristics and possible use methods; and
- Reagents under development to determine production methods, purification levels, packaging needs, shelf life, storage conditions, etc.

An IUO product is an IVD product that is being shipped or delivered for product testing that is not subject to IDE regulations under 21 CFR Part 812 (with the exception of §812.119, *Disqualification of Clinical Investigator*) prior to full commercial marketing (e.g., for testing of specimens derived from humans to compare the usefulness of the product with other products or procedures which are in current use or recognized as useful). Examples of IVD products under investigation include those that are being evaluated in comparison studies that use archived or fresh specimens to determine performance characteristics.

5.2.3 *Australia*

As with any other jurisdiction, manufacturers wishing to market therapeutic goods in Australia must first establish how their product is regulated in Australia (device, drug, biological) and then determine the risk classification according to Australian guidelines. Therapeutic products must be included in the *Australian Register for Therapeutic Goods* (ARTG) prior to being imported, supplied in or exported from Australia.

Medical device manufacturers or sponsors need to draw up an Australian Declaration of Conformity (DoC), which is a legally binding document signed by an authorized person whereby the manufacturer declares compliance of the device with the Australian requirements. DoC templates are provided on the Therapeutic Goods Administration's (TGA) website [77].

For Class 1 non-sterile, non-measuring medical devices and for Class 1 IVDs the manufacturer can self-declare compliance; hence he or she only needs to prepare the DoC and apply for inclusion in the ARTG via TGA eBusiness Services, or eBS, as mentioned in Section 5.1.2.3 in this chapter. The technical documentation has to be maintained and made available upon request.

For all other medical devices and IVDs the manufacturer must apply a conformity assessment procedure according to the Australian Therapeutic Goods (Medical Devices) Regulations and obtain TGA approval.

The manufacturer must generate and maintain product-specific documentation in accordance with regulations and guidelines, as detailed in Section 3.1.3, "Documentation Mandated by Australian Regulations".

5.2.3.1 Conformity assessment procedures

The risk classification determines which conformity assessment procedures can be applied. Conformity assessment modules applicable to the various risk classes of medical devices and IVDs are shown in Fig. 5.12, where modules are identified by the part (and section, if relevant) of the regulations.

For instance, the "Part 1.6 Design Examination" module in Fig. 5.12 refers to Section 1.6, "Examination of Design of Class 4 IVD Medical Device, Class 4 In-House IVD Medical Device, Class AIMD Medical Device or Class III Medical Device", of Part 1 of the Australian Therapeutic Goods (Medical Devices) Regulations.

Conformity assessment for high-risk devices such as Class III medical devices, AIMDs, Class 4 IVDs and Class 4 in-house IVDs requires both a design examination or a type examination and a quality system assessment. Usually, the design or type examination is done first, followed by the QMS audit or statistical verification of manufactured product, as applicable.

A condition of including AIMDs, Class III and implantable Class IIb devices in the ARTG is that the sponsor provides three consecutive annual reports to the TGA, listing the complaints received by the manufacturer over the year relating to problems with the use of the device, including complaints relating to the device supplied under a different name in other countries. Annual reports are due on October 1 each year and should cover the period July 1 of the preceding year to June 30 of the current year. If the device is included in the ARTG before April 1, then the annual report is due in October of that year; if included in the ARTG after April 1, the annual report will not be required until October 1 the following year.

Australian regulations define "in-house IVDs" as those that are developed within a laboratory or laboratory network and that are not supplied in a commercial context. Class 1, 2 and 3 in-house IVDs do not have to follow conformity procedures shown in Fig. 5.12, but laboratories making Class 1, 2 or 3 in-house IVDs must be accredited as a medical testing laboratory by the National Association of Testing Authorities (NATA) or by a Conformity Assessment Body (CAB) determined by the Australian Secretary of Health. An in-house IVD is:

- Developed de novo; or
- Developed or modified from a published source; or
- Developed or modified from any other source; or
- Used for a purpose other than that intended by the manufacturer, within the confines or scope of a laboratory or a laboratory network; and
- Not supplied for use outside the laboratory or laboratory network.

The reality is, most medical devices and IVDs placed on the Australian market come from overseas and most have a CE marking approval already. Since Australian regulations are modeled on the EU regulations, a CE marking approval will satisfy most Australian requirements, especially those related to conformity assessments of the quality systems using the ISO 13485 standard.

Certificates of Conformity issued by accredited CABs such as EU Notified Bodies can be used, with some exceptions, to obtain TGA approval; however, the TGA reserves the right to perform so-called application audits, which are mandatory for all high-risk devices and for some moderate-risk devices. Application audits ensure that

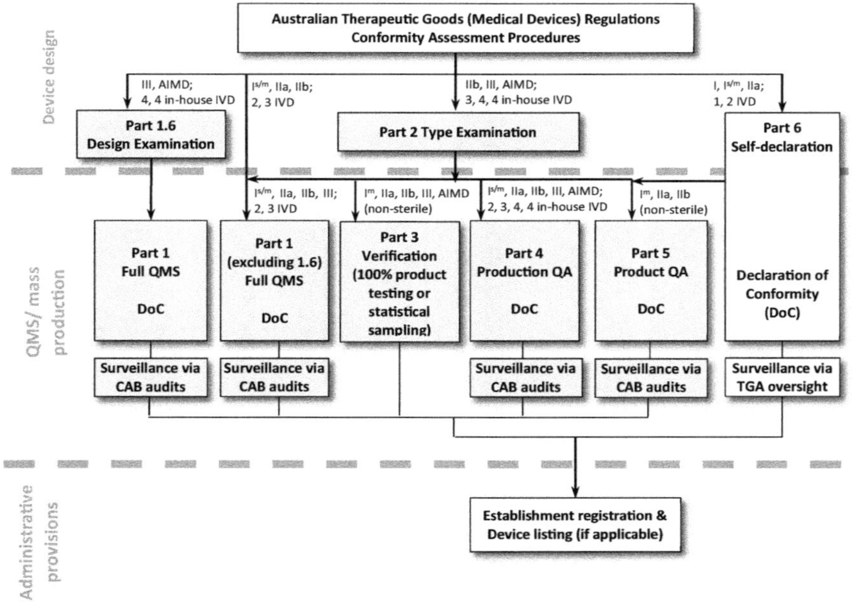

Figure 5.12 Australian Therapeutic Goods (Medical Devices) Regulations – Conformity assessment procedures. *Notes*: Shaded boxes indicate the procedures that require submission of an application to the TGA. Letters "s" and "m" in superscript indicate Class 1 devices supplied sterile and with a measuring function, respectively.

TGA reviews aspects of the device design, including correct risk classification in accordance with Australian regulations (5 pp. 136–141).

For medical devices that are manufactured overseas, except for those excluded from the Mutual Recognition Agreements (MRAs) or otherwise specified in the legislation, manufacturers may use:

- Certificates of Conformity issued by EU Notified Bodies under the EU MD and AIMD Directives, provided the correct conformity assessment procedure has been used (see Table 5.6); or
- Certificates of Conformity to Australian regulations issued under the MRAs with the EU and the European Free Trade Association (EFTA).

Table 5.6 Parallel references for the Australian and EU conformity assessment procedures for medical devices other than IVDs

Australian conformity assessment procedures for medical devices	MDD reference	AIMDD reference
Schedule 3 Part 1 – Full quality assurance procedures	Annex II	Annex 2
Schedule 3 Part 1, Clause 1.6 – Examination of design of Class AIMD or Class III	Annex II.4	Annex 2.4
Schedule 3 Part 2 – Type examination procedures	Annex III	Annex 3
Schedule 3 Part 3 – Verification procedures	Annex IV	Annex 4
Schedule 3 Part 4 – Production quality assurance procedures	Annex V	Annex 5
Schedule 3 Part 5 – Product quality assurance procedures	Annex VI	–
Schedule 3 Part 6 – Declaration of conformity procedures	Annex VII	–
Schedule 3 Part 7 – Procedures for medical devices used for a special purpose	Annex VIII and Article 12	–

For Class III, AIMD and some Class IIb devices covered by EC certificates a mandatory application audit will be conducted once the sponsor lodges an application for inclusion on the ARTG with the TGA. The application audit is to confirm that the manufacturer of a medical device has carried out conformity assessment procedures appropriate to the classification of the medical device (5 pp. 183–191).

Medical devices excluded from the MRAs are:

- Radioactive materials to the extent that these may be considered to be medical devices; and
- Medical devices incorporating tissues of animal origin; however, medical devices incorporating refined derivatives of animal-derived waxes, heparin and gelatin that conform to pharmacopoeial standards and sintered hydroxyapatite, or incorporating tissues of animal origin and where the device is intended to come into contact with intact skin only are included.

Also, the Therapeutic Goods legislation does not allow the TGA to accept an MRA certificate for medical devices that contain:

- Materials of animal, microbial or recombinant origin;
- Derivatives of human blood or plasma; or
- A medicine.

For IVDs that are manufactured overseas, except for Class 4 and Class 4 in-house IVDs, manufacturers may use:

- Conformity assessment certificates issued by EU Notified Bodies under the EU IVDD, provided the correct conformity assessment procedure has been used (see Table 5.7);
- ISO 13485 certificates issued by a EU Notified Body under the IVDD, a Canadian Medical Devices Conformity Assessment System (CMDCAS)-recognized registrar or a CAB-accredited under the International Accreditation Forum (IAF) scheme; or
- For Class 3 IVDs, a Class III or IV Medical Device Active Licence Listing (MDALL) issued by Health Canada under the Canadian Medical Devices Regulations.

Table 5.7 Parallel references for the Australian and EU conformity assessment procedures for IVDs

Australian conformity assessment procedures for IVDs	IVDD reference
Schedule 3 Part 1 - Full quality assurance procedures	Annex IV
Schedule 3 Part 1, Clause 1.6 - Examination of design of Class 4 IVD medical device and Class 4 In-house IVD medical device	Annex IV.4
Schedule 3 Part 2 - Type examination procedures	Annex V
Schedule 3 Part 4 - Production quality assurance procedures	Annex VII
Schedule 3 Part 6 - Declaration of conformity procedures	Annex III

Some Class 2 and 3 IVDs require a mandatory application audit (technical file review) by the TGA [78].

Class 4 IVDs and Class 4 in-house IVDs require conformity assessment performed by the TGA.

Further details on what manufacturers need to do to supply medical devices and IVDs in Australia are available on the TGA's website [79].

Until recently, Australian manufacturers were required to seek conformity assessment certification from the TGA in order to place medical devices or IVDs on the Australian market, whereas foreign manufacturers could use Certificates of Conformity issued by EU Notified Bodies. Historically, conformity assessment certification by EU Notified Bodies could be completed in less time and at less expense than the TGA approval, thus putting Australian manufacturers at a disadvantage, especially when Australian manufacturers needed TGA approval in order to obtain country of origin approval, which is required when applying for marketing authorization in emerging markets such as China.

Regulatory reforms introduced on November 5, 2014, allow most Australian manufacturers to use third-party CABs with the necessary expertise to undertake certification for medical devices and IVDs as well [80]. With this change, whether the medical device is manufactured in Australia or overseas the manufacturer can choose to have conformity assessment conducted either by the TGA or by an alternative CAB, such as a European Notified Body. For certain device categories an additional application audit by the TGA is required if the latter option is chosen.

TGA conformity assessment continues to be required for specified kinds of high-risk medical devices – those containing medicines or tissues of animal, biological or microbial origin or Class 4 IVD medical devices. This is already the case for such devices manufactured overseas, so all manufacturers would be on a level playing field.

5.2.3.2 Clinical trial exemptions

Australian regulations make provisions for clinical trial schemes for investigations involving devices not included in the ARTG or for using approved devices in an investigation beyond the conditions of its marketing approval. The Therapeutic Goods (Medical Devices) Regulations 2002 – Schedule 1, Part 2, Essential Principle 14 Clinical evidence states, "Every medical device requires clinical evidence, appropriate for the use and classification of the device, demonstrating that the device complies with the applicable provisions of the Essential Principles".

A properly developed risk analysis is crucial in determining what type of clinical data is required for a particular device – clinical studies, literature review and post-market data. An outcome of the analysis is the identification of any residual risks. The clinical data is expected to quantify and address those risks (5 pp. 67–72).

There are two schemes under which clinical trials involving medical devices may be conducted:

- Clinical Trial Notification (CTN) Scheme – involves a notification only to the TGA with a nominal notification fee (no approval or decision is made by the TGA); and
- Clinical Trial Exemption (CTX) Scheme – comprises an assessment by the TGA of summary data and usage guidelines for a proposed clinical development program, and if approval is granted the subsequent trials must be carried out under the terms of the approval and be notified to the TGA.

Manufacturers or sponsors may choose which clinical trial scheme to use and this low regulatory threshold for initiating a clinical study makes Australia an attractive first-world country for conducting clinical trials. Details on the CTN and CTX processes are available from the TGA website (5 pp. 267–274).

Clinical trials must be approved by a Human Research Ethics Committee (HREC). The committee must be constituted and operating in accordance with the National Health and Medical Research Council's (NHMRC) National Statement on Ethical Conduct in Human Research [81]. With respect to the conduct of a trial at a specific site, approval of the trial is required from an HREC with jurisdiction at that site. Clinical trials in which medical devices are used within the conditions of their marketing approval are not subject to CTN or CTX requirements but still need to be approved by an HREC before the trial may commence.

Medical devices used in clinical trials must be labelled with wording indicating that they are intended for pre-market clinical investigations, as required in Essential Principle §13.3 item 9, of the Therapeutic Goods (Medical Devices) Regulations 2002, Schedule 1 Essential Principles. Similarly, IVDs used for performance evaluations only must be labelled with wording to that effect.

5.2.3.3 Authorised Prescriber scheme

The TGA may grant certain medical practitioners authority to prescribe a specified unapproved medical device to recipients who have a particular medical condition. The medical practitioner becomes an Authorised Prescriber and can prescribe that product for that condition to individual patients in their immediate care without further approval from the TGA. The use of such unapproved devices is regarded as experimental.

The Authorised Prescriber is only allowed to supply the device directly to specified patients and not to other practitioners who are not authorized to prescribe/administer the device to patients. The basis for providing the approval is that the authorized medical practitioner has training and expertise appropriate for the condition being treated and the proposed use of the device and that the Authorised Prescriber is able to best determine the needs of the patient and to monitor the outcome of therapy.

Authorised Prescribers can supply individual patients with unapproved therapeutic goods under a range of circumstances, such as when:

- Devices were provided initially to patients through a clinical trial while an application for inclusion on the ARTG is being considered;
- Devices are available overseas but not in Australia; and
- No suitable alternative approved device is available in Australia.

Patients who may access unapproved medical devices prescribed by an Authorised Prescriber are those suffering from an illness or condition that is either:

- Life-threatening; or
- Serious, being generally accepted as not being appropriate to be diagnosed or evaluated and treated safely without consulting a health practitioner.

5.2.3.4 Special access scheme

The special access scheme (SAS) is a mechanism to provide for the import and/or supply of an unapproved therapeutic good for a single patient on a case-by-case basis. Applications are made by registered medical practitioners. The SAS allows individual patients, with the support of their medical practitioner, access to unapproved devices in a range of circumstances, such as when:

- Early access for terminally ill patients to almost any device, including experimental and investigational devices is needed (see Category A);
- Devices were provided initially to patients through a clinical trial while a marketing application is being considered; and
- Devices are available overseas but not in Australia.

The final responsibility for the use of an unapproved device within an institution always rests with that institution. Medical practitioners working in an institution may also need approval from the institution's Ethics Committee or Drug and Therapeutics Committee prior to using a particular device. There are two categories of patients who may use the SAS:

- Category A patients – defined in the Therapeutic Goods legislation as "persons who are seriously ill with a condition from which death is reasonably likely to occur within a matter of months, or from which premature death is reasonably likely to occur in the absence of early treatment". Medical practitioners can supply unapproved devices to some very seriously ill patients without the approval of the TGA as long as the medical practitioner notifies the TGA within 28 days.
- Category B patients – all other patients. Approval of an application to supply an unapproved device is required from a delegate in the TGA. Approval by the TGA is given on a patient-by-patient basis to reflect the needs of different patients.

The choice of classification of each patient lies with the treating medical practitioner. However, the TGA is able to review, seek clarification and request information regarding the classification of patients under Category A.

5.2.3.5 Personal importation

Personal importation occurs when an individual:

- Brings a medical device into Australia on his or her person; or
- Arranges from within Australia for a device to be sent to him or her from an overseas supplier.

The goods must be used by that individual or a member of his/her immediate family and must not be sold or supplied to any other person.

Where the device is classified as low–medium risk (Class IIa) or higher, the quantity imported must not exceed the amount required to deliver three months' treatment using the device according to a treating medical practitioner's directions. The total quantity imported per year must not exceed 15 months' treatment using the device according to a treating medical practitioner's directions.

These supply restrictions do not apply to devices used for long-term treatment, such as a hip implant.

5.2.4 *Canada*

Prior to selling medical devices and IVDs in Canada, manufacturers of Class II, III and IV devices must obtain a Medical Device Licence. Class I devices do not require a Medical Device Licence; however, manufacturers, distributors and importers are required to obtain an Establishment Licence.

5.2.4.1 Medical Device Licence

The documentation required for a Medical Device Licence application depends on the risk classification of the device involved. According to Part 1 General, Section 32, of the Medical Devices Regulations, in addition to information such as manufacturer name and address, medical device name, identifier and risk classification, the application must include the following items:

Class II devices – Section 32(2) of the Medical Devices Regulations

(a) A description of the medical conditions, purposes and uses for which the device is manufactured, sold or represented;
(b) A list of the standards complied with in the manufacture of the device to satisfy the safety and effectiveness requirements;
(c) An attestation by a senior official of the manufacturer that the manufacturer has objective evidence to establish that the device meets the safety and effectiveness requirements;
(d) An attestation by a senior official of the manufacturer that the device label meets the applicable labelling requirements of these regulations;
(e) In the case of a near patient IVD device, an attestation by a senior official of the manufacturer that investigational testing has been conducted on the device using human subjects representative of the intended users and under conditions similar to the conditions of use; and

(f) A copy of the QMS certificate certifying that the QMS under which the device is manufactured satisfies the National Standard of Canada CAN/CSA-ISO 13485:03, *Medical devices – Quality management systems – Requirements for regulatory purposes* (design control requirements are not mandatory).

Class III devices – Section 32(3) of the Medical Devices Regulations

(a) A description of the device and of the materials used in its manufacture and packaging;
(b) A description of the features of the device that permit it to be used for the medical conditions, purposes and uses for which it is manufactured, sold or represented;
(c) A list of the countries other than Canada where the device has been sold, the total number of units sold in those countries and a summary of any reported problems with the device and any recalls of the device in those countries;
(d) A list of the standards complied with in the design and manufacture of the device to satisfy the safety and effectiveness requirements;
(e) In the case of a device to be sold in a sterile condition, a description of the sterilization method used;
(f) A summary of all studies on which the manufacturer relies to ensure that the device meets the safety and effectiveness requirements, and the conclusions drawn from those studies by the manufacturer;
(g) A copy of the device label;
(h) In the case of a near patient IVD device, a summary of investigational testing conducted on the device using human subjects representative of the intended users and under conditions similar to the conditions of use;
(i) A bibliography of all published reports dealing with the use, safety and effectiveness of the device; and
(j) A copy of the QMS certificate certifying that the QMS under which the device is designed and manufactured satisfies the National Standard of Canada CAN/CSA-ISO 13485:03, *Medical devices – Quality management systems – Requirements for*

regulatory purposes (the full QMS including design controls must be covered).

Class IV devices – Section 32(4) of the Medical Devices Regulations

(a) A description of the device and of the materials used in its manufacture and packaging;
(b) A description of the features of the device that permit it to be used for the medical conditions, purposes and uses for which it is manufactured, sold or represented;
(c) A list of the countries other than Canada where the device has been sold, the total number of units sold in those countries and a summary of any reported problems with the device and any recalls of the device in those countries;
(d) A risk assessment comprising an analysis and evaluation of the risks and the risk reduction measures adopted to satisfy the safety and effectiveness requirements;
(e) A quality plan setting out the specific quality practices, resources and sequence of activities relevant to the device;
(f) The specifications of the materials used in the manufacture and packaging of the device;
(g) The manufacturing process of the device;
(h) A list of the standards complied with in the design and manufacture of the device to satisfy the safety and effectiveness requirements;
(i) Detailed information on all studies on which the manufacturer relies to ensure that the device meets the safety and effectiveness requirements, including:

 (i) Pre-clinical and clinical studies;
 (ii) Process validation studies;
 (iii) If appropriate, software validation studies; and
 (iv) Literature studies.

(j) In the case of a medical device other than an IVD device, manufactured from or incorporating animal or human tissue or their derivative, objective evidence of the biological safety of the device;

(k) In the case of a near patient IVD device, detailed information on investigational testing conducted on the device using human subjects representative of the intended users and under conditions similar to the conditions of use;
(l) A summary of the studies referred to in paragraph (i) and the conclusions drawn from those studies by the manufacturer;
(m) A summary of the investigational testing referred to in paragraph (k) and the conclusions drawn from that testing by the manufacturer;
(n) A bibliography of all published reports dealing with the use, safety and effectiveness of the device;
(o) A copy of the device label; and
(p) A copy of the QMS certificate certifying that the QMS under which the device is designed and manufactured satisfies the National Standard of Canada CAN/CSA-ISO 13485:03, *Medical devices – Quality management systems – Requirements for regulatory purposes* (the full QMS including design controls must be covered).

The Summary Technical Documentation (STED) – covered in Chapter 3 – addresses all content requirements for premarket submissions, but the actual section titles and their order in the application dossier may have to be adjusted to align with the Health Canada guidance documents listed in Section 3.1.4, "Documentation Mandated by Canadian Regulations".

Same as in Australia, most medical devices on the Canadian market are imported and already holding certificates and approvals from their country of origin. Instead of the documentation described in Sections 32(2), 32(3) and 32(4) of the Medical Devices Regulations, foreign manufacturers may use a certificate of compliance and a supporting summary report issued by a CAB recognized by the Canadian authorities, also known as CMDCAS-recognized registrars. A list of recognized registrars is available from Health Canada website [82].

A Medical Device Licence is granted bearing an issued date. There is no expiry date. However, Section 43 of the Medical Devices Regulations requires every manufacturer of a licensed medical device or their authorized regulatory correspondent to confirm annually, before November 1, that the information held by Health Canada is accurate or that amendments to correct the information will be made. Failure to do so may result in cancellation of the licence.

5.2.4.2 Custom-made and special access devices

Part 2 of the Medical Devices Regulations covers custom-made devices and medical devices that are to be imported or sold for special access. Special access means access to a medical device for emergency use or if conventional therapies have failed, are unavailable or are unsuitable.

All custom-made and special access devices must bear a statement in their labelling to specify that they are custom made or for special access, respectively.

In addition, Class III or IV custom-made devices and medical devices for special access require an authorization for sale or importation. Further details on custom-made and special access program are available from the Health Canada website [83].

The authorization will specify:

- The number of units of the device authorized to be imported;
- The number of units of the device authorized to be sold; and
- The name of the healthcare professional to whom the manufacturer or importer may sell the device.

5.2.4.3 Investigational testing

Medical Devices Regulations SOR/98-282, Section 32, Application for a Medical Device Licence, require for Class IV devices "detailed information on all studies on which the manufacturer relies to ensure that the device meets the safety and effectiveness requirements, including [. . .] clinical studies".

Part 3 of Medical Devices Regulations covers medical devices for investigational testing involving human subjects (or clinical trials), with further details provided in the guidance document *Preparation of an Application for Investigational Testing - Medical Devices* [84].

Class I medical devices may be sold to a qualified investigator for the purpose of conducting investigational testing if the manufacturer or importer possesses records that contain all the information and documents required by Section 81 of the regulations – required information includes details about the product design and manufacturing process, investigational plan and protocol.

Class II, III or IV medical devices may be sold to a qualified investigator for the purpose of conducting investigational testing if the manufacturer or importer holds an authorization and possesses records that contain all the information and documents required by Section 81 of the regulations.

Section 86 of the Medical Devices Regulations sets out the requirements of a label on a device sold for investigational testing. In addition to the name of the manufacturer and the name of the device, labels of investigational devices must include the following statements:

- "Investigational Device" and "Instrument de recherche", or any other statement, in English and French, that conveys that meaning;
- "To Be Used by Qualified Investigators Only" and "Réservé uniquement à l'usage de chercheurs compétents", or any other statement, in English and French, that conveys that meaning; and
- In the case of an IVD device, the statements "The performance specifications of this device have not been established" and "Les spécifications de rendement de l'instrument n'ont pas été établies", or any other statement, in English and French, that conveys that meaning.

The Authorization for Investigational Testing will include the following information:

- Name of the qualified investigator to whom the device may be sold;
- Type of diagnosis or treatment for which the device may be sold;
- Number of units of the device that are authorized to be sold; and

- Protocol according to which the investigational testing is to be conducted.

5.2.5 *Japan*

In Japan, the risk classification and regulatory controls applicable to a product category are specified in the Japanese Medical Device Nomenclature (JMDN) system. The JMDN is written in Japanese; therefore it is essential to engage an experienced professional fluent in Japanese for the selection of the appropriate JMDN code applicable to the medical device or IVD.

Depending on the risk classification and the novelty of the product, manufacturers need to submit one of the pre-market applications listed hereafter prior to placing medical devices or IVDs on the market.

Notification, or *Todokede* – it is a self-declaration whereby the Marketing Authorization Holder (MAH) registers the product with the PMDA; applicable to:

- Class I (extremely low risk) “general medical devices”; and
- Class I IVDs.

Certification, or *Ninsho* – this is a certification by a Registered Certification Body (RCB) to existing certification standards; applicable to:

- Class II (low risk) “specified controlled medical devices”;
- Generic/ “me too” Class III (moderate risk) “specially controlled medical devices”; and
- Class II IVDs.

Approval, or *Shonin* – it is a pre-market approval by the Pharmaceuticals and Medical Devices Agency (PMDA) using approval standards or review guidelines, where available; applicable to:

- Class II (low risk) “controlled medical devices” for which there are no standards or that do not comply with standards;
- New or improved Class III (moderate risk) “specially controlled medical devices”;

- Class IV (high risk) "specially controlled medical devices";
- Class II IVDs (low risk) for which there are no standards or that do not comply with existing standards; and
- Class III IVDs (high risk).

The STED – covered in Chapter 3 – addresses all content requirements for pre-market submissions, but the actual section titles and their order in the application dossier may have to be adjusted to align with the PMDA notifications and guidelines listed in Section 3.1.5, "Documentation Mandated by Japanese Regulations".

For Class II, III and IV medical devices, the content of the submission and the type of evaluation will depend on the type of change and novelty of the device:

- Generic ("me too") devices are either the same as, or different but substantially equivalent to, devices already approved in Japan.
- Improved devices are NSE to approved medical devices; differences may require evaluation either based on nonclinical evidence only or based on clinical trial data.
- New or novel devices are different from approved medical devices and require evaluation of clinical trial data.

Where necessary, a pre-submission consultation with the PMDA should help applicants determine the correct type of submission and evaluation applicable to their product (see Table 5.8).

Based on Table 15-5 of Fundamentals of Japanese Regulatory Affairs [85].

Under the previous J-PAL regulations the PMDA conducted quality management audits for products under pre-market approval review (*Shonin*) and RCBs conducted QMS audits under pre-market certification review (*Ninsho*) on a *facility* basis.

The recently enacted PMD Act stipulates that the QMS of an MAH, including all manufacturing facilities registered under the MAH's name, must be assessed on a *product category* basis. Foreign manufacturers holding an MAH licence and their local Designated Marketing Authorization Holder (DMAH) are subject to the QMS audit as well. Upon successful completion of a QMS audit a Certificate of QMS Conformance (*Kijun Tekigoshou*) is issued

Table 5.8 Submission and evaluation categories

Medical device risk class and novelty	Submission and evaluation categories
Generic ("me too") devices – use existing JMDN code, with submission based on a registered technical file – Class II, Class III, Class IV	• Generic device that is same as marketed devices → submission with no approval standards and no clinical trial data
	• Generic device that is substantially equivalent with marketed devices → submission with approval standards and no clinical trial data
Improved devices – use existing JMDN codes, with submission based on new technical file – Class II, Class III, Class IV	• Improved device with differences that can be evaluated using nonclinical evidence only → submission with no approval standards and no clinical trial data
	• Improved device with differences that require clinical trial data to be evaluated → submission with clinical trial data
Novel/new devices – no existing applicable JMDN codes – Class II, Class III, Class IV	• New/novel device → submission with clinical trial data

by the PMDA (for *Shonin* applications) or by an RCB (for *Ninsho* applications). Certificates of QMS Conformance must be renewed every five years [9].

5.2.5.1 Clinical evidence

Ministerial Notification or Yakushokukihatsu No. 0804001 of August 4, 2008, *Necessary Scope of Clinical Investigation Data on Medical Devices*, clarifies the circumstances in which clinical trial data is required:

When the clinical efficacy and safety of a medical device cannot be evaluated based only upon the results of nonclinical investigations such as performance tests and animal tests, or existing literature, etc., a clinical study must be conducted and technical documents on the results of the clinical investigation must be submitted.

> Whether the technical documents on clinical investigation records are necessary will be determined on a number of factors including the characteristics of the particular medical device, equivalency with an existing medical device, and nonclinical investigation results. Therefore, if necessary, use the clinical evaluation consultation or pre-application consultation service offered by the Pharmaceuticals and Medical Devices Agency (PMDA) to determine whether such technical documents are necessary [86].

This means that clinical trial data is required for Class II, III and IV medical devices that are new or improved, which are NSE to predicate products in the Japanese market (refer also to Section 1.5.2.2, "Japanese Classification System for Medical Devices, Including IVDs").

It is not mandatory for clinical trials to be performed in Japan. Data obtained from trials conducted in other countries can be used for regulatory submissions, provided the clinical trials are conducted in accordance with Japanese Good Clinical Practice, or GCP [87], or an equivalent standard such as the ICH GCP guideline [88] and that the clinical safety and efficacy for Japanese patients is evaluated and proven [89].

5.2.6 *Emerging Markets*

5.2.6.1 China

5.2.6.1.1 Overview of the regulatory regime

The first medical device regulations in China were adopted in 2000 with State Council Order 276. Since then there have been many additions and improvements, culminating with a major overhaul introduced by State Council Order 650 in 2014. The newly revised regulations include significant changes to the product classification rules and the implementation of risk-based regulatory controls, aligning thus better with the major established markets. A list of

Table 5.9 Regulations and regulatory guidelines adopted in China in 2014

Order no.	Date	Title
Order No. 650	June 1, 2014	Supervision and Administration of Medical Devices
Order No. 4	Oct. 1, 2014	Administrative Measures for Medical Device Registration
Order No. 5	Oct. 1, 2014	Administrative Measures for the Registration of IVDs
Order No. 6	Oct. 1, 2014	Administrative Rules for the Instruction and Labels of Medical Devices
Order No. 7	Oct. 1, 2014	Administrative Measures for the Supervision of Medical Device Manufacturing
Order No. 8	Oct. 1, 2014	Administrative Measures for the Supervision of Medical Device Distribution

Source: CFDA [90]

regulations and regulatory guidelines newly adopted in China for medical devices and IVDs is provided in Table 5.9.

The China Food and Drug Administration (CFDA) is the government agency responsible for the regulation of food, drugs, cosmetics and medical devices, including IVDs. It was established in 2013 by incorporating the State Food and Drug Administration (SFDA) and other government departments. The Department of Medical Device Registration is responsible for pre-market approval. The Department of Medical Device Supervision is responsible for post-market surveillance [91].

Under the new classification rules devices are classified into three risk classes, taking into consideration their indications for use, intended use, principle of operation, technology and basic design features:

- Class I – low-risk devices, for which safety and effectiveness can be ensured through routine administration;
- Class II – moderate-risk devices, for which strict control is required to ensure safety and effectiveness; and
- Class III – high-risk devices, for which special methods are required to strictly control their safety and effectiveness

The registration process of medical devices and IVDs is clearer and more streamlined than before. All medical devices and IVDs that are imported into China must be registered through the CFDA at the national level. Domestic manufacturers must register their devices with various departmental levels of the CFDA, depending on the device risk classification, as follows:

- Class I – with local municipal departments of the CFDA;
- Class II – with provincial departments of the CFDA; and
- Class III – with CFDA at the national level.

The Chinese classification system is similar to the nomenclature-based US system. The risk classification of a medical device is determined on the basis of the applicable classification code (similar to the US Product Code Classification Database) and the generic product name. When classifying a device, the manufacturer should refer to the catalogues for medical device classification. If a device does not fit into any of the existing categories in the catalogue, an application for classification should be submitted to the relevant CFDA department [92].

For imported devices applicants must submit evidence of marketing approval issued by the Regulatory Authority in the manufacturer's country of origin, such as an EC Certificate of Conformity for an EU-based manufacturer, an FDA 510(k) clearance PMA letter for a US-based manufacturer or a TGA Certificate for an Australian-based manufacturer. This is to ensure that only devices that already conform to their country of origin requirements for quality, safety and efficacy are imported into China. For lower-risk devices, country-of-origin certificates may not always list all the details such as individual model number or manufacturing sites that are required by the CFDA. Hence the applicant may need to provide an additional certificate that includes those details, for instance, a Certificate to Foreign Government (US) or a Certificate of Free Sale (Australia).

5.2.6.1.2 Regulatory pathway

The risk classification determines the regulatory pathway and the level of regulatory controls applied in the premarket phase (see Table 5.10).

Based on Figure 4 of *AusBiotech Guide* [92]

Under the newly revised regulations, manufacturers of Class I devices only need to prepare the technical documentation, including

Table 5.10 Risk classification and regulatory controls in China

Class I	Class II	Class III
Application filing with CFDA	STED for CMDE technical review Type testing reports from China accredited lab China clinical trials (unless exempt)	STED for CMDE technical review Type testing reports from China accredited lab China clinical trials (unless exempt) Clinical trial approval for selected high-risk devices

a DoC to Chinese regulations and standards and then submit a filing of Class I medical devices to the relevant CFDA office. No pre-market assessment or registration is required for Class I devices.

Once the CFDA confirms completeness of the filing dossier, it issues a Class I Medical Device Filing Certificate with an official Filing Number, which must be affixed on the product labels and instructions for use. Details for the format and content of a Class I medical device filing dossier are provided in CFDA Announcement No. 26 of May 2014.

For low- and moderate-risk devices a country-of-origin approval may not list the details required by the CFDA, such as individual model designation; hence the country-of-origin approval may have to be combined with another official document (such as an export-only certificate) to ensure that the full details of the product and the manufacturer information are provided to the CFDA.

Class II and III devices must pass type testing by a CFDA-accredited laboratory (based in China) and, unless exempt, undergo clinical trials in China. Upon completion of verification and validation (V&V) manufacturers must prepare a Chinese equivalent of the STED, including an Essential Requirements (ERs) checklist and a DoC, and submit an application to the relevant CFDA office for a pre-market assessment. Details for the format and content of a Class II and III medical device filing dossier are provided in CFDA Announcement No. 43 of September 2014 and for IVDs in Announcement No. 44 of September 2014.

The CFDA authorizes the Centre for Medical Device Evaluation (CMDE) to conduct technical reviews. Manufacturers may consult the CMDE on matters related to medical devices evaluation; the CMDE is open for consultation one day per week.

Once the pre-market assessment is completed with a positive result the CFDA grants marketing approval in form of a registration certificate. Registration certificates for Class II and III devices have a five-year validity period and require renewal if manufacturers wish to continue to market their products after the end of the validity period. An application for renewal should be submitted six months prior to certificate expiry. The application for certificate renewal must include a summary of the serious adverse events (SAEs) for the previous certification period.

While the country-of-origin approval and/or an ISO 13485 certificate would attest that imported Class II and III devices are manufactured under a compliant QMS, some manufacturers may be selected for an on-site audit if the CFDA deems appropriate during the application review [92].

5.2.6.1.3 Type testing

Most foreign manufacturers would have the complete V&V completed before initiating type testing in China. However, Class II and III devices are required to undergo type testing by a (China-based) CFDA-accredited laboratory. Currently there are 10 testing facilities in the country and they specialize in different areas of testing. The manufacturer must prepare in advance Product Technical Requirements (previously known as Product Standards) detailing the specifications of their product and how to test for those specifications.

Product Technical Requirements would typically include applicable type testing such as electrical safety, electromagnetic compatibility (EMC), biocompatibility, radio frequency (RF) testing and sterility. An example of a Master V&V Plan is provided in Section 4.4.1.5, "Master V&V Plan". Often, due to capacity or expertise limitations, it is not possible to repeat the entire set of tests in China. Manufacturers should negotiate with the relevant test centre and agree on which foreign V&V reports can be accepted without re-test.

One reason for having to repeat type testing in China is the difference between international and Chinese standards for type testing – due to a lag in adopting the most recent version of an international standard or due to variations in requirements. For example:

- The current Chinese safety standard for electrical medical devices GB9706.1-2007 is equivalent to the second edition of the international standard IEC 60601-1:1998, which was superseded by the third edition IEC 60601-1:2005; the third edition has been adopted and is currently being used in most established markets.
- The Chinese standard for EMC YY0505-2005, while similar to the international standard IEC 60601-1-2:2007, has different acceptance limits.

The applicable standards in China are, in order of precedence:

- YY Industry Standards – for example, YY 0505:2012 similar to IEC 60601-1-2:2004.
- GB China National Standards – for example, GB 9706.1:2007 standard equivalent to IEC 60601-1:1998 Ed.2; GB 16866 standard series equivalent to ISO 10993 series.
- YY/T and GB/T, are "Recommended" standards, however compliance is advisable, unless duly justifiable.

5.2.6.1.4 Clinical evidence

The requirement to provide data from clinical trials conducted in China for all Class II and III medical devices and IVDs, unless officially exempt, was introduced by the revised regulations in 2014.

Products officially exempt are listed in the CFDA exemption catalogue, which in 2014 included 488 Class II devices (Announcement No. 12 of 2014 [93]) and 79 Class III devices (Announcement No. 13 of 2014 covering [94]). As the exemption catalogue is in Chinese, it is essential to engage an experienced professional fluent in Chinese to check whether a particular product category is exempt.

Alternatively, an exemption from in-country clinical trials can be obtained by demonstrating one of the following:

- The medical device has a well-defined operating principle, an established design and mature manufacturing processes, with no record of SAEs of substantially equivalent devices, which have been marketed and in clinical use for years; without changing the conventional intended use; or
- The safety and effectiveness can be demonstrated through nonclinical assessment; or
- Safety and effectiveness can be demonstrated through analyzing and by evaluating data obtained from clinical trials or clinical application of a substantially equivalent device.

In August 2014 the CFDA issued a guidance on clinical evaluation (still in draft at the time of going to print), describing the requirements for demonstrating substantial equivalence of medical devices to one or more predicate devices available in China. The comparison should cover similarities and differences between the new device and the predicate device(s) and include justifications of why the differences do not negatively impact safety and effectiveness. The proposed guidance also details the requirements for conducting clinical evaluation, which is similar to the European MEDDEV 2.7.1 Rev3 guidance document.

Clinical trials involving moderate- and high-risk medical devices require notification to local CFDA authorities (no pre-approval required). Clinical trials involving selected high-risk Class III devices such as implantable or absorbable medical devices require CFDA approval prior to initiating the study. Key aspects related to the conduct of clinical trials in China are:

- Clinical trials are to be conducted at qualified clinical institutes;
- Two sites are required to collect data for Class II medical devices and IVDs; three sites are required for collecting data for Class III medical devices and IVDs;

- Clinical investigations must have ethics approval and type testing completed with a positive result prior to initiating the study; and
- Clinical trial monitoring and adverse events reporting are required [92].

5.2.6.1.5 Technical dossier

The STED – covered in Chapter 3 – addresses all content requirements for pre-market submissions, but the actual section titles and their order in the application dossier may have to be adjusted to align with the CFDA requirements (see Table 5.11).

5.2.6.1.6 Innovative device pathway

For novel and innovative products, the CFDA has enacted the Special Review and Approval Procedure for Innovative Medical Devices (March 2014) aimed at fast-tracking beneficial premium technology that meets the following eligibility criteria:

- The applicant holds a Chinese patent for innovative technology or be licensed to use such a patent in China; alternatively, the applicant has a patent application under review with preliminary approval from the China Patent Regulatory Authority.
- The product is a first of its kind in China, significantly superior when compared to predicate devices with regard to safety, effectiveness and clinical benefit.
- The applicant has a prototype developed under appropriate design controls [92].

5.2.6.2 ASEAN

The Association of Southeast Asian Nations (ASEAN) Medical Device Directive (AMDD) defines four risk classes of medical devices and IVDs (see Table 5.12) using generic classification rules, Essential Principles of Safety and Performance (EPs) for medical devices and IVDs, and introduces a Common Submission Dossier Template, or CSDT (see Tables 5.13 and 5.14 respectively).

Of all ASEAN member states Singapore has arguably been the most active in taking concrete steps to implement the AMDD since

Table 5.11 Table of contents for a medical device registration application

1st-level application sections	2nd-level application sections
1. Application form	-
2. Supporting documents	-
3. Basic requirements for safety & effectiveness of the medical device	-
4. Summary	4.1 Overview
	4.2 Device description
	4.3 Model and specification
	4.4 Packaging description
	4.5 Indications for use and contraindications
	4.6 Reference to similar or predicate devices (if applicable)
	4.7 Other essential information
5. Product verification and validation (V&V)	5.1 Product performance
	5.2 Biocompatibility assessment
	5.3 Biological safety
	5.4 Sterilization and disinfection processes
	5.5 Shelf life and packaging
	5.6 Animal studies
	5.7 Software
	5.8 Other
6. Manufacturing information	6.1 Manufacturing process description
	6.2 Manufacturing site
7. Clinical evaluation	-
8. Risk analysis	-
9. Product Technical Re uirement (formerly Product Standard)	-
10. Type testing reports issued by CFDA-accredited lab in China	10.1 Type-testing reports
	10.2 Pre-evaluation comments
11. User manual and label samples	
11.1 User manual	
	11.2 Minimum sales unit label sample
12. Declaration of Conformity (DoC)	-

Source: English translation of CFDA Order No. 43

Table 5.12 Risk classification for medical devices and IVDs under the AMDD

Risk class	Medical devices	IVDs
A	Low risk	Low individual risk and low public risk
B	Low to moderate risk	Moderate individual risk and/or low public health risk
C	Moderate to high risk	High individual risk and/or moderate public health risk
D	High risk	High individual risk and/or high public health risk

Table 5.13 Table of contents of an ASEAN CSDT for medical devices other than IVDs

Sections	Section title and description
4.1	Relevant Essential Principles and method used to demonstrate conformity
4.1.1	Essential Principles (EPs) and evidence of conformity
4.2	Device description
4.2.1	Device description and features
4.2.2	Intended use
4.2.3	Indications
4.2.4	Instructions for use
4.2.5	Contraindications
4.2.6	Warnings
4.2.7	Precautions
4.2.8	Potential adverse effects
4.2.9	Alternative therapy
4.2.10	Materials
4.2.11	Other relevant specifications
4.3	Summary of design verification and validation (V&V) documents
4.3.1	Pre-clinical studies
4.3.1.1	Software V&V studies
4.3.1.2	Devices containing biological material
4.3.2	Clinical evidence
4.3.2.1	Use of existing bibliography
4.4	Device labelling
4.4.1	Samples of labels on the device and its packaging
4.4.2	Instructions for use (IFUs)
4.5	Risk analysis
4.5.1	Results of risk analysis
4.6	Manufacturer information
4.6.1	Manufacturing process

Source: HSA [95]

Table 5.14 Table of Contents of an ASEAN CSDT for IVDs

Sections	Section title and description
4.1	Relevant Essential Principles and method used to demonstrate conformity
4.1.1	Essential Principles (EPs) and evidence of conformity
4.2	Device description
4.2.1	Device description and features
4.2.2	Intended use
4.2.3	Instructions for use
4.2.4	Limitations
4.2.5	Warnings
4.2.6	Precautions
4.2.7	Materials
4.2.8	Other relevant specifications
4.2.9	Other descriptive information
4.3	Product verification and validation (V&V)
4.3.1	Pre-clinical studies
4.3.2	Clinical evidence
4.3.2.1	Use of existing bibliography
4.4	Device labelling
4.4.1	Samples of labels on the device and its packaging
4.4.2	Instructions for use (IFUs)
4.5	Risk analysis
4.5.1	Results of risk analysis
4.6	Manufacturer information
4.6.1	Manufacturing process

Source: HSA [95]

it was first drafted in 2012; hence the Singapore model is likely to be adopted by other ASEAN countries as well. The Health Sciences Authority (HSA), Singapore's regulatory agency responsible for regulating drugs, biologics, medical devices and IVDs, has published consultations and regulatory guidelines on its website [96].

Under HAS regulations, dealers of medical devices and IVDs must be licensed by the HSA. Dealers include manufacturers, importers and wholesalers. HSA GN-15 *Guidance on Medical Device Product Registration* defines conformity assessment procedures applicable to medical devices and IVDs in the four risk classes. Regulatory controls are applied proportionately with the level of risk [97].

Class A devices supplied non-sterile do not require product registration, but dealers must provide product lists to be included in the *Singapore Medical Device Register*, or SMDR, and must comply with regulatory provisions for advertising, keeping distribution records and complaint records and adverse event reporting and notification. Manufacturers and importers are, in addition, responsible for ensuring product compliance with the EPs of safety and performance prior to placing the devices on the market.

Class A sterile, Class B, Class C and Class D devices require product registration. Acceptable evidence of QMS compliance includes certification and/or compliance with the following standards and regulations:

- ISO 13485 standard;
- US FDA QSR; and
- Japan MHLW Ordinance 169.

Submissions for Class B, C and D must be in CSDT format and include a EPs checklist and a DoC. Once the pre-market assessment is completed with a positive result the HSA grants marketing approval and the product is listed in the SMDR. Providing evidence of approval from one or more independent reference regulatory agencies – EU Notified Bodies, US FDA, Australia TGA, Health Canada and/or Japan MHLW – will help accelerate the evaluation process.

For Class B devices – evidence supporting an abridged, expedited or immediate evaluation:

- EC Certificates of Conformity issued by EU Notified Bodies, as applicable:
  - √ MDD Annex II Section 3 or Annex V for Class IIa medical devices; or
  - √ IVDD Annex IV or Annex V with Annex VII for List B and self-testing IVDs.
- US FDA 510(k) or PMA – as applicable;
- Australian TGA device registration licence;
- Health Canada device registration licence; and
- Japan MHLW pre-market certification (*Ninsho*) from an RCB or premarket approval (*Shonin*) from MHLW – as applicable.

For Class C and Class D devices – evidence supporting an abridged or expedited evaluation:

- EC Certificates of Conformity issued by EU Notified Bodies, as applicable:
  - √ MDD Annex II Section 3 or Annex III coupled with Annex V for Class IIb medical devices; or
  - √ MDD Annex II Sections 3 and 4 for Class III; or
  - √ AIMDD Annex 2 Sections 3 and 4 for AIMDs; or
  - √ IVDD Annex IV, including Sections 4 and 6 for List A IVDs; or
  - √ IVDD Annex IV or Annex V with Annex VII for List B and self-testing IVDs.
- US FDA 510(k) or PMA– as applicable;
- Australian TGA device registration licence;
- Health Canada device registration licence; and
- Japan MHLW pre-market certification (*Ninsho*) from an RCB or pre-market approval (*Shonin*) from the MHLW – as applicable.

Approvals from the EU and the TGA will qualify as an independent reference regulatory agency's approval for Class C and D applications only if the devices have been reviewed and approved by the respective agencies and the devices are not registered on the basis of the MRA.

5.2.6.3 Brazil

Manufacturers of medical devices and IVDs must obtain a marketing authorization from Agência Nacional de Vigilância Sanitária (ANVISA) prior to placing products on the market. Foreign manufacturers without a local subsidiary need to appoint a Brazil Registration Holder (BRH) to handle applications on their behalf. The BRH can be a local distributor or an independent agent, the latter option affording the foreign manufacturer more control over registration ownership and better protection of intellectual property but potentially at a higher cost.

Medical device regulations are similar to the EU MDD and the level of regulatory control depends on the product risk classification. Medical devices and IVDs are classified into four risk classes – Class I, II, III, or IV – according to their level of risk (see Table 5.15).

Table 5.15 Risk classification for medical devices and IVDs under Brazil regulations

Risk class	Medical devices	IVDs
I	Low risk	Low individual risk and low public risk
II	Low to moderate risk	Moderate individual risk and/or low public health risk
III	Moderate to high risk	High individual risk and/or moderate public health risk
IV	High risk	High individual risk and/or high public health risk

Higher-risk devices require the *registro* submission route; lower-risk devices require the abbreviated *cadastro* submission route.

Medical devices are classified using the classification rules in Annex II of Resolution RDC No. 185/2001, *Registration of medical products*, which mirror closely those in EU MEDDEV Guidance 2.4/1. All Class III and IV medical devices and certain Class I and II devices require a *registro* application. Most Class I and II medical devices are exempt from *registro* application and only require a *cadastro* application. Technical documentation requirements are also defined in Resolution No. 185/2001 [98].

All medical devices must comply with the applicable essential requirements for safety and effectiveness defined in Resolution RDC No. 56/2001 [99]. In addition, most electrical and some non-electrical medical devices must obtain National Institute of Metrology, Quality and Technology (INMETRO) certification before they can be registered with ANVISA. This involves testing and certification by an organization accredited by INMETRO or by members of international accreditation schemes EA, IAAC, IAF or ILAC (see also Table 1.3 in Chapter 1). An INMETRO certificate authorizes the certificate holder to affix the INMETRO certification mark on its products. INMETRO certificates are valid for five years and require annual factory inspections.

IVDs are classified using the nine classification rules in Resolution No. 61 on requirements for IVD product classification. Class II, III and IV IVDs require a *registro* application; Class I IVDs require a *cadastro* application [100]. Technical and documentation requirements are defined in Resolution RDC No. 206/2006 [101].

Manufacturers of medical devices and IVDs must also comply with the Good Manufacturing Practice (GMP) regulations defined in Resolution RDC No. 16/2013 [102]. Resolution No. 15/2014 introduced an exemption from GMP certification for Class I and II devices; Class III and IV devices still require GMP certification in order to obtain marketing authorization. At the time of going to print ANVISA was in the process of reviewing additional draft resolutions aimed at simplifying the pre-market process for medical devices and IVDs, including requirements for clinical trials [103].

For imported devices applicants must also provide the approval issued by the Regulatory Authority in the manufacturer's country of origin or an acceptable substitute, such as an INMETRO certificate or proof of marketing approval in two other countries.

Cadastro and *registro* applications must follow the content and format defined in Resolutions RDC No. 185/2001 for medical devices and RDC No. 206/2006 for IVDs. They must be submitted to ANVISA for review. Upon granting marketing authorization (regulatory approval), ANVISA will publish the registration number in the official registry *Diário Oficial da União* (DOU). Registrations are valid for five years and require renewal if manufacturers wish to continue to market their devices after registration expiry.

5.3 Case Study: Out of Sync

A medical device manufacturer rolled out design control procedures that failed to define a clear content and structure for the Design History File (DHF). There was also no check to make sure that the procedures would enable the delivery of important technical documentation required for regulatory submissions worldwide.

As a consequence, design and development (D&D) project teams repeatedly failed to generate certain documents required for most regulatory submissions such as V&V summary reports with discussions and conclusions on how safety and effectiveness requirements were met. Many documents that the project teams did generate did not follow fundamental best practices such as structure, clarity and complete and accurate content. Summary reports were mere lists of associated documents to which the reviewers were expected to refer without drawing any conclusions or making any explanations. Overall it was difficult to understand the information presented without prior insider knowledge.

A large volume of detailed documents would usually be "dumped" in a hurry on the overseas affiliate regulatory teams, one or two days before submission deadline, without any structure or organization. The overseas affiliates would then "write the submission" to try and fill in the gaps left by the missing summaries, depending on whatever available information was available. Because of the time pressure, there was little or no quality control done on the submission as a whole to check that the submission content was complete, that individual documents were released versions rather than drafts and that the cross-references within documents were correct.

Communication and time zone challenges meant that regional submissions prepared by the affiliate teams occasionally contained information that was materially different from what it should have been. Sometimes the regulatory submissions were written directly in a different language (Chinese, Japanese or Korean) without being translated back into English; hence the head office could not check what was actually being submitted.

Some changes that had been agreed upon with regulatory agencies as a condition for obtaining regulatory approval were neither implemented nor documented in the DHF by revising relevant documents. This meant effectively that the view the company had about the product was different from the view the agency had about the same product. These errors were causing confusion and delays during the course of subsequent submissions for product modifications, as well as resulting in audit findings during quality system audits.

5.4 Concluding Summary

Chapter 5 explains basic terminology related to entities responsible for placing medical devices on the market. The processes of submitting applications and obtaining regulatory approvals, including administrative provisions such as registration, are described for each major market. The level of the regulatory scrutiny and oversight for each type of submission is directly proportionate with the risk classification of the medical device for which approval is sought. The chapter covers:

- Definition and terminology related to legal manufacturer and in-country representative; key responsibilities of in-country representatives in the established jurisdictions – EEA, including Switzerland and Turkey, the United States, Australia, Canada and Japan;
- Administrative provisions for establishment registration and product listing in the established markets;
- Processes for submitting regulatory applications and obtaining marketing authorization (regulatory approval) in the established markets;
- Processes for making available unapproved devices – clinical investigations and special access schemes – in the established markets; and
- Overview of regulatory processes in key emerging markets – China, ASEAN (represented by Singapore) and Brazil.

References

1. Health Canada. Medical Device Regulations SOR/98-282) – Establishment Licence – Section 44. Prohibition. *laws-lois.justice.gc.ca.* [Online] December 16, 2011. [Cited: May 31, 2014.] http://laws-lois.justice.gc.ca/eng/regulations/SOR-98-282/page-10.html# docCont.
2. Gross, A. Japan: Designated Marketing Authorization Holder (DMAH). *www.pacificbridgemedical.com.* [Online] August 14, 2012. [Cited: May 31, 2014.] http://www.pacificbridgemedical.com/publications/japan-designated-marketing-authorization-holder-dmah/.
3. European Commission. MEDDEV 2.5/10 Guideline for Authorised Representatives. *ec.europa.eu.* [Online] January 2012. [Cited: May 31, 2014.] http://ec.europa.eu/health/medical-devices/files/meddev/2_5_10_ol_en.pdf.
4. Food and Drug Administration. U.S. Agents. *www.fda.gov.* [Online] October 5, 2012. [Cited: May 31, 2014.] http://www.fda.gov/Medical

Devices/DeviceRegulationandguidance/HowtoMarketYourDevice/RegistrationandListing/ucm053196.htm.

5. Therapeutic Goods Administration. *Australian Regulatory Guidelines for Medical Devices* (ARGMD). *www.tga.gov.au.* [Online] May 2011. [Cited: May 31, 2014.] http://www.tga.gov.au/pdf/devices-argmd-p2.pdf.
6. Health Canada. Medical Device Regulations (SOR/98-282) - Establishment Licence - Sections 52–56 Distribution Records; 57–58 Complaint Handling; 59–61 Mandatory Problem Reporting; 64–65 Recall. *laws-lois.justice.gc.ca.* [Online] December 16, 2011. [Cited: May 31, 2014.] http://laws-lois.justice.gc.ca/eng/regulations/SOR-98-282/page-12.html#docCont.
7. Pharmaceuticals and Medical Devices Agency. Ministerial Ordinances. *www.pmda.go.jp.* [Online] 2014. [Cited: November 1, 2014.] http://www.pmda.go.jp/english/service/ministerial.html.
8. Regulatory Affairs Professionals Society. *Fundamentals of Japanese Regulatory Affairs, First Edition.* Rockville, MD 20852 : Regulatory Affairs Professionals Society, 2010.
9. Miyahara, M., Eisenhart. S. *An Overview of Japan's new Pharmaceutical and Medical Devices Law (PMDL) Introduced in November 2014.* November, s.l. : Emergo, 2014.
10. European Commission. List of contact points within the national competent authorities. *ec.europa.eu.* [Online] [Cited: October 3, 2014.] http://ec.europa.eu/health/medical-devices/links/contact_points_en.htm.
11. MHRA. Registration of medical devices. *www.mhra.gov.uk.* [Online] October 28, 2013. [Cited: May 31, 2014.] http://www.mhra.gov.uk/Howweregulate/Devices/Registrationofmedicaldevices/.
12. European Commissions. List of contact points within national competent authorities. *ec.europa.eu.* [Online] [Cited: May 31, 2014.] http://ec.europa.eu/health/medical-devices/links/contact_points_en.htm.
13. Food and Drug Administration. Who Must Register, List and Pay the Fee. *www.fda.gov.* [Online] March 18, 2014. [Cited: May 31, 2014.] http://www.fda.gov/MedicalDevices/DeviceRegulationandGuidance/HowtoMarketYourDevice/RegistrationandListing/ucm053165.htm#definitions.
14. Food and Drug Administration. How to Register and List. *www.fda.gov.* [Online] September 25, 2013. [Cited: May 31, 2014.] http://www.fda.

gov/MedicalDevices/DeviceRegulationandGuidance/HowtoMarketYourDevice/RegistrationandListing/ucm053185.htm.

15. Therapeutic Goods Administration. Client details form. *www.tga.gov.au.* [Online] October 28, 2014. [Cited: October 30, 2014.] http://www.tga.gov.au/form/client-details-form.
16. Therapeutic Goods Administration. What do I need to do to supply a medical device in Australia? *www.tga.gov.au.* [Online] July 28, 2008. [Cited: October 30, 2014.] http://www.tga.gov.au/what-do-i-need-do-supply-medical-device-australia.
17. Health Canada. Guidance on Medical Device Establishment Licensing and Medical Device Establishment License Fees (GUI-0016). *www.hc-sc.gc.ca.* [Online] April 1, 2013. [Cited: October 30, 2014.] http://www.hc-sc.gc.ca/dhp-mps/compli-conform/licences/directives/gui-0016-eng.php#a72.
18. Pharmaceuticals and Medical Devices Agency. Accreditation of Foreign Manufacturers. *www.pmda.go.jp.* [Online] [Cited: October 30, 2014.] http://www.pmda.go.jp/english/service/acc_foreign.html.
19. Food and Drug Administration. Medical Device User Fee and Modernization Act (MDUFMA). *www.fda.gov.* [Online] September 30, 2014. [Cited: October 3, 2014.] http://www.fda.gov/MedicalDevices/DeviceRegulationandGuidance/Overview/MedicalDeviceUserFeeandModernizationActMDUFMA/.
20. Health Canada. Establishment Licences. *www.hc-sc.gc.ca.* [Online] April 29, 2014. [Cited: May 31, 2014.] http://www.hc-sc.gc.ca/dhp-mps/compli-conform/licences/index-eng.php.
21. Health Canada. Fees. *www.hc-sc.gc.ca.* [Online] July 21, 2011. [Cited: May 31, 2014.] http://www.hc-sc.gc.ca/dhp-mps/md-im/fees-frais/index-eng.php.
22. Therapeutic Goods Administration. Fees & payments. *www.tga.com.au.* [Online] October 28, 2014. [Cited: November 18, 2014.] https://www.tga.gov.au/fees-payments.
23. Therapeutic Goods Administration. ARGMD – Section 2. Fees and charges for medical devices. *www.tga.gov.au.* [Online] May 2011. [Cited: May 31, 2014.] http://www.tga.gov.au/pdf/devices-argmd-p1-01.pdf.
24. Pharmaceuticals and Medical Devices Agency. The Pharmaceuticals and medical devices agency annual report FY 2012. *www.pmda.go.jp.* [Online] [Cited: October 3, 2014.] http://www.pmda.go.jp/english/about/pdf/2012/annual_report_FY2012.pdf.

25. Cohen, D. *How a Fake Hip Showed Up Failings in European Device Regulation.* London : BMJ, 2012.
26. European Commission. Nando (New Approach Notified and Designated Organisations) Information System. *ec.europa.eu.* [Online] June 17, 2014. [Cited: June 18, 2014.] http://ec.europa.eu/enterprise/newapproach/nando/index.cfm.
27. Maxwell, A. Notified Bodies dropping like flies? New-style authority audits cause near-50% cull. *www.team-nb.org.* [Online] February 10, 2012. [Cited: May 31, 2014.] http://www.team-nb.org/documents/2013/Clinica-Notified-bodies-dropping-like-flies-20131017.pdf.
28. European Commission. Restoring confidence in medical devices. Action Plan after the PIP scandal tightened control in Europe. *ec.europa.eu.* [Online] June 20, 2014. [Cited: October 3, 2014.] http://europa.eu/rapid/press-release_IP-14-699_en.htm.
29. European Commission. How to reproduce the CE mark. *ec.europa.eu.* [Online] November 19, 2007. [Cited: May 31, 2014.] http://ec.europa.eu/enterprise/faq/ce-mark.htm.
30. NBOG. Certificates issued by Notified Bodies with reference to MDD, AIMDD and IVDD. *www.nbog.eu.* [Online] March 2010. [Cited: October 3, 2014.] http://www.nbog.eu/resources/NBOG_BPG_2010_3.pdf.
31. European Commission. Implementation of the Joint Plan for Immediate Actions under the existing Medical Devices legilation. *ec.europa.eu.* [Online] June 13, 2014. [Cited: October 3, 2014.] http://ec.europa.eu/health/medical-devices/files/swd_pip_14_en.pdf.
32. European Commission. Commission Recommendation on the audits and assessments performed by Notified Bodies in the field of medical devices. [Online] September 24, 2013. [Cited: October 3, 2014.] http://eur-lex.europa.eu/legal-content/EN/TXT/?uri=uriserv:OJ.L_.2013.253.01.0027.01.ENG.
33. NBOG. BPG 2014-1 Renewal of EC Design-Examination and Type-Examination Certificates: Conformity assessment procedures and general rules. *www.nbog.eu.* [Online] November 2014. [Cited: November 18, 2014.] http://www.nbog.eu/resources/NBOG_BPG_2014_1.pdf.
34. NBOG. Best Practice Guide – Change of Notified Body. *www.nbog.eu.* [Online] November 2008. [Cited: May 31, 2014.]
35. MHRA. Custom-made devices. *www.mhra.gov.uk.* [Online] August 16, 2013. [Cited: May 31, 2014.] http://www.mhra.gov.uk/Howweregulate/Devices/Complyingwithlegislation/ActiveImplantableMedicalDevicesDirective/Custommadedevices/index.htm.

36. European Commission. MEDDEV 2.7/4 Guidelines on clinical investigation. *ec.europa.eu.* [Online] December 2010. [Cited: October 3, 2014.] http://ec.europa.eu/health/medical-devices/files/meddev/2_7_4_en.pdf.

37. European Commission. MEDDEV 2.7.2 Guide for Competent Authorities in making an assessment of clinical investigation notification. *ec.europa.eu.* [Online] December 2008. [Cited: October 3, 2014.] http://ec.europa.eu/health/medical-devices/files/meddev/guidelines2008_en.pdf.

38. MHRA. Clinical investigations of medical devices – guidance for manufacturers. *www.mhra.gov.uk.* [Online] November 2013. [Cited: May 31, 2014.] http://www.mhra.gov.uk/home/groups/es-era/documents/publication/con007504.pdf.

39. MHRA. Exceptional use of non-complyingdevices. *www.mhra.gov.uk.* [Online] April 9, 2014. [Cited: October 30, 2014.] http://www.mhra.gov.uk/Howweregulate/Devices/Enforcementpolicy-Complianceinspectionandaction-Yourrights/index.htm#4.

40. Food and Drug Administration. MDUFA Performance Goals and Procedures. *www.fda.gov.* [Online] April 18, 2012. [Cited: October 3, 2014.] http://www.fda.gov/downloads/MedicalDevices/NewsEvents/WorkshopsConferences/UCM295454.pdf.

41. Food and Drug Administration. Third Party Review. *www.fda.gov.* [Online] June 25, 2014. [Cited: July 1, 2014.] http://www.fda.gov/MedicalDevices/DeviceRegulationandGuidance/HowtoMarketYourDevice/PremarketSubmissions/ThirdParyReview/default.htm.

42. Food and Drug Administration. Intent to Exempt Certain Class II and Class I Reserved Medical Devices from Premarket Notification Requirements. *www.fda.gov.* [Online] August 1, 2014. [Cited: October 3, 2014.] http://www.fda.gov/downloads/MedicalDevices/DeviceRegulationandGuidance/GuidanceDocuments/UCM407292.pdf.

43. Food and Drug Administration. FDA Guidance – eCopy Program for Medical Device. *www.fda.gov.* [Online] October 10, 2013. [Cited: October 3, 2014.] http://www.fda.gov/downloads/MedicalDevices/DeviceRegulationandGuidance/GuidanceDocuments/UCM313794.pdf.

44. Food and Drug Administration. MDUFA III Guidance Documents. *www.fda.gov.* [Online] October 30, 2014. [Cited: November 1, 2014.] http://www.fda.gov/MedicalDevices/DeviceRegulationandGuidance/Overview/MDUFAIII/ucm313674.htm.

45. Food and Drug Administration. Requests for Feedback on Medical Device Submissions: The Pre-Submission Program and Meetings with FDA Staff. *www.fda.gov.* [Online] February 18, 2014. [Cited: October 3, 2014.] http://www.fda.gov/downloads/MedicalDevices/DeviceRegulationandGuidance/GuidanceDocuments/UCM311176.pdf.
46. Food and Drug Administration. Types of Communication During the Review of Medical Device Submissions. *www.fda.gov.* [Online] April 4, 2014. [Cited: October 3, 2014.] http://www.fda.gov/MedicalDevices/DeviceRegulationandGuidance/GuidanceDocuments/ucm341918.htm.
47. Food and Drug Administration. Refuse to Accept Policy for 510(k)s. *www.fda.gov.* [Online] December 31, 2012. [Cited: July 1, 2014.] http://www.fda.gov/downloads/MedicalDevices/DeviceRegulationandGuidance/GuidanceDocuments/ucm315014.pdf.
48. Food and Drug Administration. FDA and Industry Actions onPremarket Notification (510(k)) Submissions: Effect on FDA Review Clock and Goals. *www.fda.gov.* [Online] October 15, 2012. [Cited: October 3, 2014.] http://www.fda.gov/MedicalDevices/DeviceRegulationandGuidance/GuidanceDocuments/ucm089735.htm.
49. Food and Drug Administration. Acceptance and Filing Reviews for Premarket Approval Applications (PMAs). *www.fda.gov.* [Online] December 31, 2012. [Cited: October 3, 2014.] http://www.fda.gov/downloads/MedicalDevices/DeviceRegulationandGuidance/GuidanceDocuments/UCM313368.pdf.
50. Food and Drug Administration. FDA and Industry Actions on Premarket Approval Applications (PMAs): Effect on FDA Review Clock and Goals. *www.fda.gov.* [Online] October 15, 2012. [Cited: October 3, 2014.] http://www.fda.gov/MedicalDevices/DeviceRegulationandGuidance/GuidanceDocuments/ucm089733.htm.
51. Food and Drug Administration. Factors to Consider When Making Benefit-Risk Determinations in Medical Device Premarket Approvals and De Novo Classifications. *www.fda.gov.* [Online] March 28, 2012. [Cited: October 3, 2014.] http://www.fda.gov/MedicalDevices/DeviceRegulationandGuidance/GuidanceDocuments/ucm267829.htm.
52. Food and Drug Administration. How To Find A Predicate Device. *www.fda.gov.* [Online] December 20, 2013. [Cited: May 31, 2014.] http://www.fda.gov/MedicalDevices/DeviceRegulationandGuidance/HowtoMarketYourDevice/PremarketSubmissions/PremarketNotification510k/ucm134571.htm.

53. Food and Drug Administration. 21 CFR Subpart E – Premarket Notification Procedures. *www.accessdata.fda.gov.* [Online] June 1, 2013. [Cited: May 31, 2014.] http://www.accessdata.fda.gov/scripts/cdrh/cfdocs/cfcfr/CFRSearch.cfm?CFRPart=807&showFR=1&subpartNode=21:8.0.1.1.5.5.
54. Food and Drug Administration. Content of a 510(k). *www.fda.gov.* [Online] March 18, 2014. [Cited: July 1, 2014.] http://www.fda.gov/MedicalDevices/DeviceRegulationandGuidance/HowtoMarketYourDevice/PremarketSubmissions/PremarketNotification510k/ucm142651.htm.
55. Food and Drug Administration. 510(k) Submision Process. *www.fda.gov.* [Online] January 3, 2013. [Cited: July 1, 2014.] http://www.fda.gov/MedicalDevices/DeviceRegulationandGuidance/HowtoMarketYourDevice/PremarketSubmissions/PremarketNotification510k/ucm070201.htm.
56. Food and Drug Administration. The New 510(k) Paradigm – Alternate Approaches to Demonstrating Substantial Equivalence in Premarket Notifications. *www.fda.gov.* [Online] March 20, 1998. [Cited: July 1, 2014.] http://www.fda.gov/MedicalDevices/DeviceRegulationandGuidance/GuidanceDocuments/ucm080187.htm.
57. Food and Drug Administration. 21 CFR Part 814 – Premarket Approval of medical devices. *www.fda.gov.* [Online] June 1, 2013. [Cited: July 1, 2014.] http://www.accessdata.fda.gov/scripts/cdrh/cfdocs/cfcfr/CFRSearch.cfm?CFRPart=814&showFR=1.
58. Food and Drug Administration. Premarket Approval (PMA). *www.fda.gov.* [Online] January 24, 2012. [Cited: July 1, 2014.] http://www.fda.gov/MedicalDevices/DeviceRegulationandGuidance/HowtoMarketYourDevice/PremarketSubmissions/PremarketApprovalPMA/default.htm.
59. Food and Drug Administration. PMA Review Process. *www.fda.gov.* [Online] September 4, 2014. [Cited: October 3, 2014.] http://www.fda.gov/MedicalDevices/DeviceRegulationandGuidance/HowtoMarketYourDevice/PremarketSubmissions/PremarketApprovalPMA/ucm047991.htm.
60. Food and Drug Administration. FDA guidance on PMA Interactive Procedures for Day-100 Meetings and Subsequent Deficiencies. *www.fda.gov.* [Online] February 19, 1998. [Cited: July 1, 2014.] http://www.fda.gov/MedicalDevices/DeviceRegulationandGuidance/GuidanceDocuments/ucm080190.htm.

61. Food and Drug Administration. 21 CFR 814.40 Time frames for reviewing a PMA. *www.accessdata.fda.gov.* [Online] June 1, 2013. [Cited: July 1, 2014.] http://www.accessdata.fda.gov/scripts/cdrh/cfdocs/cfcfr/CFRSearch.cfm?fr=814.40.
62. Food and Drug Administration. 21 CFR Part 814.37 PMA amendments and resubmitted PMAs. *www.fda.gov.* [Online] June 1, 2013. [Cited: July 1, 2014.] http://www.accessdata.fda.gov/scripts/cdrh/cfdocs/cfcfr/CFRSearch.cfm?fr=814.37.
63. Food and Drug Administration. Panel review of Premarket Approval Applications #P91-2 (blue book memo). *www.fda.gov.* [Online] May 3, 1991. [Cited: July 1, 2014.] http://www.fda.gov/MedicalDevices/DeviceRegulationandGuidance/GuidanceDocuments/ucm081363.htm.
64. Food and Drug Administration. PMA Approvals. *www.fda.gov.* [Online] January 16, 2014. [Cited: July 1, 2014.] http://www.fda.gov/MedicalDevices/ProductsandMedicalProcedures/DeviceApprovalsandClearancesPMAApprovals/default.htm.
65. Food and Drug Administration. Premarket Approval Application Modular Review. *www.fda.com.* [Online] November 3, 2003. [Cited: July 1, 2014.] http://www.fda.gov/MedicalDevices/DeviceRegulationandGuidance/GuidanceDocuments/ucm089764.htm.
66. Food and Drug Administration. FDA Guidance (draft) – Expedited Access for Premarket Approval Medical Devices Intended for Unmet Medical Need for Life Threatening or Irreversibly Debilitating Diseases or Conditions. *www.fda.gov.* [Online] April 23, 2014. [Cited: October 3, 2014.] http://www.fda.gov/medicaldevices/deviceregulationandguidance/guidancedocuments/ucm393879.htm.
67. Food and Drug Administration. Evaluation of Automatic Class III Designation (De Novo) Summaries. *www.fda.gov.* [Online] June 16, 2014. [Cited: July 1, 2014.] http://www.fda.gov/AboutFDA/CentersOffices/OfficeofMedicalProductsandTobacco/CDRH/CDRH-Transparency/ucm232269.htm.
68. Food and Drug Administration. 21 CFR Part 814 – Subpart H Humanitarian Use Devcies. *www.accessdata.fda.gov.* [Online] June 1, 2013. [Cited: July 1, 2014.] http://www.accessdata.fda.gov/scripts/cdrh/cfdocs/cfcfr/CFRSearch.cfm?CFRPart=814&showFR=1&subpartNode=21:8.0.1.1.11.7.
69. Food and Drug Administration. Humanitarian Devcie Exemption. *www.fda.gov.* [Online] June 26, 2014. [Cited: July 1, 2014.] http://www.fda.gov/MedicalDevices/DeviceRegulationandGuidance/HowtoMarket

YourDevice/PremarketSubmissions/HumanitarianDeviceExemption/default.htm.

70. Faris, O., Food and Drug Administration. Clinical trials for medical devices: FDA and the IDE process. *www.fda.gov.* [Online] November 12, 2013. [Cited: October 3, 2014.] http://www.fda.gov/downloads/Training/ClinicalInvestigatorTrainingCourse/UCM378265.pdf.
71. Food and Drug Administration. Device Advice: Investigational Device Exemption (IDE). *www.fda.gov.* [Online] June 19, 2014. [Cited: October 3, 2014.] http://www.fda.gov/MedicalDevices/DeviceRegulationandGuidance/HowtoMarketYourDevice/InvestigationalDeviceExemptionIDE/default.htm.
72. Food and Drug Administration. FDA Decisions for Investigational Device Exemption Clinical Investigations. *www.fda.gov.* [Online] August 19, 2014. [Cited: October 3, 2014.] http://www.fda.gov/downloads/MedicalDevices/DeviceRegulationandGuidance/GuidanceDocuments/UCM279107.pdf.
73. Food and Drug Administration. IDE Application. *www.fda.gov.* [Online] June 30, 2014. [Cited: October 10, 2014.] http://www.fda.gov/MedicalDevices/DeviceRegulationandGuidance/HowtoMarketYourDevice/InvestigationalDeviceExemptionIDE/ucm046706.htm.
74. Food and Drug Administration. IDE Early/ Expanded Access. *www.fda.gov.* [Online] June 27, 2014. [Cited: October 3, 2014.] http://www.fda.gov/MedicalDevices/DeviceRegulationandGuidance/HowtoMarketYourDevice/InvestigationalDeviceExemptionIDE/ucm051345.htm.
75. Food and Drug Administration. Custom Device Exemption. *www.fda.gov.* [Online] September 24, 2014. [Cited: October 3, 2014.] http://www.fda.gov/downloads/MedicalDevices/DeviceRegulationandGuidance/GuidanceDocuments/UCM415799.pdf.
76. Food and Drug Administration. Distribution of In Vitro Diagnostic Products Labeled for Research Use Only or Investigational Use Only. *www.fda.gov.* [Online] November 25, 2013. [Cited: October 3, 2014.] http://www.fda.gov/medicaldevices/deviceregulationandguidance/guidancedocuments/ucm253307.htm.
77. Therapeutic Goods Administration. Declaration of conformity templates (medical devices). *www.tga.gov.au.* [Online] February 5, 2014. [Cited: October 3, 2014.] https://www.tga.gov.au/form/declaration-conformity-templates-medical-devices.

78. Therapeutic Goods Administration. What a sponsor needs to know about conformity assessment and manufaturer's evidence for IVDs. *www.tga.gov.au.* [Online] March 7, 2011. [Cited: October 3, 2014.] http://www.tga.gov.au/publication/what-sponsor-needs-know-about-conformity-assessment-and-manufacturers-evidence-ivds#evidence.
79. Therapeutic Goods Administration. What do I need to do to supply a medical device in Australia? *www.tga.gov.au.* [Online] July 28, 2008. [Cited: October 3, 2014.] https://www.tga.gov.au/what-do-i-need-do-supply-medical-device-australia.
80. Therapeutic Goods Administration. Medical devices reforms. *www.tga.gov.au.* [Online] October 15, 2014. [Cited: November 1, 2014.] https://www.tga.gov.au/medical-devices-reforms.
81. National Health and Medical Research Council (NHMRC). National Statement on Ethical Conduct in Human Research. *www.nhmrc.gov.au.* [Online] March 2014. [Cited: October 3, 2014.] https://www.nhmrc.gov.au/guidelines/publications/e72.
82. Health Canada. List of Registrars Recognized by Health Canada under section 32.1 of the Medical Devices Regulations (MDR). *www.hc-sc.gc.ca.* [Online] December 4, 2013. [Cited: August 10, 2014.] http://www.hc-sc.gc.ca/dhp-mps/md-im/qualsys/list_liste_regist-eng.php.
83. Health Canada. Medical Devices – Special Access Programme. *www.hc-sc.gc.ca.* [Online] March 13, 2013. [Cited: October 3, 2014.] http://www.hc-sc.gc.ca/dhp-mps/acces/md-im/index-eng.php.
84. Health Canada. Preparation of an Application for Investigational Testing – Medical Devices. *www.hc-sc.gc.ca.* [Online] February 22, 1999. [Cited: October 3, 2014.] http://www.hc-sc.gc.ca/dhp-mps/md-im/applic-demande/guide-ld/md_gd_ita_im_ld_aee-eng.php.
85. Regulatory Affairs Professionals Society. *Fundamentals of Japanese Regulatory Affairs, First Edition.* Rockville, MD 20852 : Regulatory Affairs Professionals Society, 2010.
86. Emergo Group. Clinical Data Evaluation for Foreign Medical Device Companies Seeking Japanese PMDA Approval. *www.emergogroup.com.* [Online] [Cited: September 1, 2014.] http://www.emergogroup.com/services/japan/clinical-data-management-japan.
87. MHLW. Ministerial Ordinance No. 36 on Good Clinical Practice. *www.pmda.go.jp.* [Online] March 23, 2005. [Cited: September 1, 2014.] http://www.pmda.go.jp/english/service/pdf/ministerial/20110307No_36.pdf.

88. ICH. Efficacy Guidelines – Good Clinical Practice. *www.ich.org.* [Online] May 1996. [Cited: September 1, 2014.] http://www.ich.org/products/guidelines/efficacy/efficacy-single/article/good-clinical-practice.html.
89. MHLW. Notification No. 0928010 Basic principles on Global Clinical Trials. *www.pmda.go.jp.* [Online] September 28, 2007. [Cited: September 1, 2014.] http://www.pmda.go.jp/english/service/pdf/notifications/PFSB-ELD-0928010.pdf.
90. China Food and Drug Administration. China Food and Drug Administration. *www.sfda.gov.cn.* [Online] [Cited: November 1, 2014.] http://www.cfda.gov.cn/WS01/CL0001/.
91. China Food and Drug Administration. China – Update on medical device regulations. *www.imdrf.org.* [Online] November 2013. [Cited: October 3, 2014.] http://www.imdrf.org/docs/imdrf/final/meetings/imdrf-meet-131112-belgium-presentation-china-regulatory-update.pdf.
92. Xiao, L. Guide for Australian medical technology companies seeking to engage in China (First Edition – draft). *www.ausbiotech.org.* [Online] [Cited: November 18, 2014.] www.ausbiotech.org/data/downloads/V9_Draft%20China%20Guide.docx.
93. China Food and Drug Administration. CFDA Announcement No. 12. *www.cfda.gov.cn.* [Online] August 21, 2014. [Cited: November 1, 2014.] http://www.cfda.gov.cn/WS01/CL0087/105225.html.
94. China Food and Drug Administration. CFDA Announcement No. 13. *www.cfda.gov.cn.* [Online] August 21, 2014. [Cited: November 1, 2014.] http://www.cfda.gov.cn/WS01/CL0087/105224.html.
95. Health Sciences Authority. GN-18: Guidance on Preparation of a Product Registration Submission for IVDs using the ASEAN CSDT. *www.hsa.gov.sg.* [Online] May 2014. [Cited: November 18, 2014.] http://www.hsa.gov.sg/content/dam/HSA/HPRG/Medical_Devices/Overview_Framework_Policies/Guidances_for_Medical_Device_Registration/GN-18-D1.1%20Guidance%20on%20Preparation%20of%20a%20Product%20Registration%20Submission%20for%20IVD%20MD%20using%20the%20ASEAN.
96. Health Sciences Authority. Regulatory Updates. *www.hsa.gov.sg.* [Online] [Cited: November 1, 2014.] http://www.hsa.gov.sg/content/hsa/en/Health_Products_Regulation/Medical_Devices/Regulatory_Updates.html.

97. Health Sciences Authority. GN-15: Guidance on Medical Device Product Registration. *www.hsa.gov.sg.* [Online] May 2014. [Cited: November 1, 2014.] http://www.hsa.gov.sg/content/dam/HSA/HPRG/Medical_Devices/Overview_Framework_Policies/Guidances_for_Medical_Device_Registration/GN-15-R6.1%20Guidance%20on%20Medical%20Device%20Product%20Registration.pdf.
98. ANVISA (English translation provided by Emergo). Resolution RDC No. 185 Registration of medical products. *www.emergogroup.com.* [Online] October 22, 2001. [Cited: November 1, 2014.] http://www.emergogroup.com/sites/default/files/file/rdc_185_2001_classification_and_registration_requirements_of_medical_products_0.pdf.
99. ANVISA. Resolution RDC No. 56 on the essential requirements for safety and effectiveness of medical devices. *www.emergogroup.com.* [Online] April 6, 2001. [Cited: November 1, 2014.] http://www.emergogroup.com/sites/default/files/file/rdc_56_2001_safety_and_efficacy_requirements.pdf.
100. ANVISA. Resolution RDC No. 61 Requirements for in-vitro diagnostic product classification. *www.emergogroup.com.* [Online] November 18, 2011. [Cited: November 1, 2014.] http://www.emergogroup.com/sites/default/files/file/rdc_61_2011_classification_rules_in-vitro_dianostic_products.pdf.
101. ANVISA. Resolution RDC No. 206 Technical regulation on IVDs and their registro and cadastro registration. *www.emergogroup.com.* [Online] November 17, 2006. [Cited: November 1, 2014.] http://www.emergogroup.com/sites/default/files/file/rdc_206_2006_technical_regulation_on_in-vitro_diagnostic_products.pdf.
102. ANVISA. Resolution RDC No. 16 Good Manufacturing Practices of Medical Devices and IVDs. *www.emergogroup.com.* [Online] March 28, 2013. [Cited: November 1, 2014.] http://www.emergogroup.com/sites/default/files/file/rdc_16_2013_gmp_requirements_for_md_and_ivd.pdf.
103. ANVISA. Update on the Brazilian regulatory aspects on medical devices – IMDRF meeting. *www.imdrf.org.* [Online] September 17, 2014. [Cited: November 18, 2014.] http://www.imdrf.org/docs/imdrf/final/meetings/imdrf-meet-140829-washington-brazil-update.pdf.

Chapter 6

Post-Market Phase

This chapter deals with regulatory controls in the post-market phase, which commences once a therapeutic product obtains marketing authorization (regulatory approval). Topics covered include preparing for a product launch, maintaining continued compliance for the established markets, change controls and vigilance and adverse event reporting. This chapter concludes with a discussion of key performance indicators relevant to regulatory processes.

6.1 Product Launch

A product launch may mean different things to different parts of an organization, but it certainly denotes an event, a point in time when a product is presented to the external audience - the target market. Although one might assume that a product launch is only about printing colourful brochures and running ad campaigns, in reality preparations for a product launch start with defining the user needs (refer also to Section 4.4.1.1, "User Needs").

Unfortunately too many products come to market without a clear purpose. They manifest through the excitement of "we can build it", a technical road-map perspective. This differs greatly from an

Medical Device Regulatory Practices: An International Perspective
Val Theisz

ISBN 978-981-4669-10-8 (Hardcover), 978-981-4669-11-5 (eBook)
www.panstanford.com

approach that says, "Just because we can build it, should we?" The two approaches could not be further apart.

Too often, products are introduced that have undergone extensive investment in research and development but offer no real innovation or unique purpose for the target market. These products are built because they offer a step-wise improvement. But given the large regulatory and clinical efforts needed to support these products throughout their lifetime, are they the most effective use of a medical device organization's limited resources?

Technology is certainly the driving enabler for product innovation and development. However, if it is the leading, or only, consideration in the product development process, the product is often developed through a "bigger and better" (or "smaller and better" in the case of miniaturization) approach rather than focusing on addressing the user needs.

This approach may also suffer from trying to be all things to all people, and in the end there may be too many features yet not enough prioritization of the functionalities that really matter to the end user. A product without a (Regulatory Authority–approved) marketing claim can only be sold on its features, not its benefits.

Bringing a medical device to market globally requires highly skilled people, can take years and is very expensive. These high costs need to be weighed against the projected return on investment. Although there are no hard and fast rules, a medical device company should limit the number of product upgrades (consisting of incremental improvements only) to one or maximum two per year.

6.1.1 *Elements of a Product Launch*

Elements of a product launch include, but are not limited to:

(1) Communication plan – internal and external – describes the stages and level of information disclosure and the target audience – within the organization as well as to healthcare professionals, patients and other stakeholders; and
(2) Launch event – introduces the product to the marketplace and communicates what the product benefits are and why it will meet user needs.

6.1.1.1 Communication plan

One model for a communication plan that describes the stages of disclosing information about the product is outlined hereafter.

Stage 1: Release for internal planning – consists of limited internal disclosure, whereby senior and strategic management support incorporation of product impact on long-term strategic planning activities.

Stage 2: Release for clinicals – consists of clinical engagement disclosure, whereby communications and actions support the recruitment and interactions with potential clinical study centres; requires confidentiality agreements to be put in place.

Stage 3: Release for internal discussion – represents an operational disclosure, whereby communication is initiated across the marketing, sales and customer support functions within the organization on the strategic importance, planning and operational aspects of launching the product.

Stage 4: Release for external discussion – consists of external communications, initiated on a market-by-market basis after obtaining the formal marketing authorization (regulatory approval) and prior to the formal product launch; external communications may begin with key opinion leaders (KOLs) and strategic accounts (customers).

Stage 5: Release for (limited) sale – represents the external promotion of the product, whereby formal promotional activities are initiated to the general target audience; at this stage, the final, approved product documentation (labels, instructions for use, advertising materials) are finalized; however, the manufacturing line may or may not be fully ramped up for a large-scale product release.

6.1.1.2 Launch event

In today's interconnected world, it is unclear if a product needs a launch event in the traditional form of this activity. However, a product does need to be properly introduced to the marketplace. So by whichever channels the company chooses to promote a product, sell the product and support the product, it does need to be communicated. The target audience needs to know what the product benefits are and why this product will meet their needs like no other.

Product launch activities typically include the preparation of brochures, sales aids, demo kits, advertising and email campaigns, setting up and/or updating of websites, product training and other promotional tasks.

Any claims made about the product during a product launch and beyond in a particular market must be consistent with the product indications for use and intended use that were approved by the Regulatory Authority in that market.

6.1.2 *Regulations Covering Advertising*

Regulations in established markets are consistent in their core message about advertising of medical devices. Any promotion of a medical device must be limited to the use for which the device is intended according to its approved labelling (instructions for use). False, misleading or deceptive claims are in violation of the law and subject to enforcement actions, including mandatory recalls and fines.

6.1.2.1 The EU

Although the European Union (EU) medical devices directives do not have specific requirements on promotion and advertising, this does not mean that these activities are not regulated in the EU. Article 2 of each directive states, "Devices may be placed on the market and/or put into service only if they comply with the requirements laid down in [these Directives] when duly supplied and properly installed, maintained and used in accordance with their intended purpose". *Intended purpose* means, according to definitions in Article 1 of the directives, "the use for which the device is intended according to the data supplied by the manufacturer on the labelling, in the instructions for use and/or in promotional materials".

Another provision against deceiving product claims is defined in Article 17 of the Medical Devices Directive (MDD), Article 12 of the Active Implantable Medical Device Directive (AIMDD) and

Article 16 of the In Vitro Diagnostics Directive (IVDD), which says, "It is prohibited to affix marks or inscriptions which are likely to mislead third parties with regard to the meaning or the graphics of the Conformité Européenne (CE) marking. Any other mark may be affixed to the device, to the packaging or the instruction leaflet accompanying the device provided that the visibility and legibility of the CE marking is not thereby reduced".

Direct-to-consumer promotion of prescription-only medical devices is largely banned in the EU. Directive 2005/29/EC prohibits unfair business-to-consumer commercial practices in the internal market [1]. According to this directive, "Unfair commercial practices shall be prohibited. A commercial practice shall be unfair if:

(a) It is contrary to the requirements of professional diligence, and
(b) It materially distorts or is likely to materially distort the economic behavior with regard to the product of the average consumer whom it reaches or to whom it is addressed, or of the average member of the group when a commercial practice is directed to a particular group of consumers".

Article 6 of the Unfair Commercial Practices Directive defines *misleading commercial practice* as any action that "contains false information and is therefore untruthful or in any way, including overall presentation, deceives or is likely to deceive the average consumer, even if the information is factually correct" and also if "it causes or is likely to cause the average consumer to take a transactional decision that he would not have taken otherwise". Misleading omissions are defined in Article 7 as commercial practices omitting, hiding or providing material information in an unclear, unintelligible, ambiguous or untimely manner.

For example, a foot massager claiming to "improve circulation" in its labelling or promotion materials is classified as a medical device. Without supporting evidence and without a valid MDD certificate, the claim is misleading and the promotion of the product is in violation of the law.

Thanks to the Unfair Commercial Practices Directive national enforcers have been able to curb a broad range of unfair business practices, such as providing untruthful information to consumers or using aggressive marketing techniques to influence their choices.

Its legal framework is proving well suited to assess the fairness of the new online practices that are developing in parallel with the evolution of advertising sales techniques [2].

Directive 2006/114/EC is aimed at protecting businesses (competitors, distributors, traders) against misleading and comparative advertising [3]. According to this directive, misleading advertising is any advertising that, in any way, including in its presentation, is capable of:

- Deceiving the persons to whom it is addressed;
- Distorting their economic behavior; or
- As a consequence, harming the interests of competitors.

When determining whether advertising is misleading, several factors shall be taken into account. These are:

- The characteristics of the goods or services concerned;
- The price;
- The conditions of delivery of the goods or provision of the services involved; and
- The nature, attributes and rights of the advertiser.

The Misleading and Comparative Advertising Directive also lays down the conditions under which comparative advertising is allowed. In particular, it requires traders to ensure that their advertisements:

- Are not misleading;
- Compare "like with like"– goods and services meeting same needs or intended for the same purpose;
- Objectively compare important features of the products or services concerned;
- Do not discredit other companies trademarks; and
- Do not create confusion among traders.

Legislation pertaining to promotion and advertising is enforced by the competent authorities and courts in the EU member states [4]. Note, however, that most EU member states and European Economic Area (EEA) countries have separate national regulations regarding advertising of medical devices.

6.1.2.2 The United States

According to an US appellate court decision, "Most, if not all advertising, is labeling. The term 'labeling' is defined in the federal FD&C Act as including all printed matter accompanying any article. Congress did not, and we cannot, exclude from the definition printed matter which constitutes advertising" [5].

Section 201(k) of the federal Food, Drug, and Cosmetic Act (FD&C Act) defines a *label* as a "display of written, printed, or graphic matter upon the immediate container of any article".

The term "immediate container" does not include package liners. Any word, statement or other information appearing on the immediate container must also appear "on the outside container or wrapper, if any there be, of the retain package of such article, or is easily legible through the outside container of wrapper".

Section 201(m) of the FD&C Act defines *labelling* as:

- "all labels and other written, printed, or graphic matter
  - (a) upon any article or any of its containers or wrappers, or
  - (b) accompanying such article" at any time while a device is held for sale after shipment or delivery for shipment in interstate commerce

The term "accompanying" is interpreted liberally to mean more than physical association with the product. It extends to posters, tags, pamphlets, circulars, booklets, brochures, instruction books, direction sheets, fillers, etc. *Accompanying* also includes labelling that is brought together with the device after shipment or delivery for shipment in interstate commerce.

According to the general controls defined in Section 502 of the FD&C Act, a device is considered to be misbranded if:

- Its labeling is false or misleading in any particular;
- It is in package form and its label fails to contain the name and place of business of the manufacturer, packer or distributor and an accurate statement of the quantity of the contents in terms of weight, measure or numerical count;

- Any required wording is not prominently displayed as compared with other wording on the device or is not clearly stated;
- Its label does not bear adequate directions for use, including warnings against use in certain pathological conditions or by children where its use may be dangerous in health or against unsafe dosage or methods or duration of administration or application;
- It is dangerous to health when used in the dosage or manner or with the frequency or duration prescribed, recommended or suggested in the labeling; or
- It does not comply with the colour additives provisions listed under Section 706 of the Act.
- If the device's established name (if it has one) its name in an official compendium or any common or usual name is not prominently printed in type at least half as large as that used for any proprietary name;
- If the establishment is not registered with the Food and Drug Administration (FDA) as per Section 510, has not listed the device as per Section 510(j) or obtained applicable premarket notification clearance as per Section 510(k);
- If the device is subject to a performance standard and it does not bear the labelling prescribed in that standard;
- If there is a failure or refusal to comply with any requirement prescribed under the Act, Section 518 on notification and other remedies or failure to furnish any materials or information requested by or under Section 519 on reports and records or under Section 522; or
- If there is any representation that created an impression of official approval because of the possession by the firm of an FDA registration number.

This phrase "false or misleading" is not confined in meaning to untrue, forged, fraudulent or deceptive. In fact, the word, statement or illustration may be true in the strict sense of the word; however, the labelling can be deemed by the FDA to be in violation of the law if it proves deceptive to the customer.

It is not a necessary condition that the labelling should be flatly and baldly false; the work "misleading" in the Act means that labelling is deceptive if it is such as to create or lead to a false impression in the mind of the reader. A false impression not only may result from a false deceptive statement but may also be instilled in the mind of the purchaser by ambiguity or misdirection. It may also be caused by failure to inform the consumer of facts that are relevant to those statements actually made. In other words, the label that remains silent as to certain consequences may be as deceptive as the label that contains extravagant claims [6].

Examples of false labelling include:

- Incorrect, inadequate or incomplete identification;
- Unsubstantiated claims of therapeutic value;
- Inaccuracies concerning condition, state, treatment, size, shape or style; and
- Substitution of parts or material.

Examples of misleading labelling include:

- Ambiguity, half-truths and trade puffery;
- Expressions of opinion or subjective statements; and
- Failure to reveal material facts, consequences that may result from use or the existence of difference of opinion.

Examples of other objectionable labelling practices include:

- Deceptive pictorial matter;
- Misleading testimonials;
- Misleading list of parts or components; and
- Use of brand or trade names instead of "established names" [6].

The following are FDA regulations relevant to labelling:

- 21 CFR Part 801, *General Device Labeling*
- 21 CFR Part 809, *IVD Products*
- 21 CFR Part 812, *Investigational Device Exemptions*
- 21 CFR Part 820, *Good Manufacturing Practices*
- 21 CFR Part 1010, *General Electronic Products*

Additional details on labelling topics are provided in FDA guidance documents available on the FDA's website [5].

FDA compliance and enforcement actions in the case of misbranded medical devices include the issue of warning letters, administrative detention, seizure and injunction [7].

6.1.2.3 Australia

In Australia, the advertising of therapeutic goods to consumers and health practitioners is controlled by a combination of statutory measures administered by the Therapeutic Goods Administration (TGA) and self-regulation through Codes of Practice administered by the relevant therapeutic goods industry associations.

The laws and regulations governing advertising of therapeutic goods include the Therapeutic Goods Act of 1989 and Regulations and the Competition and Consumer Act of 2010. A summary of the regulation of advertising of medical devices in Australia is provided in Table 6.1.

Table 6.1 Summary of the regulation of advertising of therapeutic goods in Australia

	Medical devices	
	Direct-to-consumer ads	Ads to healthcare professionals
Permitted?	Yes	Yes
Regulated by	Therapeutic Goods Act Therapeutic Goods Regulations Therapeutic Goods Advertising Code Trade Practices Act	Therapeutic Goods Act Therapeutic Goods Regulations
Prior approval required?	No	No
Complaint-handling process	Complaints Resolution Panel (for broadcast media, mainstream print media, billboards, cinema films) TGA	TGA

Source: TGA [8]

Medical devices may be advertised directly to consumers and the regulatory requirements are similar to those applying to direct-to-consumer advertising of non-prescription medicines. However, there is no requirement for prior approval of these advertisements. Further details relating to advertising of therapeutic goods are available on the TGA's website [9].

The Complaints Resolution Panel considers complaints about advertisements for medical devices and therapeutic devices appearing in broadcast and mainstream print media, billboards, cinema films, the Internet, etc.

TGA enforcement actions in case of non-compliance with legislative and regulatory provisions include restrictions/warnings, suspensions/sanctions and cancellation/prosecution [10].

6.1.2.4 Canada

In Canada, only health products that are authorized for sale by Health Canada may be advertised.

Section 26 of the Medical Devices Regulations prohibits the promotion of Class II, III and IV medical devices for the purpose of sale unless:

(a) The manufacturer of the device holds a licence in respect of that device or, if the device has been subjected to a change described in Section 34, an amended medical device licence; or
(b) The advertisement is placed only in a catalogue that includes a clear and visible warning that the devices advertised in the catalogue may not have been licensed in accordance with Canadian law.

Advertisements for investigational devices (used in clinical trials) are also prohibited, according to Section 87 of the Medical Devices Regulations, unless:

(a) The clinical trial sponsor holds an authorization to sell or import the device for the purpose of conducting investigational testing; and

(b) The advertisement clearly indicates that the device is the subject of investigational testing, and the purpose of the investigational testing.

Section 24 of the Medical Devices Regulations is dedicated to advertising of contraceptive devices, which says:

(1) Condoms may be advertised and sold to the general public for the purpose of preventing the transmission of sexually transmitted diseases if the advertisement and the label of the condom claim only that the condom reduces the risk of transmitting sexually transmitted diseases.
(2) Contraceptive devices, other than intrauterine devices, may be advertised to the general public by any means other than by the distribution of samples of the devices door to door or through the mail.

Advertisements are subject to the provisions of the Foods and Drugs Act, in particular:

- Section 9(1): Prohibits health product advertising that is false, misleading or deceptive or is likely to create an erroneous impression regarding its character, value, quantity, composition, merit or safety. Examples of possible Section 9(1) contraventions: messages that emphasize only product benefits without including safety information and messages discussing off-label use of a product.
- Section 20(1): Prohibits false, misleading or deceptive advertising of medical devices.
- Section 3(1): Prohibits consumer-directed ads for health products (including medical devices) that make claims to treat, prevent or cure any of the serious diseases listed in Schedule A to the Act (although Schedule A prevention claims are now permitted by regulation for over-the-counter drugs and natural health products).

Guidelines containing further details pertaining to health products advertising are available on Health Canada's website [11].

6.1.2.5 Japan

In Japan, the rules governing advertising of healthcare products are defined in *Notification on Standards for Fair Advertising Practice of Drug Products, etc.* (Yakuhatsu No. 1339 of 1980). The aim of these standards is "to prevent false or exaggerated advertisements (of drug products, quasi-drugs and cosmetics) and to ensure that advertisements are appropriate" [12].

The standards specifically prohibit the following activities:

(1) **Exaggerated advertisements** – this covers false or exaggerated advertisements regarding manufacturing methods, efficacy, benefits or performance and advertisements in which doctors or others guarantee such qualities.
(2) **Direct-to-consumer advertisements for medical devices intended for professional users only** – this covers TV, radio, newspapers and Internet advertisements for medical devices other than those intended for the general public.
(3) **Advertisements for unapproved medical devices** – this covers any advertisements for medical devices that do not have (yet) regulatory approval; limited promotion during exhibitions, trade fairs or academic conferences is allowed provided the organizer grants permission [12]

In addition, there are industry self-regulation rules that industry associations members commit to adhere to. For medical devices these are:

- Promotion Code in the Medical Device Industry of the Japan Federation of Medical Devices Association; and
- Fair Competition Code for the Medical Devices Industry, which is based on Article 11 of the Pharmaceutical and Medical Device (PMD) Act against Unjustifiable Premiums and Misleading Representations [13].

6.1.3 *Translation Procedure*

Selling medical devices in countries with different official languages involves providing translations of product labelling and accompanying documentation such as instructions for use, training, marketing and promotional materials. Accurate translations are essential to ensure that the medical device is installed and used correctly and that the safety and performance of the device are not compromised.

The importance of having a robust translation procedure in place is perhaps nowhere more evident than in Europe. Article 4(4) of the MDD, AIMDD and IVDD states that EU member states may require that information accompanying the medical device or the in vitro diagnostics (IVD) is provided in their national language(s). The 28 EU member states and 4 European Free Trade Association (EFTA) countries that have adopted the medical devices directives into their national legislation have specific, legally enforceable language requirements. Currently there are 24 official languages in the EU member states (see Table 6.2).

Some countries may allow instructions for use to be provided in English for professional use only, but unless a specific derogation has been obtained from the national Competent Authority, the manufacturer should always provide the product accompanying documentation in the national language(s), as required by law.

Failure to comply with the language requirements may result in product shipments being held at customs at the first point of entry in the EU, recall of products already on the market or inability to obtain product liability insurance. In the event that an incident and near incident is linked to the misuse of a device that might have been caused by confusing or poorly translated labelling and instructions for use, the manufacturer and, if applicable, its EU Authorised Representative are liable for any related deaths or injuries.

Elements of a good translation procedure include, but are not limited to, the following:

- Use professional, accredited translation providers that are familiar with the medical and technical terminology.
- Maintain a master labelling document as the baseline containing the product information, installation and use instructions, warnings and precautions that are common for all country variants.
- Identify for each product the country-by-country differences in indications for use, intended use, official medical terminology, specific wording and symbols required by regulations, etc.

Table 6.2 European countries and their official languages

Countries	EU/EFTA membership (Status: December 2014)	Official language(s)
Albania	EU candidate country	Albanian
Austria	EU	German
Belgium	EU	Dutch, French and German
Bosnia and Herzegovina	EU potential candidate	Bosnian, Croatian, Serbian
Bulgaria	EU	Bulgarian
Croatia	EU	Croatian
Cyprus	EU	Greek
Czech Republic	EU	Czech
Denmark	EU	Danish
Estonia	EU	Estonian
Finland	EU	Finnish, Swedish
France	EU	French
Germany	EU	German
Greece	EU	Greek
Hungary	EU	Hungarian
Iceland	EFTA; EU candidate country	Icelandic
Ireland	EU	Irish, English
Italy	EU	Italian
Kosovo	EU potential candidate	Albanian, Serbian
Latvia	EU	Latvian
Liechtenstein	EFTA	German
Lithuania	EU	Lithuanian
Luxembourg	EU	French, German
(The former Yugoslav republic of) Macedonia	EU candidate country	Macedonian
Malta	EU	Maltese, English
Montenegro	EU candidate country	Montenegrin
Netherlands	EU	Dutch
Norway	EFTA	Norwegian
Poland	EU	Polish
Portugal	EU	Portuguese
Romania	EU	Romanian
Serbia	EU candidate country	Serbian
Slovakia	EU	Slovak
Slovenia	EU	Slovenian
Spain	EU	Spanish
Sweden	EU	Swedish

(*Contd.*)

Table 6.2 (*Contd.*)

Countries	EU/EFTA membership (Status: December 2014)	Official language(s)
Switzerland	EFTA	German, French, Italian, Romansh (Romansh is not mandatory for the government's legal documents or medical device labelling.)
Turkey	EU candidate country	Turkish
United Kingdom	EU	English

Sources: European Commission [14], European Free Trade Association [15]

- Include a translation validation step in the translation process, whereby a different translator validates the translation against the original (English) version.
- Maintain records of who did the translation and when and what was the original (English) version and revision used.
- Include in the translation procedure a requirement for adherence to the national laws pertaining to official language(s) of each country where the product is being marketed.
- Use internationally recognized symbols (according to ISO 15223-1 and EN 980 standards) on product labels and packaging where space is limited) and include an explanation of symbols used in the accompanying documentation (instructions for use, product leaflet, package insert etc.).

An example of a translation process is shown in Fig. 6.1.

6.1.4 *Distribution of Medical Devices*

To be able to manage the multitude and complexity of situations arising during distribution and maintenance of medical devices, a manufacturer must understand the legal terminology related to placing medical devices on the market.

6.1.4.1 Distributing medical devices in US interstate commerce

In the United States, a manufacturer or importer must meet the applicable provisions of the federal FD&C Act and of the

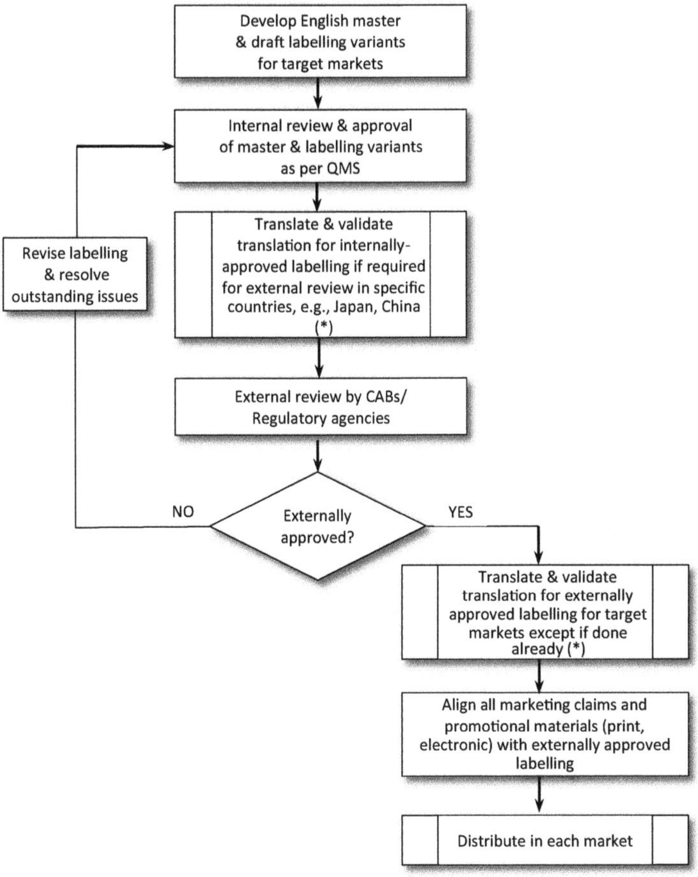

Figure 6.1 Example of a typical translation process.

FDA regulations before distributing a medical device in *interstate* commerce. Section 201(b) of the FD&C Act tells what circumstances place a product in interstate commerce:

(1) commerce between any State or Territory and any place outside thereof; and
(2) commerce within the District of Columbia or within any other Territory not organized with a legislative body".

Interstate commerce applies to all steps in a product's manufacture, packaging and distribution. It is very rare that a product on the US market is not in interstate commerce under the law. For example, at least some of a product's components are likely to originate from out of state, or even out of the United States, and it is foreseeable that a product will leave the state it has been made in. Hence the requirements of the federal FD&C Act and the FDA regulations are likely to apply to most, if not all, medical devices distributed in the United States.

6.1.4.2 Placing medical devices on the EU market

In the EU, the concept of "placing on the market" is fundamental for the application of the medical devices directives. Article 1(2)(h) of the MDD and AIMDD, and Article 1(2)(i) of the IVDD define the term "placing on the market" as follows:

> "Placing on the market" means the first making available in return for payment or free of charge of a device [. . .], with a view to distribution and/or use on the Community market, regardless of whether it is new or fully refurbished.

Blue Guide on the Implementation of EU Product Rules (*Blue Guide*) [16] states the following:

> The placing on the market is the most decisive point in time concerning the application of the Union harmonized legislation. When made available on the market, products must be in compliance with the Union harmonization legislation applicable at the time of placing on the market.
>
> As for "making available", the concept of placing on the market refers to each individual product, not to a type of product, and whether it was manufactured as an individual unit or in series. Consequently, even though a product model or type has been supplied before new Union harmonization legislation laying down new mandatory requirements entered into force, individual units of the same model or type, which are placed on the market after the new requirements have become applicable, must comply with these new requirements.

> The making available of a product supposes an offer or an agreement (written or verbal) between two or more legal or natural persons for the transfer of ownership, possession or any other right concerning the product in question after the stage of manufacture has taken place. The transfer does not necessarily require the physical handover of the product.
>
> This transfer can be for payment or free of charge, and it can be based on any type of legal instrument. Thus, a transfer of a product is considered to have taken place, for instance, in the circumstances of sale, loan, hire, leasing and gift. Transfer of ownership implies that the product is intended to be placed at the disposal of another legal or natural person.

The *Blue Guide* also specifies that placing on the market is considered *not* to take place where a product is "in the stocks of the manufacturer (or the authorised representative established in the Union) or the importer, where the product is not yet made available, unless otherwise provided for in the applicable Union harmonization legislation". The aim of this provision is to discourage manufacturers to produce quantities of products according to "old" legal requirements, stockpile them in their warehouse and sell them over a long period of time. However, if the ownership of a product has been transferred to either a distributor or the end user but the product is still stored by the manufacturer on their behalf, the product can be considered as placed on the market [17].

6.1.4.3 Distribution records

Each manufacturer, importer and distributor of medical devices is required to ensure that its distribution records are maintained so as to enable their timely retrieval upon request by Regulatory Authorities and to accommodate the company's own post-market activities regardless of where the records are physically located. It is recommended that in most circumstances distribution records be retrievable within one to two business days. There may be situations where a company needs more time to access records that are in archived databases. If, in the event of a product recall, a company needs more time to access the distribution records this should be identified in the recall strategy.

Both paper and electronic records should be stored in circumstances that will maintain their integrity, and made available upon request to the relevant authorities. The retention period for the distribution records must comply with the statutory requirements defined in the medical device regulations.

Sponsors are not required to maintain records of the individual users of medical devices; however, a sponsor should have records of distribution centres, hospitals and export countries the device has been supplied to.

For implanted devices, traceability to individual patients, for example, through implant registries, should be maintained, while maintaining patient confidentiality and personal data protection.

6.2 Continued Regulatory Compliance

6.2.1 *Device History Records*

Marketing authorizations are granted for the version of design and manufacturing specifications that were assessed and approved at the time. For each batch, lot or unit of manufactured product, manufacturers must maintain production records to demonstrate that the device is manufactured in accordance with the approved design specifications. This is a requirement defined in the ISO 13485:2009 standard, Section 7.5.1, Control of production and service provision, as well as in the FDA quality system regulations (QSR), Section 820.184, *Device History Record* (DHR).

According to FDA regulation 21 CFR 820.184, *Device History Record*, "Each manufacturer shall establish and maintain procedures to ensure that DHR's for each batch, lot, or unit are maintained to demonstrate that the device is manufactured in accordance with the DMR [refer also to Section 4.4.4, "Design Transfer"]. The DHR shall include, or refer to the location of, the following information:

(a) The dates of manufacture;
(b) The quantity manufactured;
(c) The quantity released for distribution;
(d) The acceptance records which demonstrate the device is manufactured in accordance with the DMR;

(e) The primary identification label and labeling used for each production unit; and
(f) Any unique device identifier (UDI) or universal product code (UPC), and any other device identification(s) and control number(s) used" [18].

DHRs should be traceable to the product model designation and (production) part number to facilitate information retrieval, field corrections and recalls, when necessary. For information on various product identifiers refer to Section 4.5.1, "Product Identifiers".

6.2.2 *Regulatory Requirements in the Post-Market Phase*

A synopsis of regulatory requirements in the established markets and recent developments in international harmonization is provided in the following sub-sections.

6.2.2.1 The EU

In Europe, medical device regulations require that substantial changes to the design and quality system must be notified to the Notified Body and approved prior to implementation. These requirements are found in:

- MDD Annex II, Sections 3.4 and 4.4; Annex III, Section 6; Annex V, Section 3.4; and Annex VI, Section 3.4;
- AIMDD Annex 2, Sections 3.4 and 4.4; Annex 3, Section 6; and Annex 5, Section 3.4; and
- IVDD Annex III, Section 6.3; Annex IV, Sections 3.4, 4.4 and 4.5; Annex V, Sections 6 and 6.1; and Annex VII, Section 3.4.

The first guidance document assisting manufacturers to determine whether a change is "substantial" or not was Recommendation NB-MED/2/5/2, *Reporting of design changes and changes of the quality System*, issued first in in 1997 and revised to Revision 8 in 2008 [22].

A more recent guidance issued in November 2014 by the Notified Bodies Oversight Group (NBOG) – the Best Practice Guide BPG 2014-3, *Guidance for manufacturers and Notified Bodies on reporting of design changes and changes of the quality system*. The criteria for

Table 6.3 MDD: horizontal "criteria for notification", "criteria for new approval" and "criteria to be assessed"

Conformity assessment annex	Criteria for notification	Criteria for a new (supplementary) approval	Criteria to be assessed
Annex II Section 4.4	Any changes made to the approved design	Changes could affect conformity with the Essential Requirements.	Conformity with the requirements of the MDD
Annex III Section 6	Any significant change made to the approved product	Changes may affect conformity with the Essential Requirements or with the conditions prescribed for use of the product.	Conformity with the requirements of the MDD
Annex II Section 3.4	Any plan for substantial changes to the quality system or the product range covered	-	Requirements referred to in Annex II, Section 3.2
Annex V Section 3.4	Any plan for substantial changes to the quality system	-	Requirements referred to in Annex II, Section 3.2
Annex VI Section 3.4	Any plan for substantial changes to the quality system	-	Requirements referred to in Annex II, Section 3.2

notification, the criteria for a new (supplementary) approval and the criteria to be assessed are summarized for each of the three medical devices directives in Tables 6.3, 6.4 and 6.5 [23].

In a nutshell, changes to the design that affect compliance with the Essential Requirements (ERs) and/or changes in the indications for use, contraindications or warnings determined by the manufacturer to be appropriate to ensure the clinical performance of the device are considered substantial or significant.

Changes to the quality system that affect compliance of the devices covered by the quality system with the ERs or the approved type/design, and changes that affect the compliance of the quality system with its own regulatory requirements, such as switching from paper to electronic archiving, are also considered substantial or significant.

Table 6.4 AIMDD: horizontal "criteria for notification", "criteria for new approval" and "criteria to be assessed"

Conformity assessment annex	Criteria for notification	Criteria for a new (supplementary) approval	Criteria to be assessed
Annex 2 Section 4.4	Any modification made to the approved design	Modifications may affect conformity with the Essential Requirements.	Conformity with the requirements of the AIMDD
Annex 3 Section 6	Any modification made to the approved product	Modifications may affect conformity with the Essential Requirements or with the conditions of use specified for the product.	Satisfy the requirements of the AIMDD
Annex 2 Section 3.4	Any plan to alter the quality system	-	Requirements referred to in Annex 2, Section 3.2
Annex 5 Section 3.4	Any plan to alter the quality system	-	Requirements referred to in Annex 2, Section 3.2

Examples of design changes that would be considered significant:

- Changes to built-in control mechanisms (means of verifying or checking that the specifications or outputs of the device meet a standard or predetermined result, put in place to maintain ongoing control or regulate the output of a device);
- Changes to operating principles, including changes in the source of energy (means by which a device produces or brings about an intended or appropriate effect); and
- Changes to design specifications that may affect the indications for use or the performance of the device or raise new safety and performance issues, including but not limited to changes in expiration date, primary packaging or energy type, physical, dimensional and environmental specifications and ergonomics of the patient/user interface.

Table 6.5 Table 6.5 IVDD: horizontal “criteria for notification”, “criteria for new approval” and “criteria to be assessed”

Conformity assessment annex	Criteria for notification	Criteria for a new (supplementary) approval	Criteria to be assessed
Annex III Section 6.3	Any significant change made to the approved design	Changes could affect conformity with the Essential Requirements of the IVDD or with the conditions prescribed for use of the product.	Conformity with the design-related requirements of the IVDD
Annex IV Section 4.4	Any changes made to the approved design	Changes could affect conformity with the Essential Requirements of the IVDD or with the conditions prescribed for use of the product.	Conformity with the requirements of the IVDD
Annex IV Section 4.5	Any changes to the pathogen and markers of infections to be tested, in particular as a consequence of biological complexity and variability	-	Conformity with the requirements of the IVDD
Annex V Section 6	Any changes to the pathogen and markers of infections to be tested, in particular as a consequence of biological complexity and variability	-	Meet the Essential Requirements of the IVDD
Annex V Section 6.1	Any changes to the approved device	Wherever the changes may affect conformity with the Essential Requirements of the IVDD or with the conditions prescribed for use of the device	Meet the Essential Requirements of the IVDD
Annex IV Section 3.4	Any plan for substantial changes to the quality system or the product-range covered	-	Requirements referred to in Annex IV, Section 3.2
Annex VII Section 3.4	Any plan for substantial changes to the quality system	-	Requirements referred to in Annex VII, Section 3.2

Example of software changes that would be considered significant:

- A software change, which impacts the control of the device, that may alter the diagnosis or therapy delivered to the patient;
- An alteration in software that modifies an algorithm impacting the diagnosis or the therapy delivered;
- A software change that impacts the way data is read or interpreted by the user such that the treatment or diagnosis of the patient may be altered when compared to the previous
- A version of the software;
- A software change that replaces previously required user input to a closed-loop decision;
- Addition of a new feature to the software that may change the diagnosis or the therapy delivered to the patient;
- Introduction to or removal of a new alarm function from the software such that a response to the new configuration may change the treatment of the patient in comparison to the previous version of the software; and
- A software change that incorporates a significant change to the operating system on which the software runs.

Examples of changes to materials that would be considered significant:

- Changes to the sourcing or processing of materials of human origin or substances, which, if used separately, may be considered to be a medicinal product;
- For materials of animal origin, changes of the geographical source of animals, the raw materials of animal origin and the processes for selection, collection, handling, control and inactivation/elimination that may modify viral safety;
- For tissues (or derivatives) of animal origin, changes regarding tissues (or derivatives), processes for selection, collection, processing, handling, inactivation and elimination or any new data collected by the manufacturer and relevant to the medical device with regard to transmissible spongiform encephalopathy (TSE) risk; and

- Changes within a single generic material type or changes in formulation that can affect the chemistry, metallurgy or other property, such as stability, of the device.

Examples of changes to materials for IVDs that would be considered significant:

- Changes to materials that affect the IVD's performance characteristics, including specificity or sensitivity;
- Changes to materials that require additional testing to determine the performance characteristics of the IVD, unless the additional performance testing only confirms that the altered IVD still conforms to the certified performance specifications and no labelling changes are necessary;
- Changes to the materials of an IVD that result in a change to the operating principle of the product, for example, change from immunofluorescence assay (IFA) to enzyme-linked immunosorbent assay (ELISA); and
- Changes to materials that potentially affect the operating principle of an IVD, including changes in reaction components or materials, such as calibration materials, or changes in methods such as specimen pre-treatment, incubation times and temperatures, that result in altered performance characteristics that are reflected in the labelling.

Examples of changes to labelling that would be considered significant:

- Changes to the intended use or indications for use, unless the changes are within the already approved set of indications;
- Adding of a contraindication as a result of concerns associated with the safe and effective use of the device;
- Removing of a contraindication, warning or precaution; and
- Changes in the shelf life and/or the protocols and methods for determining the shelf life.

Examples of changes to manufacturing processes, facility or equipment that would be considered significant:

- Changes to the manufacturing process, facility or equipment that affect the safety or performance of a device, including changes to the packaging process;
- Adding or moving of manufacturing facilities;
- Changes in the manufacturing process, facility or equipment of a critical supplier (subcontractors in charge of processes that are essential for ensuring compliance with legal requirements or suppliers of crucial components or of the entire devices);
- Changes to test/inspection acceptance criteria or methods; and
- Removal of test acceptance criteria, in-process inspection or final inspection.

Examples of changes to sterilization that would be considered significant:

- Change to the sterilization method or process or change to the packaging for the sterilization of a medical device;
- Changes that increase the bioburden alert or action levels or that introduce an organism that is more difficult to kill;
- Changes in the manufacturing location;
- Device design and material changes that introduce a feature that is more difficult to sterilize;
- Changes in the sterilization process or equipment or cycle parameter;
- Change of the sterilization service provider;
- Changes in the density or configuration of the sterilization load;
- Changes to the quality control verification and validation (V&V) process, such as introducing parametric release; and
- Reductions in conventional incubation durations.

6.2.2.2 The United States

In the United States, changes that could significantly affect the safety and effectiveness of the device must be submitted for review and approval prior to implementation. These requirements are defined in the following FDA regulations:

- For devices cleared under a 510(k): 21 CFR §807.81 when a pre-market notification submission is required;
- For devices approved under a Premarket Approval (PMA): 21 CFR §814.39, *PMA Supplements*, and §814.84, *(Annual) Reports*; and
- For devices undergoing a review under a PMA or a PMA supplement: 21 CFR §814.37, *PMA Amendments and Resubmitted PMAs*.

The FDA has published the following guidelines to assist manufacturers in determining whether a change is significant or not and what regulatory action is required for different types of significant changes:

- *Deciding When to Submit a 510(k) for a Change to an Existing Device* – contains detailed flowcharts providing direction to manufacturers on deciding when to submit a 510(k) for a change to an existing device [24];
- *How to Prepare a Special 510(k)* – describes the streamlined 510(k) process for modifications to a device cleared under 510(k) [25];
- *PMA Supplements and Amendments* – provides an overview of the methods of notifications and FDA involvement of changes to a PMA-approved medical device [26];
- *Real-Time Premarket Approval Application (PMA) Supplements* – describes the real-time review (RTR) process applicable to changes validated according to accepted test methods or procedures for devices of that type and involving review within a single scientific discipline [27];
- *30-Day Notices, 135-Day Premarket Approval (PMA) Supplements and 75-Day Humanitarian Device Exemption (HDE) Supplements for Manufacturing Method or Process Changes* – covers the methods of notifications for manufacturing changes [28]; and
- *Supplements to Approved Applications for Class III Medical Devices: Use of Published Literature, Use of Previously Submitted Materials, and Priority Review* – provides examples of how the use of published literature may be used in support of a

PMA, Product Development Protocol (PDP) or Humanitarian Device Exemption (HDE) supplement [29].

In general, if changes do not affect the device's safety or effectiveness they are considered non-significant and do not require the FDA's approval prior to implementation. However, for devices approved under a PMA such changes need to be included in the periodic (annual) reports to the FDA as a condition to approval of the device, for example, an editorial change in labelling that does not affect the safety or effectiveness of the device.

Part of the assessment for all changes should include a risk analysis and validation (or, where appropriate, verification) of the changes to the design or manufacturing process and subsequent assessment of the need for regulatory submission. For devices approved under a PMA, if risk analysis for the change determines that additional verification or validation testing is required to establish that the device remains safe and effective, a regulatory submission is likely to be required.

The type of changes and criteria for regulatory submission are summarized in Table 6.6 for devices cleared under 510(k) and in Table 6.7 for devices approved under PMA.

The standard conditions of approval for a PMA include typically:

- A requirement to submit periodic reports at intervals of one year (unless specified otherwise) from the date of approval of the original PMA application, hence their name – "Annual Reports"; the periodic reports should list changes in a tabular format with reference to which PMAs are impacted by the changes, and should include a summary description (what was changed) and the rationale for each change (why was the change made and why no PMA supplement was required).
- A requirement to submit a PMA supplement when unanticipated adverse events, increases in the incidence of anticipated adverse events or device failures necessitate a labelling, manufacturing or device modification.
- A requirement to submit a PMA supplement if the device is to be modified and the modified device should be subjected

Table 6.6 Devices cleared under 510(k): criteria for change assessment and regulatory action

Regulation/guideline	Types of changes/criteria for notification	Regulatory action/submission type
Deciding When to Submit a 510(k) for a Change to an Existing Device	Changes to a legally marketed device that is the subject of a recall – proposed fixes	New 510(k)
Deciding When to Submit a 510(k) for a Change to an Existing Device Flowchart A	**A. Labelling changes:** A1: a change that affects indications for use A2: a change in warnings or precautions A3: a change that adds a contraindication A4: a change that deletes a contraindication A5: labelling being revised for clarity to insure safer or more effective use; changes do not impact safety and effectiveness	A1, A4: new 510(k) A2, A5: document to file A3: new 510(k) changes being effected
Deciding When to Submit a 510(k) for a Change to an Existing Device Flowchart B	**B. Technology or performance changes:** B1: a change to the control mechanism B2: a change in the operating principle B3: a change in energy type B4: a change in environmental specifications + additional conditions B5: a change in performance specifications + additional conditions B6: a change in ergonomics of the patient/user interface + additional conditions B7: a change in dimensional specifications + additional conditions B8: a change in software or firmware + additional conditions Additional conditions for B4–B8 changes:	B1, B2, B3: new 510(k) B4, B5, B6, B7, B8, B10, B10.1: new 510(k) B9 and other design changes: document to file

	• Affect indications for use; or • Require clinical data for establishing safety and effectiveness for purposes of substantial equivalence; or • Design validation raises new questions of safety and effectiveness. B9: a change in packaging or expiration dating B10: a change in sterilization B10.1: change in performance specification or decrease in sterility assurance level (SAL)	
Deciding When to Submit a 510(k) for a Change to an Existing Device Flowchart C	**C. Materials changes:** C1: if an IVD, use flowchart D C2: a change in material type and if device is an implant or likely to come in direct contact with tissue or body fluids, and/or additional testing to ISO 10993-1 required C3: a change in material formulation and if device is an implant or likely to come in direct contact with tissue or body fluids, and/or additional testing to ISO 10993-1 required C2–C3 changes in material type or formulation that change device performance specifications and:	C1: flowchart D C2, C3, C4: new 510(k) Other changes: document to file

(*Contd.*)

Table 6.6 (*Contd.*)

Regulation/guideline	Types of changes/criteria for notification	Regulatory action/submission type
	• Affect indications for use; or • Require clinical data for establishing safety and effectiveness for purposes of substantial equivalence; or • Design validation raises new questions of safety and effectiveness. C4: a change in material supplier and material is not ordered to a spec	
Deciding When to Submit a 510(k) for a Change to an Existing Device Flowchart D	**D. Materials changes for IVDs:** D1: a change in performance specification and D1.1 clinical data necessary to establish safety and effectiveness for purposes of substantial equivalence, and/or D1.3 design validation raises new questions of safety and effectiveness D1.2: clinical data necessary to show conformance to a recognized standard D2: a change in the operating principle	D1, D1.1, D1.3, D2: new 510(k) D1.2 and other changes: document to file

Table 6.7 Devices cleared under PMA: criteria for change assessment and regulatory action

Regulation/guideline	Types of changes/criteria for notification	Regulatory action/submission type
FD&C Act Section 737(4)(B)	Changes in indications for use, design or performance of the device for which substantial clinical data is generally necessary	Panel-Track Supplement (new clinical and potentially some new preclinical data)
21 CFR §814.39(a)	**Changes that affect the safety or effectiveness of the device:** • New indication for use of the device; • Labelling changes; • The use of a different facility or establishment to manufacture, process, sterilize or package the device; • Changes in manufacturing facilities, methods or quality control procedures; • Changes in sterilization procedures; • Changes in packaging; • Changes in the performance or design specifications, circuits, components, ingredients, principles of operation or physical layout of the device; and • Extension of the expiration date of the device based on data obtained under a new or revised stability or sterility testing protocol that has not been approved by the FDA. [If the protocol has been previously approved by the FDA, a supplement is not submitted but the change must be reported to the FDA in the post-approval periodic reports, as described in §814.39(b).]	180-Day PMA Supplement (pre-clinical and potentially limited confirmatory clinical data) – same process as PMA Or Real-time review, or RTR (pre-clinical data only) – only for minor changes that can be reviewed by a reviewer in one scientific discipline; for which there is an FDA-accepted test methods or procedures for devices of that type, such as an FDA-recognized standard or guidance document, and for which the applicant has requested and the FDA has granted a meeting or similar forum to jointly review and determine the status of the supplement

(*Contd.*)

Table 6.7 *(Contd.)*

Regulation/ guideline	Types of changes/criteria for notification	Regulatory action/submission type
21 CFR §814.39(d)	**Changes that enhance the safety of the device or the safety in the use of the device:** • Labelling changes that add or strengthen a contraindication, warning, precaution or information about an adverse reaction; • Labelling changes that add or strengthen an instruction that is intended to enhance the safe use of the device; • Labelling changes that delete misleading, false or unsupported indications; and • Changes in quality controls or the manufacturing process that add a new specification or test method or otherwise provide additional assurance of purity, identity, strength or reliability of the device.	Special PMA Supplement Changes Being Effected – may be implemented by the applicant prior to the receipt of a written FDA order approving the PMA supplement, but after the applicant receives specific acknowledgement that the application qualifies for review under §814.39(d)(2)
21 CFR §814.39(f)	**Changes to manufacturing procedures or methods of manufacture that affect the safety or effectiveness of the device, *except* changes in a manufacturing/sterilization site or to design or performance specifications:** • Sterilization process parameters within the same facility; • Automating existing processes;; • Joining processes; • Cleaning methods used to remove manufacturing materials; • Manufacturing materials; • Environmental conditions of the manufacturing, storage or distribution facilities; • Suppliers of components, materials or services, where specifications are unchanged; • Quality control testing; and • Type of manufacturing process.	30-Day Notice and 135 PMA Supplement – If the change qualifies as a 30-Day Notice, the change may be made 30 days after the FDA receives the 30-Day Notice unless the FDA informs the PMA holder that the 30-Day Notice is not adequate and describes the additional information or action required. If the 30-Day Notice was not adequate, but contained data meeting appropriate content requirements for a PMA supplement, then the 30-Day Notice will become a 135-Day PMA Supplement.

21 CFR §814.39	**Change in the manufacturing site:** • Use of a different facility or establishment to manufacture, process or package the device – certain conditions apply, that is, the manufacturing site must have received a quality system/GMP inspection within the last two years.	PMA Manufacturing Site Change Supplement – If requirements are not met, a 180-Day PMA Supplement must be submitted.
21 CFR §814.39(e) §814.84	**Changes that do not affect safety or effectiveness of the device**	Annual Report – periodic report listing changes described in §814.39(a) and §814.39(b)

to animal or laboratory or clinical testing designed to determine if the modified device remains safe and effective.

Annual Reports are not to be taken lightly, as deficiencies found in Annual Reports may result in violations of the FD&C Act. This is for example an excerpt from an FDA Annual Report Deficiency Letter:

> The "Conditions of Approval" that accompanied the FDA approval order for the above referenced PMA require your submission, under receipt for FDA approval, of a PMA supplement before commercial distribution of the device with changes and modifications affecting its safety or effectiveness. The FDA approval order advised that commercial distribution of a device that is not in compliance with these conditions of approval is a violation of the Federal Food, Drug, and Cosmetic Act (the Act).
>
> It may be possible that the above changes were implemented without your submission, and receipt of prior FDA approval, of the required PMA supplements based upon your firm's misunderstanding of the PMA supplement requirements under 21 CFR §814.39. We hope that this letter and the changes identified above will provide you with appropriate guidance in this matter and thereby enable you to implement remedial measures to avoid noncompliance with these requirements in the future.
>
> Following receipt of the above requested PMA supplements we will determine whether further FDA action is necessary.

6.2.2.3 Australia

In Australia, medical device regulations require that substantial changes to the design and quality system be notified to the TGA and approved prior to implementation. These requirements are covered in the following sections of the medical device regulations, Schedule 3 of conformity assessment procedures (Table 6.8):

- Part 1 Full quality assurance procedures, Section 1.5, Changes to quality management system or kinds of medical device to which system is to be applied, and Section 1.6, Examination of design of Class 4 IVD, Class 4 in-house IVD, Class AIMD or Class III medical device;
- Part 2 Type examination procedures, Section 2.4, Changes to design of medical device after examination;

Table 6.8 Australian conformity assessment procedures (Schedule 3): "criteria for notification" and "criteria to be assessed"

Conformity assessment procedure	Criteria for notification	Criteria to be assessed
Part 1 Section 1.5	A substantial change to the quality system or A change to the kinds of medical devices to which the quality system is applied	After any change to the quality management system, the changed system continues to meet the requirements of Clause 1.4 of Schedule 3. Have available, in writing, details of any consequential changes to the information and documentation required in Sub-clause 1.3(2) of Schedule 3 in relation to the system or kinds of devices.
Part 1 Section 1.6	A substantial change to the design, or the intended performance, of the kind of device	The design, or the intended performance, of the medical device, as changed, complies with the applicable provisions of the Essential Principles. Have available, in writing, details of any consequential changes to the documentation in relation to the design of the device mentioned in Paragraph 1.4(5)(c) of Schedule 3.
Part 2 Section 2.4	A substantial change to the design, or intended performance, of the kind of medical device to which the type relates	The type, as changed, meets the requirements of Clause 2.3 of Schedule 3. Have available, in writing, details of any consequential changes to the documentation required under Sub-clause 2.3(3) of Schedule 3 in relation to the type.

(*Contd.*)

Table 6.8 *(Contd.)*

Conformity assessment procedure	Criteria for notification	Criteria to be assessed
Part 4 Section 4.5	A substantial change to the quality system	After any change to the quality management system, the changed system continues to meet the requirements of Clause 4.4 of Schedule 3. Have available, in writing, details of any consequential changes to the information and documentation required under Sub-clause 4.3(2) of Schedule 3 in relation to the system.
Part 5 Section 5.5	A substantial change to the quality system or A change to the kinds of medical devices to which the quality system is applied	After any change to the quality management system, the changed system continues to meet the requirements of Clause 5.4 of Schedule 3. Have available, in writing, details of any consequential changes to the information and documentation required under Sub-clause 5.3(2) of Schedule 3 in relation to the system or kinds of devices.

- Part 4 Production quality assurance procedures, Section 4.5, Changes to production quality management system; and
- Part 5 Product quality assurance procedures, Section 5.5, Changes to product quality management system or kinds of medical device.

At the time of going to print the TGA guidelines for change controls (Section 21, Changes to ARTG Inclusions of the *Australian Regulatory Guidelines for Medical Devices*, or ARGMD) are yet to be drafted.

6.2.2.4 Canada

In Canada, medical device regulations require that significant changes be submitted to Health Canada for approval prior to implementation. Significant change means a change that could reasonably be expected to affect the safety or effectiveness of a medical device. It includes a change to any of the following:

(a) The manufacturing process, facility or equipment;
(b) The manufacturing quality control procedures, including the methods, tests or procedures used to control the quality, purity and sterility of the device or of the materials used in its manufacture;
(c) The design of the device, including its performance characteristics, principles of operation and specifications of materials, energy source, software or accessories; and
(d) The intended use of the device, including any new or extended use, any addition or deletion of a contraindication for the device and any change to the period used to establish its expiry date.

According to Section 34, Application for a Medical Device Licence Amendment, the following changes must be submitted for assessment:

(a) In the case of a Class III or IV medical device, a significant change;
(b) A change that would affect the class of the device;
(c) A change in the name of the manufacturer;
(d) A change in the name of the device;

(e) A change in the identifier of the device, including the identifier of any medical device that is part of a system, test kit, medical device group, medical device family or medical device group family; and

(f) In the case of a Class II medical device, a change in the medical conditions, purposes or uses for which the device is manufactured, sold or represented.

Health Canada's *Guidance for the Interpretation of Significant Changes* contains detailed step-by-step flowcharts and examples covering medical devices and IVDs that will assist manufacturers in determining whether a change is significant or not (see also Table 6.9).

According to this guideline, "For any change contemplated, a manufacturer must consider the device in question, the impact of the change on the patient, practitioner and/or user of the device, and the impact of the change on the specifications of the device, and decide whether the change could reasonably be expected to impact the safety and effectiveness of the device. When considering several simultaneous changes, this guidance document should be used to assess each change separately, as well as the collective impact of the changes".

Furthermore, "All changes must be documented in the Quality Management System by the manufacturer. If changes have been found not to be significant by applying the principles of this guidance document and these changes are related to the information and/or documents originally submitted by the manufacturer with respect to the device licence application, then the changes must be reported to Health Canada at the time of annual licence renewal. These changes should be briefly itemized, in a tabular form with appropriate dates and with any necessary attachments" [30].

6.2.2.5 Japan

In Japan, certain changes to the device design and quality system require submission and, if applicable, approval prior to implementation (see Table 6.10).

Table 6.9 Devices approved under a Canadian Medical Device Licence: criteria for change assessment and regulatory action

Regulation/guideline	Types of changes/criteria for notification	Regulatory action/submission type
Guidance for the Interpretation of Significant Change of a Medical Device Flowchart A	**A. Changes in manufacturing processes, facility or equipment:** A1: a change in manufacturing process, facility or Equipment that impacts the safety and effectiveness of the device A2: adding a new manufacturing facility (same manufacturer's name and address on the labelling) A3: a change in a supplier's manufacturing process, facility or equipment that results in a change in the device specification and/or a change in the incoming inspections to evaluate the material/equipment provided by the supplier A4: a change to the manufacturing process, facility or equipment for a combination product A5: a change in sterilization procedures or methods	A1, A2, A3: licence amendment A4: as per policy Drug/ medical device combination products Other changes: document to file A5: flowchart D
Guidance for the Interpretation of Significant Change of a Medical Device Flowchart B	**B. Changes in manufacturing quality control procedures:** B1: a change due to removal of test acceptance criteria, in-process inspections or final inspections without replacement of these activities B2: a change to the manufacturing quality control procedure (the methods, tests and procedures used to control the quality, purity and sterility of the material or the device) that alters the design specification of the device	B1: licence amendment B2: flowchart C Other changes: document to file
Guidance for the Interpretation of Significant Change of a Medical Device Flowchart C	**C. Changes in design:** C1: a change to the control mechanism (i.e., mechanisms maintaining ongoing control or regulating the output of a device) C2: a change to the operating principles, including a change in the source of energy used by the device C3: a change to the design specification, physical description, patient or user interface, software or firmware that affect the indications for use C4: a change requiring clinical data to support the safety and effectiveness of the altered device C5: changes resulting in design validation that raises new issues of safety and effectiveness	C1, C2, C3, C4, C5: licence amendment Other changes: document to file

(Contd.)

Table 6.9 *(Contd.)*

Regulation/ guideline	Types of changes/criteria for notification	Regulatory action/submission type
Guidance for the Interpretation of Significant Change of a Medical Device Flowchart D	**D. Changes to sterilization:** D1: a change that increases the bioburden alert or action levels or that introduces a more difficult-to-kill organism D2: a change to the device design or material that introduces a more difficult-to-sterilize feature D3: a change in sterilization process (e.g., cycle parameters, equipment, density or configuration of load), with additional new test acceptance criteria or test method and test methodology is not an accepted or recognized test method by Health Canada; and/or the change in sterilization method hasn't been reviewed in a previous application for similar devices and/or is more difficult to sterilize than the previously licensed device D4: a change in the device packaging that hasn't been reviewed in a previous application for similar devices and/or is more difficult to sterilize than the previously licensed device D5: a change made from non-parametric release to a parametric release	D1, D2, D3, D4, D5: licence amendment Other changes: document to file
Guidance for the Interpretation of Significant Change of a Medical Device Flowchart E	**E. Changes to software:** E1: a change that impacts the control of the device in a manner that might alter the diagnosis or therapy delivered E2: a change that modifies an algorithm that impacts the diagnosis or therapy delivered E3: a change that impacts the way data is read and/or interpreted, such that the treatment or diagnosis of the patient may be altered when compared to previous version of the software E4: a change that modifies a decision point from requiring user input to fully automated (e.g., closed-loop decision) E5: a change that adds a new feature that may change the diagnosis or therapy delivered E6: a change that introduces or removes an alarm function, and a response to the new alarm may change the treatment of the patient in comparison to the previous version of the software E7: a change in software that incorporates a change in the operating system on which the software is running E8: a change that corrects an error for which there is a safety risk to the patient is the error is not fixed	E1, E2, E3, E4, E5, E6, E7: licence amendment E8: requires clarification from Health Canada If E8 corrects an inadvertent logic error to bring the system back to specification or introduces only non-therapeutic/non-diagnostic features or modifies only the user interface with negligible risk of impacting diagnostic or therapy delivered or disables a feature that does not interact with other features: document to file

Guidance for the Interpretation of Significant Change of a Medical Device Flowchart F	**F. Changes in materials for medical devices other than IVDs:** F1: if an IVD, use flowchart G F2: a change in material of animal origin F3: a change in the supplier or vendor of the material, and the material does not meet the manufacturer's previously reviewed acceptance criteria F4 –the device is surgically invasive or intended to be absorbed by the body or to remain in the body for at least 30 consecutive days, and the altered material will be in contact with body tissues or fluids F5: the device is surgically invasive or intended to be absorbed by the body or to remain in the body for at least 30 consecutive days, and the altered material will not be in contact with body tissues or fluids, but there are changes to the design specification required; use flowchart C F6: the device is not intended to be absorbed by the body or to remain in the body for at least 30 consecutive days, but the altered material is in contact with body tissues and fluids and the specifications have changed	F1: flowchart G F2, F3, F4, F6: licence amendment F5: flowchart C Other changes: document to file
Guidance for the Interpretation of Significant Change of a Medical Device Flowchart G	**G. Changes in materials for IVDs:** G1: a change that requires testing of additional clinical samples to determine the performance characteristics of the IVD, and the additional clinical testing confirms that the altered IVD still meets the licensed performance specifications and no labelling changes are necessary G2: a change that requires testing of additional clinical samples to determine the performance characteristics of the IVD, but the additional clinical testing does not confirm that the altered IVD still meets the licensed performance specifications and labelling changes are necessary	G1: document to file G2: licence amendment

(*Contd.*)

Table 6.9 *(Contd.)*

Regulation/guideline	Types of changes/criteria for notification	Regulatory action/submission type
Guidance for the Interpretation of Significant Change of a Medical Device Flowchart H	**H. Changes to labelling:** H1: a change in the indications for use that is not within an approved set of indications H2 –a change to the existing warning and precautions that adds or removes a contraindication H3: deletion of a warning or precaution H4: a change in the shelf life of an IVD	H1, H2, H3, H4: licence amendment
Guidance for the Interpretation of Significant Change of a Medical Device	**Non-significant changes:** Changes related to the information and/or documents originally submitted by the manufacturer with respect to the device licence application	Included in reports submitted with the annual licence renewal

Table 6.10 Japan medical device regulations: types of changes and submissions

Type of change	Type of application
Changes with no effect on product safety, effectiveness or quality	Notification of minor changes; must be submitted within 30 days after the change
Changes limited within a specific scope, for example: • Raw materials of parts/ components coming into contact with tissue or blood • Sterilization methods, methods of determining sterilization doses or methods of sterilization validation	Application for specific changes
Changes qualifying for accelerated assessment according to official notifications, for example: • Shelf life extension • Changes to or addition of manufacturing sites	Accelerated application for changes
Changes other than above	Standard application for changes

Based on Table 15-7 of *Fundamentals of Japanese Regulatory Affairs* [12]

6.2.2.6 Emerging markets

As existing regulations in emerging markets are being revised and new ones adopted, manufacturers are should expect newly or better defined requirements for changes in the post-market phase.

In China, for instance, the new regulations require that changes to the device be submitted to the relevant China Food and Drug Administration (CFDA) department. Significant changes that are technical in nature require CFDA approval prior to implementation; changes that are administrative in nature require filing with the CFDA (see Table 6.11). For imported devices, changes must be first approved in the country of origin before they can be approved in China [31].

In December 2014 the Singapore Health Sciences Authority has updated its *Guidance on Licensing for manufacturers, Importers and Wholesalers of Medical Devices*, which includes the types of changes that require regulatory action (see Table 6.12) [32].

Table 6.11 Variations requiring regulatory action in China

Type of changes	Regulatory action/type of submission
Variations to approved items (technical in nature): Product name Model designation Specifications Structure and components Indications for use Technical requirements Manufacturing site changes	Approval by the CFDA – may require supporting data such as type testing and/or clinical trials
Variations to registered items (administrative in nature): Manufacturer (applicant) name and address Sponsor name and address	Filing with the CFDA

6.3 Change Management

6.3.1 *Change Controls*

The quality management system (QMS) must have controls in place to ensure that any changes made to the device or its manufacturing processes are assessed and implemented only if compliance is maintained. This requirement is defined in ISO 13485:2009, Section 7.3.7, Control of design and development changes, as follows:

> Design and development changes shall be identified and records maintained. The changes shall be reviewed, verified and validated, as appropriate, and approved before implementation. The review of design and development changes shall include evaluation of the effect of the changes on constituent parts and product already delivered. Records of the results of the review of changes and any necessary actions shall be maintained.

Similarly, in Section 820.30(i), Design changes of FDA's quality system regulations (QSR), it is stated that "each manufacturer shall establish and maintain procedures for the identification, documentation, validation or where appropriate verification, review, and approval of design changes before their implementation".

Table 6.12 Changes requiring regulatory action in Singapore

Type of changes	Regulatory action/type of submission
1. Change in applicant information	Global update of applicant details in E-service
2 Change in licence information: 2.1 Type of dealer's licence 2.2 Risk classification 2.3 Certification - quality system 2.4 Certification body 2.5 QMS expiry date 2.6 Scope of operations 2.7 Cold-chain management for Good Distribution Practice for Medical Devices (GDPMDS) - addition/removal 2.8 Operating site address(es)/premises of third-party logistics service providers/outsourced activities related to GDPMDS or ISO 13495 activities - addition/removal	2.1: New application 2.2–2.8: licence amendment
3 Company information 3.1 Name, business address, contact person details 3.2 Legal entity, Unique Entity Number (UEN)	3.1: change in business information 3.2: new application
4 Class A Exemption List - exempted Class A medical devices imported or manufactured - addition/removal	Submission of update of Class A medical device exemption list

The FDA identifies two principal administrative elements involved in controlling design changes:

- Document control-enumeration of design documents, and tracking their status and revision history (design documents, drawings and other items of design input or output that characterize the design or some aspect of it); and
- Change control-enumeration of deficiencies and corrective actions arising from verification and review of the design and tracking their resolution prior to design transfer [19].

Changes in a product design and/or manufacturing processes would typically result in the revision of relevant design outputs

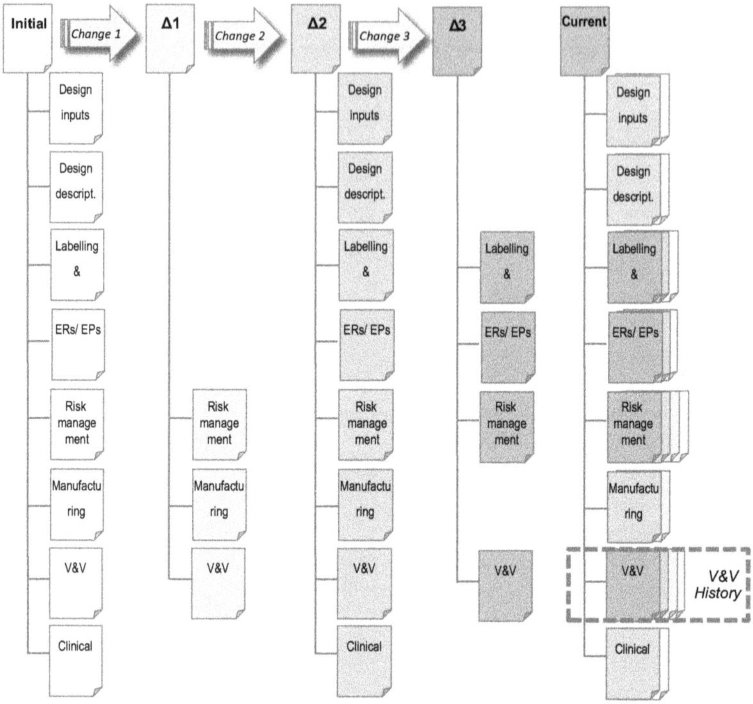

Figure 6.2 Example of managing the technical documentation as changes are made to the product design and/or manufacturing process.

(specifications, design descriptions, labelling) and V&V documentation (protocols and reports), as applicable. The product technical documentation (Design Dossier) is comprised of controlled documents uniquely identified by document and revision numbers. The technical documentation reflects the current status of the product design and manufacturing processes at any point in time, and if properly managed, it should enable the quick and easy retrieval of the product history as well (see Fig. 6.2).

Changes must be documented – what was changed and why – and must reference the documentary evidence – risk analysis, failure mode and effects analysis (FMEA), V&V – demonstrating that the changed product still conforms to approved specifications, including requirements for safety and effectiveness. Every change to a product

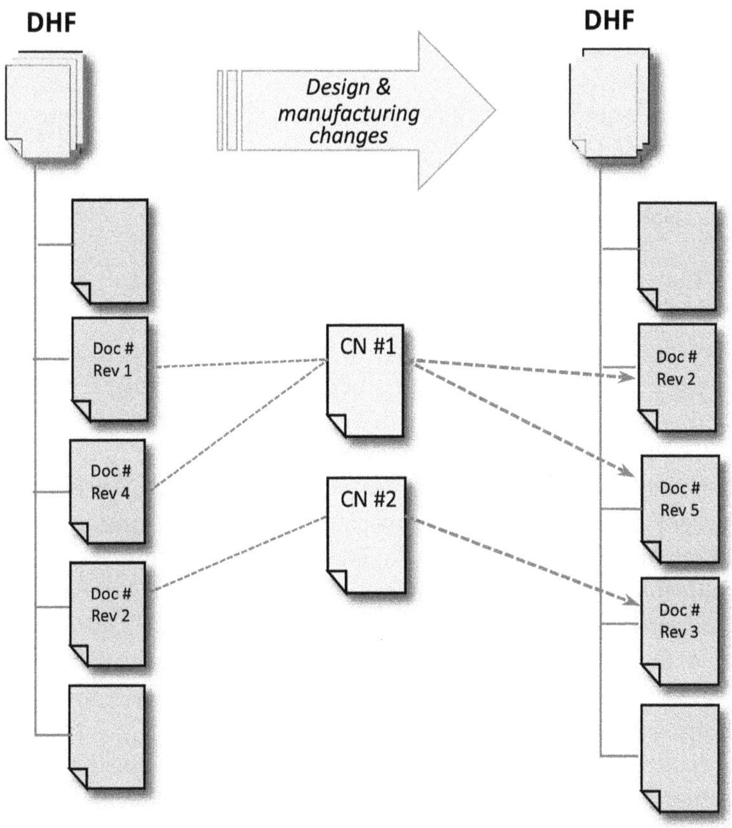

Figure 6.3 Example of traceability between change control enumeration and document control enumeration.

in post-market phase must be assigned a change control number to uniquely identify the change.

Changes resulting in the revision of Design History File (DHF) documents should reference the revised DHF documents by their number and revision, establishing thus clear traceability between the change and the DHF documentation affected by the change and revised as a result of the change (see example in Fig. 6.3).

In this example, the product undergoes multiple related changes in its design and manufacturing process requiring partial re-test

(ΔV&V). Changes are consolidated and grouped into two significant changes:

- One significant design change documented in Change Note CN #1; and
- One significant manufacturing change documented in Change Note CN #2.

The revised DHF documents (specifications, V&V reports) identified by document number and (new) revision number are referenced in the Change Notes, establishing thus clear traceability between the change control numbers (CN #) and the DHF documentation control numbers (Document #, Revision #).

The FDA has strict requirements for changes made in the post-market phase and for a good reason. In its *Medical Device Recall Report FY2003 to FY2012*, the FDA concluded that "the most frequent causes for recalls are related to device design, software, and non-conforming material or component issues". For each recall, the FDA determines the associated regulatory violations. All top 10 regulatory violations for the period covered in the report were related to *Quality System Regulations* (21 CFR Part 820), with design controls (21 CFR 820.30) being the first on the list.

In terms of reasons for recalls, 36% of recalls were due to design-related failures, 28% due to material or component failure, 17% due to process control failures, 13% due to packaging and labelling problems and 6% due to change control failures [20].

Change controls apply to software as well. According to the FDA:

> Combined with a lack of understanding of software, it can lead managers to believe that tightly controlled engineering is not needed as much for software as it is for hardware. In fact, the opposite is true. Because of its complexity, the development process for software should be even more tightly controlled than for hardware, in order to prevent problems that cannot be easily detected later in the development process.
>
> Due to the complexity of software, a seemingly small local change may have a significant global system impact. When any change (even a small change) is made to the software, the validation status of the software needs to be re-established.

Whenever software is changed, a validation analysis should be conducted not just for validation of the individual change, but also to determine the extent and impact of that change on the entire software system [21].

6.3.2 *Change Management Process*

A typical change management process for medical devices is represented in Fig. 6.4. The main process steps and sub-processes are explained thereafter.

1. **Change requests** – Change requests can be raised by any function, but they should not be put through the formal change control process without receiving the go-ahead from a change planning group, usually comprised of representatives from design and development (D&D), manufacturing, marketing, communications, regulatory and quality assurance, tasked with triaging proposals and requests for modifications to the product design or manufacturing processes. A change request should contain a clear summary description of proposed change and the rationale for the change.
2. **Change planning** – Modifications to the product design or manufacturing process during the post-market phase requires careful and systematic planning. The purpose of change planning is to avoid duplicate or contradictory change requests going through the formal review and approval system and also to consolidate similar or related change requests into one change, wherever possible.

   In the pre-market phase the manufacturer has more flexibility to modify the design and manufacturing processes, but during the post-market phase controls tighten; hence it is advisable to balance the need to make changes with the need to avoid spending excessive amount of time, effort and money on many separate post-market changes, including regulatory submissions required for each significant change. Considering that it may take around six months or even more to implement changes in production and/or product labelling and obtain necessary regulatory approvals, it is perhaps recommendable to have no

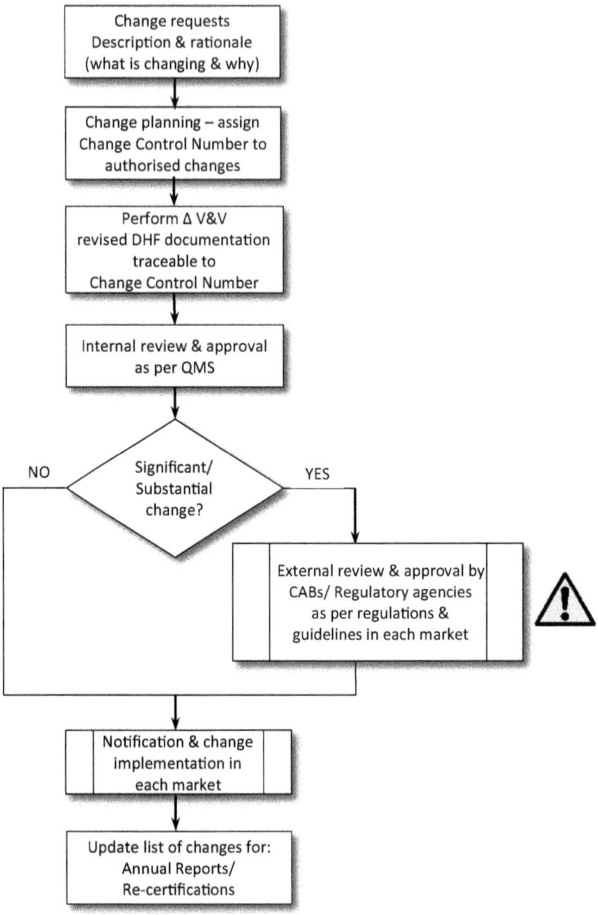

Figure 6.4 Change management process: simplified representation.

more than two product upgrades or significant changes per year for the same product.

The change planning group should assess the potential technical, regulatory and financial implications of proposed changes. A change request authorized to proceed through the formal change control process becomes a Change Note (sometimes also referred to as "Engineering Change Order" or "Engineering Change

Notice") and it is assigned a unique Change Control Number, for example, CN #, for traceability purposes.

3. **Verification and validation** – Most changes require some form of V&V, from minimal visual inspection to product type testing, process validation and clinical investigations. The requirements affected by the change should be identified, for example, using the company's requirements traceability database (see also example in Section 4.4.3, Fig. 4.8, illustrating requirements traceability and V&V).
   The impact of the change should be analyzed by asking pertinent questions, for instance, What V&V is required to establish continued compliance with state-of-the art requirements of safety and effectiveness? Are there any new risks introduced by the change, and if so, what are the (new) risk mitigations? Does the risk profile change? If so, is a clinical evaluation necessary?
   As V&V testing is performed, relevant parts of the DHF are revised accordingly. The change control documentation must establish clear traceability between changes and the related revised documentation, for example, by using Change Control Numbers and a change tracking database where all Change Notes are stored.
4. **Formal review and approval** – The Change Note with the change description and rationale and supporting documentation (revised specifications, labelling, V&V protocols and reports, etc.) is circulated for internal review and approval. If the information package is unsatisfactory (incomplete, unclear, contradictory information), internal reviewers provide comments in writing and reject the change.
   Typically a review leader with appropriate qualifications and expertise (usually a systems engineering, risk management or regulatory subject matter expert) makes the final decision, depending on all reviewers' comments, to approve the change or to reject it until all outstanding issues are addressed. The review lead's decision must be documented; it should include a rationale if the decision goes against any of the reviewers' comments.
   Depending on whether the change is significant or not, the next step is implementation or regulatory submission(s):

- Non-significant changes may proceed to implementation. Part of implementation may include filing of administrative changes to Regulatory Authorities (if applicable).
- Significant changes require additional external review and approval by the relevant Conformity Assessment Bodies (CABs) or regulatory agencies in accordance with relevant regulatory guidelines (detailed in Section 6.2.2 of this chapter). Any requests for corrections, clarifications or additional information must be addressed by the change originator(s) and the relevant project team. Upon receiving external approval, significant changes may proceed to implementation.

5. **Change notification and implementation** – Once approved, changes are notified as ready for implementation to stakeholders within the company, for example, manufacturing, marketing, sales and distribution. A typical implementation plan consists of staggered releases of modified product to target markets, as regulatory approvals are obtained in various jurisdictions.
   If the product labelling (labels, instructions for use/user manual) have changed, the implementation plan should include actions such as notifying patients and health professionals of the change and its impact, as appropriate.
6. **Updating of list of changes** – Manufacturers have statutory obligations to demonstrate continued compliance with regulatory requirements. To this end most CABs and regulatory agencies expect to see an updated list of changes either as part of post-market approval conditions (PMA Annual Reports in the United States) or at the time of re-certification and licence renewal (renewal of EC certificate in the EU and annual licence renewal in Canada). Systematic maintenance of such lists for each product or product family will facilitate preparation of periodic reports and applications for certification renewal with minimum time and effort.

6.3.3 *Change Management Process KPIs*

To measure how effective and agile a company's change controls really are, a manufacturer should collect process data at critical steps in the change management process and put in place key performance indicators, or KPIs. This can be done irrespective of whether the company is small and has a paper-based system or whether it is large and employs an electronic document management system (EDMS) to track changes.

The following data should be recorded for process KPI measurements:

- Date of authorizing the work for the change to proceed (performing V&V, revising documentation) by the change planning group – status of the change is "change initiated/work authorized to proceed";
- Date of initiating internal review – status of the change is "change sent for internal review";
- Number of rejections by internal reviewers due to review package being incomplete or otherwise unsatisfactory – status of the change is "change internally rejected – iteration #");
- Date of internal approval – status of the change is "change internally approved";
- Date(s) of regulatory submission(s) for change approval in relevant markets – status of the (significant) change branches to "change submitted in market X", "change submitted to market Y", etc.;
- Date(s) of regulatory approval(s) – status of the (significant) change is "change approved in market X", "change approved in market Y", etc.;
- Number of iterations with the assessing authority (rounds of questions and answers); and
- Date(s) of implementation in relevant markets – status of the change is "change implemented in market X", "change implemented in market Y" and it runs in parallel for applicable markets.

KPIs can be defined using best practice timelines between change initiation and change approval, maximum number of iterations with internal reviewers and with assessing authorities (CABs/regulatory agencies) (see Fig. 6.5). By measuring how the change management process is actually doing, a company can identify the outliers and

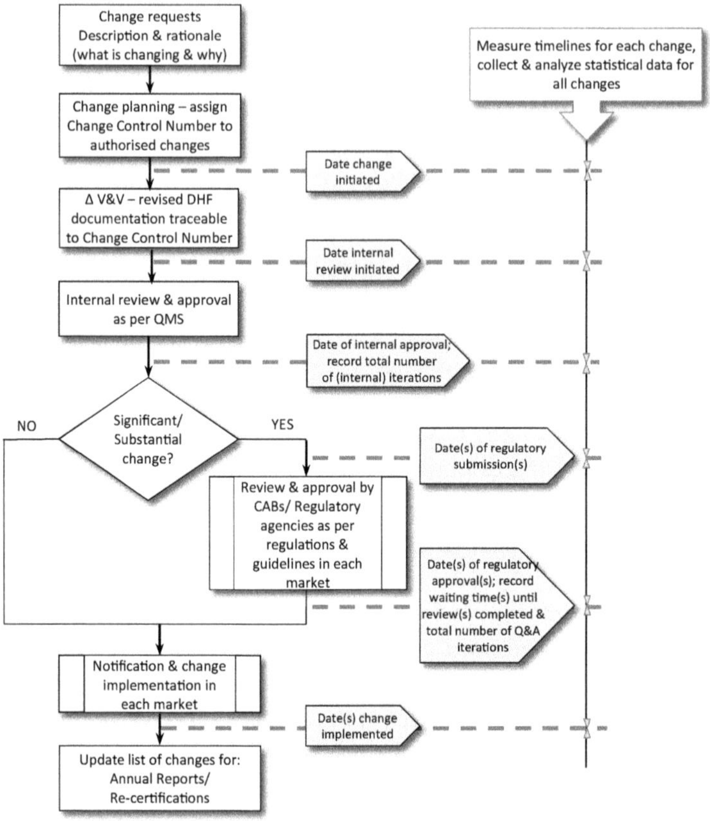

Figure 6.5 Measuring the performance of the change management process.

weak spots in the process and implement targeted corrective actions and preventive actions (CAPAs). Certain timelines, such as waiting for the assessing authority to complete its review, are independent of manufacturers' processes and outside their influence; hence they should be factored in when measuring change management process performance.

6.3.4 *Configuration Management*

Maintaining regulatory compliance in the post-market phase is intrinsically linked with managing the configuration of medical devices. Robust configuration management is a necessity for higher-risk, complex products such as active implantables and other electrical medical devices.

There are many definitions for *configuration* and *configuration management*, but perhaps the ones most widely used are those provided in the international standard ISO 10007:2003, *Quality management systems – Guidelines for configuration management*:

> **Configuration** – interrelated functional and physical characteristics of a product defined in product configuration information (requirements for product design, realization, verification, operation and support)
>
> **Configuration management** – coordinated activities to direct and control configuration

A widespread problem that causes unnecessary delays in obtaining marketing approvals is the inadequate identification and control of various product configurations. Applicants don't seem to be able to quickly and clearly demonstrate:

- What design version(s) were used for V&V?
- If different versions of the build standard were used for the various V&V tests, what is the version that meets all requirements and what evidence is there to prove it?
- What is the justification for the selection of test items as representative of a whole product family?

This section is not intended to be a tutorial in configuration management and examples presented here are for reference only. The aim is not to counsel perfection; however, there are a few important aspects that manufacturers of medical devices need to consider when putting in place a configuration management system:

- The different types of product identifiers and how they relate to each other should be clearly defined and managed according to their purpose – model designation, catalogue number, (production) part number and serial or lot/batch number (for more details refer also to Section 4.5.1, "Product Identifiers").

There must be full traceability between the model number, catalogue number, (production) part number and serial or batch/lot number of the same product.

- The product configuration and the configuration management rules should be clearly defined using the form, fit and function decision process.
- The configuration management process should be managed consistently, throughout the product life cycle, and using the valid product information in the relevant documentation repositories (DHF, Device Master Record [DMR], Device History Record [DHR]).

6.3.4.1 Product build configuration

The most common representation for a product build configuration (or build standard) is a multi-level bill of materials, or BOM (see example in Fig. 6.6). Part numbers are production identifiers that are allocated to components, assemblies and finished products.

In addition to part numbers, saleable items (finished products, accessories and spare parts that are packed and sold separately) are assigned catalogue numbers; ready-to-use medical devices with specific indications for use, intended use, design and performance characteristics are assigned model designations as well.

Critical parts and materials should be identified in the BOM, as applicable, so that changes to those parts trigger appropriate regulatory assessment and action. Critical parts and materials (sometimes referred to as "high integrity") would typically require separate certification to relevant component or material standards to ensure compliance with Essential Requirements (ERs)/Essential Principles (EPs) (e.g., mains power cord and plug, X-/Y-capacitors, material coming in direct contact with blood or tissue, material requiring a minimum low flammability grade, etc.).

6.3.4.2 Configuration management rules

Configuration management rules specify under what circumstances product identifiers need to change. For instance, configuration man-

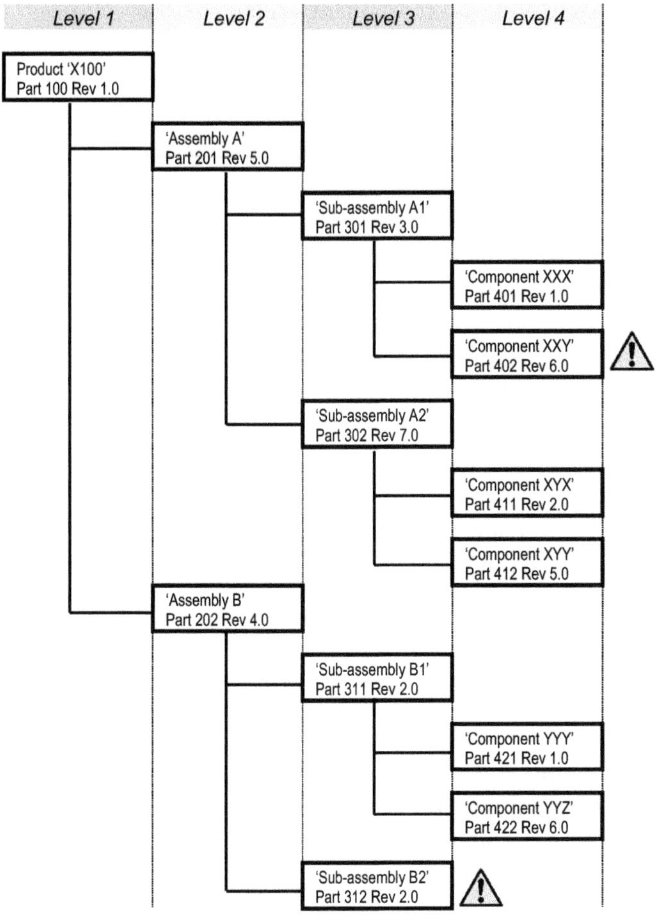

Figure 6.6 Example of a multiple-level BOM structure.
Note: Parts marked with the "!" symbol in a triangle are critical components requiring separate certification to relevant component/material standards to ensure compliance with ERs/EPs (e.g., mains power cord and plug, X/Y capacitors, material coming in direct contact with blood or tissue, enclosure material requiring a minimum low flammability grade, etc.).

agement rules for (production) part numbers, catalogue numbers and model designations can be defined as follows:

- The (production) **part number** changes when the form, fit or function of the part changes, for example, adding or removing a component, changing the supplier of a critical component (i.e., requiring separate certification to relevant component standard for regulatory compliance with ERs/EPs) or sub*contracting the manufacturing of an assembly to a different contract manufacturer.

- The **catalogue number** changes when adding a new variant of the same product, such as a new regional variant (EU, US, etc.) or a new colour variant or a new dimensional variant to accommodate variations in patient or user anatomy – that is, when form, fit or function changes without changing the indications for use, intended use or principle of operation.
- The **model designation** changes when the product form, fit or function *at the user level* changes, which generally corresponds with situations when the instructions for use must be changed significantly; for example, a different indication for use and intended use, adding or removing of product functionalities or changing of the principle of operation.

An example of the decision process and how it might be implemented in the product BOM when a change is made to the product specification is shown in Figs. 6.7, 6.8 and 6.9. At the core of the decision-making process is assessing whether, after each change, the resulting product configuration is valid and meets the requirements, including regulatory requirements.

- If form, fit or function is not affected by the change, that is, if the new or changed part is interchangeable/compatible with the old or unchanged part, only a revision change is applied to the (production) part numbers of all parent parts of the changed part.
- If form, fit or function is affected, that is, the new or changed part is not interchangeable/compatible with the old or unchanged part, a new part number is assigned to the (production) part numbers of all parent parts of the changed part; a new catalogue number and/or model designation would be assigned as well if required by the configuration management rules.

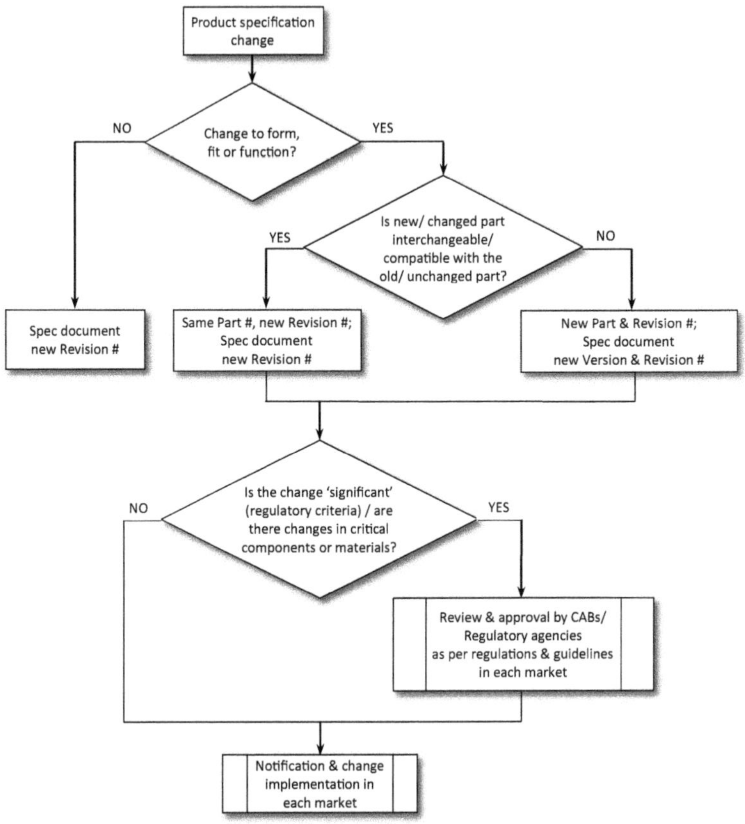

Figure 6.7 Example of the decision-making process when product specification is being changed.

Furthermore, if form, fit or function is affected by one change, other changes may have to be made as well in order to maintain interoperability/compatibility between assemblies or system components. For example, changes made to a male female connector used to attach the percutaneous lead of a ventricular assist device to the implantable blood pump may require changes to the percutaneous lead itself and/or changes to the design of the blood pump (refer also to Fig. 4.5 in Section 4.4.1.4, "Multi-Level Requirements").

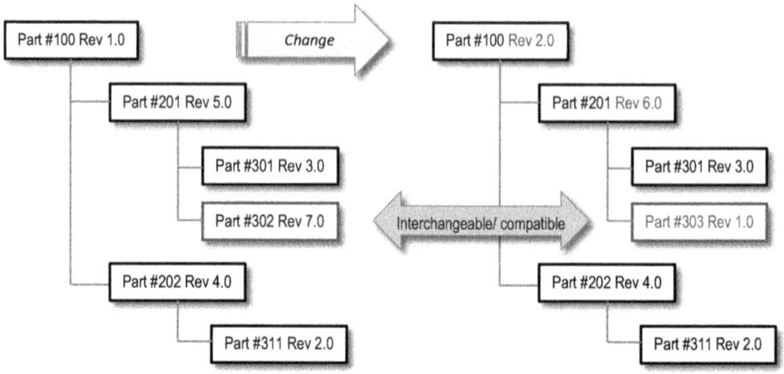

Figure 6.8 Part #302 Rev 7.0 is replaced with another part – #303 Rev 1.0 – that is interchangeable with Part #302 Rev 7.0. A new revision number is applied to all the parent parts of the changed part.

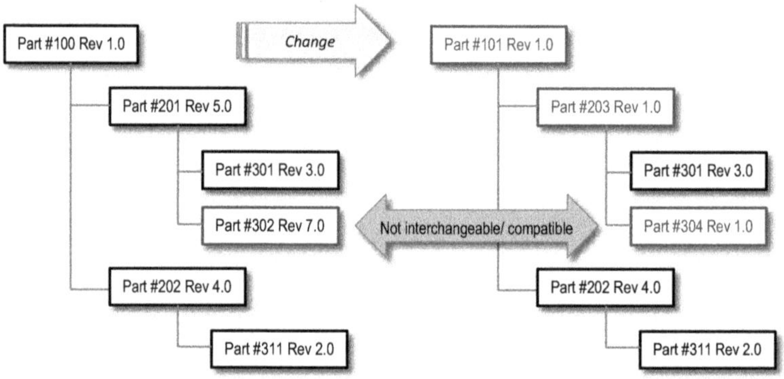

Figure 6.9 Part #302 Rev 7.0 is replaced with another part – #304 Rev 1.0 – that is *not* interchangeable with Part #302 Rev 7.0. A new part number is applied to all the parent parts of the changed part.

6.3.4.3 Configuration management process

According to the Institute of Configuration Management, configuration management "serves to ensure that as-built configurations conform to their documented requirements and are built to the correct versions of those documents" [33].

Product configuration needs to be managed throughout the product life cycle (see Fig. 6.10). During each life cycle stage,

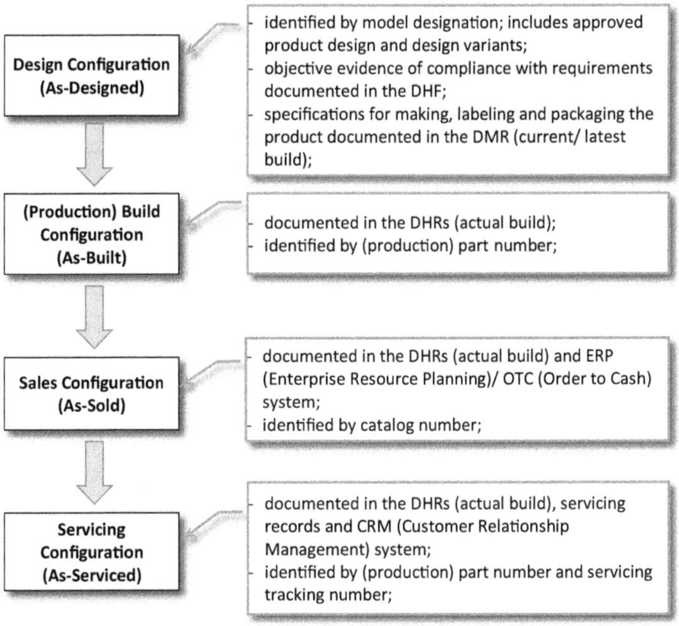

Figure 6.10 Product configuration management throughout the product life cycle.

manufacturers must check that the product configuration is valid and in compliance with the approved product configuration in each jurisdiction where the device is marketed.

6.3.5 *Regulatory Strategy in the Post-Market Phase*

As mentioned earlier, the regulatory function should be represented in the change planning group to advise on the possible regulatory impact of proposed changes, such as applicable regulatory submissions required in key markets if changes are potentially significant, expected timelines for approvals and application fees. During the change planning stage, only a minimum amount of work is done to assess the potential technical, regulatory and business impact.

The preliminary regulatory assessment during the change planning stage would typically be made on the basis of initial information available at the time; hence it is important that the change summary description and rationale be clear and accurate. Quick-reference checklists, covering the main criteria for significant product and QMS changes, are provided hereafter.

Significant changes to product design and manufacturing processes are those that could reasonably be expected to affect the safety and effectiveness of a medical device, considering the impact of the change on the patient or user and the impact of the change on the specifications of the device. They include, but are not limited to, the following:

- New or changed indications for use, intended use of the medical device;
- Labelling changes (other than editorial);
- Changes in the performance or design specifications, software, circuits, components, ingredients or materials, principles of operation or physical layout of the device and any other changes that may affect the safety and effectiveness of the device;
- Extension of the expiration date of the device on the basis of data obtained under a new/revised stability/sterility testing protocol that has not been approved by the regulator;
- Changes made to correct a failure mode, as a result of a new failure mode or as a result of an increase in product failures rates;
- The use of a different facility or establishment to manufacture, process, sterilize or package the device; and
- Changes in manufacturing facilities, new test methods, acceptance criteria or quality control procedures, sterilization, packaging and suppliers of critical components or services.

Significant changes to the QMS affecting compliance of the devices covered by the quality system with the requirements for safety and effectiveness, as well as affecting compliance of the QMS with its own regulatory requirements include, but are not limited to, the following:

- Additions to the product range covered by the quality system;
- Changes to the manufacturing quality control procedures, including test methods, tests or procedures used to control

the quality, purity and sterility of the device or of the materials used;

- Changes in roles and responsibilities of the legal manufacturer and in-country authorized agents/representatives;
- Changes in the process for ensuring compliance with conditions of approval (e.g., periodic reporting); and
- Changes in the process notification to/approval by regulatory agencies of changes and their subsequent implementation for marketed medical devices.

An important element of the change assessment is the risk analysis and any V&V required. If the change introduces potential new risks that require additional V&V testing, the change is likely to be significant.

Significant changes are likely to require major submissions in established and other key markets such as China; hence it is recommendable to document the market access strategy for such changes, for example, by using the template provided in Section 4.3.2, "Example of a Market Access Strategy Template". The market access strategy covers the regulatory, clinical and reimbursement strategies.

The regulatory strategy should, for instance, specify whether the applications for regulatory approvals will be submitted simultaneously or in a staggered manner and, if staggered, in what order. For example, changes for imported devices must be first approved in the country of origin before they can be approved in China.

The clinical strategy would have to specify whether new/additional clinical investigations are required or whether existing clinical evaluation data can be used. Where clinical evaluation is based on the rationale of equivalence with existing, previously marketed models, the equivalence must be demonstrated using side-by-side comparisons, including bench test results.

The reimbursement strategy would specify, for instance, whether new or enhanced design features or functionalities can qualify for a higher reimbursement rate – and higher pricing – and if an application for higher reimbursement rate is made what data is required. Marketing pricing strategy should be aligned with the reimbursement and the overall market access strategy.

Although some changes may initially be assessed as potentially non-significant, this preliminary assessment may change as more information becomes available and it may subsequently be determined that the change is significant after all. If needed, the manufacturer should consult with the CAB or the relevant regulatory agencies, for instance, using the FDA Presubmission Process or a requesting EU Notified Body's formal opinion.

The regulatory professional needs to be included in the internal review and approval of the DHF documents that are being revised as a result of the change, as these documents may have to be included in the submission for significant change approval or may need to be made available for review if requested by the CAB/regulatory agency.

It is strongly recommendable to organize the review of documentation in groups of related documents so that the internal reviewers, including the regulatory professional, can pick up and correct inconsistencies, gaps or contradictions in the information presented, before the submission is sent to the CAB/regulatory agency (refer also to Fig. 3.4 showing the Summary Technical Documentation (STED) as a sub-set of the DHF, in Chapter 3).

An often-encountered problem is the constant pressure to implement changes quickly by avoiding external approval by CABs/regulatory agencies. Change originators are pressured by their managers to "demonstrate a can-do attitude", "be creative" and other euphemisms for cutting corners. They in turn put pressure on regulatory professionals to convince them that the proposed change is non-significant. For example, a change described as "minor editorial changes to the work instruction for in-process testing of [parameter], for the purpose of improving clarity" may turn out to be a change in pass/fail acceptance criteria for a critical parameter and hence a significant change.

Another issue is the intentional splitting of a change into many, seemingly minor, changes in the hope that, if considered in isolation, would be assessed as being non-significant, avoiding thus submissions for external approval by CABs/regulatory agencies. Other than causing excessive administrative burden due to multiple change notes, review and approval workflows, this pseudo-strategy is more likely to result in internal confusion, gaps and errors in managing changes rather than avoid regulatory scrutiny.

Good planning, governance and leadership are needed to balance regulatory compliance and commercial imperatives. Here are a few things that if followed should avoid unnecessary stressful situations and willful non-compliance:

(1) Do not submit applications for marketing authorizations before the D&D of the product is finished. Only submit the version of the product that the company actually intends to commercialize. Adding functionalities or changing the design and manufacturing process in any substantial way after the application for initial approval was submitted or immediately after obtaining approval of an interim design version that was not intended for commercialization will result in delaying the initial market release.
(2) Consolidate similar or related changes into one change and limit the number or significant changes for the same product to a maximum of two per year, wherever possible.
(3) Maintain good documentation that enables quick assessment and approval of changes and easy retrieval of historical information on changes.
(4) Train and educate stakeholders and personnel involved in the change management process on applicable regulatory requirements in the post-market phase.

6.4 Post-Market Surveillance

A condition of maintaining regulatory approval is to conduct post-market surveillance throughout the medical device lifetime and implement appropriate corrective and preventive actions, where necessary. Post-market surveillance consists of systems and processes put in place to monitor the safety and performance of medical devices in real-life situations. Information obtained from user input and feedback is used to detect and provide early warning of potential product-related problems and reduce their recurrence through corrective and preventive actions. Any newly identified risks and trends are fed back into the risk management process for the ongoing risk–benefit assessment.

Table 6.13 Regulatory Authorities' websites and databases providing post-market information on product-related safety warnings, alerts and recalls

Regulatory Authorities' databases and official websites		Jurisdiction
MHRA	Safety Information	U.K.
BfArM	Information on risk	Germany
ANSM	Surveiller	France
SwissMedic	Materiovigilance – Liste Rückrufe	Switzerland
FDA	MAUDE – Manufacturer and User Facility Device Experience Medical Device Recalls Database – containing data on recalls since November 1, 2012	United States

Post-market surveillance incorporates both proactive and reactive feedback, with typical examples of each provided hereafter.

Proactive post-market surveillance activities include:

- Post-Market Clinical Follow-Up (PMCF);
- Clinical investigations performed as part of conditions of regulatory approvals;
- Manufacturer's implant registries and other device tracking databases; and
- Customer surveys and focus groups.

Reactive post-market surveillance – also known as vigilance – includes:

- Customer complaints and other unsolicited feedback (e.g., through social media);
- Servicing of returned devices;
- Failure mode and effects analysis (FMEA);
- Routine in-house testing;
- Scientific literature reviews;
- Device registries and third-party-sponsored clinical trials; and
- Regulatory Authorities databases with reported serious adverse events and product recalls (refer to Table 6.13).

Reporting of incidents involving medical devices and IVDs represents an important element of post-market surveillance.

Manufacturers need to ensure that they have robust systems and processes in place for complaint handling and reporting of product-related serious adverse events in accordance with statutory requirements in each market where the products are being marketed.

In situations where manufacturers rely on distributors for timely reporting of serious adverse events, they may need to put contractual agreements in place that specify roles and responsibilities for ensuring compliance with regulations, such as timelines for mandatory reporting of serious adverse events, to ensure that key activities are in fact being carried out. Failure to report serious adverse events can result in the cancellation of a distributor licence under Medical Devices Regulations.

Product-related incidents that fulfill the criteria for reportable events must be reported within the statutory timelines in each jurisdiction where the device is being marketed. When a hazard is considered unacceptable, corrective actions may have to include the removal of affected devices from the market.

It should be noted that the same action has to take place identically in all markets if the same lot can be found on several markets. In addition, manufacturers can expect that regulatory agencies worldwide monitor/screen the public web pages of agencies which publish adverse incidents and/or field safety corrective actions (FSCAs).

A recall strategy should address the following elements regarding the conduct of the recall:

i. Identifying, from the DHRs, the product batch/lot numbers and/or serial numbers affected;
ii. Identifying, from the distribution records, where the affected devices have been distributed; for active implantable medical devices, tracking the patients being implanted with devices related to the incident;
iii. Determining the appropriate depth of the recall:
    - Distributors/importers;
    - Professional users (healthcare facilities, healthcare professionals);
    - Retail; and
    - General public (consumers and patients).

iv. Planning the timelines of recall actions in accordance with statutory requirements in each jurisdiction affected by the recall;

v. Communications:

- To regulatory agencies – initial, progress and final reports;
- To distributors/importers;
- To professional users ("Dear Doctor" letters);
- To retailers; and
- To the general public (via websites, newspaper ads, TV news, social media).

vi. Performing effectiveness checks, as appropriate:

- 100% of consignees to be contacted;
- Percentage of the total number of consignees to be contacted to be determined on a case-by-case basis – greater than 10% but less than 100% of the total number of consignees;
- 10% or less of the total number of consignees to be contacted, percentage is to be determined on a case-by-case basis; and
- No effectiveness checks.

Terminology related to post-market regulatory actions such as "product recall", "withdrawal", "field correction", "upgrade notice", etc., may mean different things in different jurisdictions. Manufacturers, sponsors and distributors need to examine closely the type of action undertaken and apply the correct definition in each market. For instance, the term "product withdrawal" is synonymous with "systematic product recall" in the EU according to the AIMDD, but it denotes a non-recall voluntary action in Australia.

Authorities in key jurisdictions have been working towards harmonization of reporting requirements and the establishment of an international alert system for sharing information on serious adverse events and coordinate actions to minimize risks to patients, users and the community at large [34]. A synopsis of the relevant regulatory requirements in the established markets is provided hereafter.

6.4.1 *EU Statutory Requirements*

In the EU, requirements for conducting systematic post-market surveillance are defined in the medical devices directives, as follows:

- MDD Annex II, Section 3.1; Annex IV, Section 3; Annex V, Section 3.1; Annex VI, Section 3.1 – the manufacturer must implement a "systematic procedure to review experience gained from devices in the post-production phase", including "an obligation to notify the competent authorities" of serious adverse events; the clinical evaluation and its documentation "must be actively updated with data obtained from the post-market surveillance", unless duly justified not to do so.
- AIMDD Annex 2, Section 3.1; Annex 4, Section 4; Annex 5, Section 3.1 – the manufacturer must implement "a post-marketing surveillance system", including "an obligation to notify the competent authorities" of serious adverse events; the clinical evaluation and its documentation "must be actively updated with data obtained from the post-market surveillance", unless duly justified not to do so.
- IVDD Annex III, Section 5; Annex IV, Section 3.1; Annex VI, Section 3 – the manufacturer must implement "a systematic procedure to review experience gained from devices in the post-production phase" and "notify the competent authorities" of serious adverse events.

There are two major EU guidelines that provide detailed guidance for post-market statutory requirements:

- MEDDEV 2.12/1, *Medical Device Vigilance System*; and
- MEDDEV 2.12/2, *Post-Market Clinical Follow-Up Studies.*

6.4.1.1 Vigilance system

Medical device regulations define incidents (serious adverse events) as:

i. Any malfunction or deterioration in the characteristics and/or performance of a device, as well as any inadequacy in the instructions for use that might lead or might have led to the death of a patient or user or to a serious deterioration in his state of health; and

ii. Any technical or medical reason connected with the characteristics or performance of a device, leading for the reasons referred in point (i) above to a systematic recall of devices of the same type by the manufacturer.

MEDDEV guidance 2.12/1, *Medical Device Vigilance System* [35], describes the actions to be taken by manufacturers and national Competent Authorities when a serious adverse event occurs, and includes examples of reportable incidents. The vigilance procedure applies to:

(a) Devices carrying the CE marking;
(b) Devices without a CE marking but falling under the scope of one of the medical devices directives, for example, custom-made devices;
(c) Devices without a CE marking placed on the market before the entry into force of the medical devices directives; and
(d) Devices without a CE marking but where an incident leads to corrective action relevant to the devices mentioned in (a), (b) and (c) above;

To be reportable, an incident must fulfill all these three conditions:

A. An event has occurred – even if no death or serious injury occurred, it is sufficient that the incident associated with the device happened, and the incident was such that, if it occurred again, it *might* lead to death or serious injury.
B. The manufacturer's device is suspected to be a contributory cause of the incident.
C. The event led, or *might* have led, to death or serious injury (life-threatening illness, permanent impairment of a body function or damage to a body structure, condition necessitating medical or surgical intervention, any direct harm as a consequence of an incorrect diagnostic or IVD test result or as a consequence of the use of an IVF/ART device, foetal distress, foetal death or any congenital abnormality or birth defects).

Table 6.14 Timelines for reporting incidents in the EU

Reporter	Reportable incident	To whom	Timeline
Manufacturer/ Authorised Representative	Serious public health threat	National Competent Authority	Immediately but no later than **2 calendar days** of becoming aware
Manufacturer/ Authorised Representative	Death or unanticipated serious injury	National Competent Authority	Immediately but no later than **10 calendar days** of becoming aware
Manufacturer/ Authorised Representative	Other	National Competent Authority	Immediately but no later than **30 calendar days** of becoming aware

Adverse events that usually do not need to be reported become reportable if there is a change in trend, usually an increase in frequency of occurrence, or a change in pattern of an issue that can potentially lead to death or serious injury or public health concern.

The corrective action undertaken by the manufacturer in the event of an incident usually includes the following:

- Notifying the relevant national Competent Authority of the incident and any applicable field safety corrective action (FSCA), within the timelines provided in Table 6.14; the list of EU national Competent Authorities is available from the official website of the European Commission.
- Implementing an FSCA, which may include the following actions:
  - The return of product to the supplier;
  - Device modification, for example, permanent or temporary changes to the labelling or instructions for use or software upgrades following the identification of a fault in the software version already in the field, regardless of who implements the update – customers, field service engineers or by remote access;
  - Device exchange;
  - Device destruction;
  - Retrofit by purchaser to manufacturer's modification or design change; and

  - Advice given by the manufacturer regarding the use of the device and/or the follow-up of patients, users or others, such as modification to the clinical management of patients/samples to address a risk of death or serious deterioration in state of health related specifically to the characteristics of the device, for example, special patient follow-up for implantable devices or recall of patients or patient samples for re-testing or the review of previous results in the case of diagnostic devices (IVDs, imaging equipment or devices).
- Sending a field safety notice (FSN) to customers and/or users, in relation to an FSCA.

In the EU, a "field safety corrective action" is synonymous with "systematic recall of devices of the same type" referred to in MDD Article 10 §1.(b) and IVDD Article 11 §1.(b), as well as with the term "withdrawal" used in the AIMDD. Product removals for purely commercial non-safety-related reasons are not considered recalls.

Written reports may carry a disclaimer with words to this effect: "This incident report to [national Competent Authority] is not to be construed as an admission of liability for the incident and its consequences."

Incidents that occurred outside the European Economic Area (EEA), Switzerland and Turkey that did not require an FSCA relevant to these geographic areas do not need to be reported. Incidents that occurred outside the EEA, Switzerland and Turkey that required an FSCA relevant to the above-mentioned geographical areas must be reported as an FSCA.

6.4.1.2 Post-market clinical follow-up studies

A PMCF study is carried out following the CE marking of a device and intended to answer specific questions relating to clinical safety or performance (i.e., residual risks) of a device when used in accordance with its approved labelling.

PMCF studies must be planned in advance. A Post-Market Surveillance Plan (or PMFC Plan) describes the methods for collecting clinical data during the post-market phase for a product or product family. The objective is to confirm clinical performance and safety throughout the expected lifetime of the medical device, the acceptability of identified risks and to detect emerging risks on the basis of factual evidence. The PMCF Plan would typically be required as part of the CE marking submission.

MEDDEV guidance 2.12/2, *Post-Market Clinical Follow-Up Studies* [36] provides examples of circumstances that may require PMCF studies, including the following:

- Innovation, for example, where the design of the device, materials, substances, principles of operation, technology or medical indications are novel;
- Significant changes to the products or to its intended use for which pre-market clinical evaluation and re-certification have been completed;
- High product-related risk, for example, based on design, materials, components, invasiveness or clinical procedures;
- High-risk anatomical locations;
- High-risk target populations, for example, paediatrics and the elderly;
- Severity of disease/treatment challenges;
- Unanswered questions of long-term safety and performance;
- Results from any previous clinical investigation, including adverse events or post-market surveillance activities;
- Identification of previously unstudied subpopulations that may show a different benefit–risk ratio, for example, hip implants in different ethnic populations;
- Continued validation in cases of discrepancy between reasonable pre-market follow-up time scales and the expected life of the product;
- Risks identified from the literature or other data sources for similar marketed devices;
- Interaction with other medical products or treatments;
- Verification of safety and performance of device when exposed to a larger and more varied population of clinical users;
- Emergence of new information on safety or performance; and
- Where the regulatory approval was based on equivalence.

The data and conclusions derived from PMCF studies are used to provide clinical evidence for the clinical evaluation of the device and continued compliance with applicable ERs. The assessment may result in corrective or preventive actions, for example, changes to the product design or manufacturing processes, changes to the device labelling or public health notifications.

6.4.2 *US Statutory Requirements*

6.4.2.1 Post-market surveillance

Under Section 522 of the FD&C Act the FDA may by order "require a manufacturer to conduct post-market surveillance for any device of the manufacturer which is a class II or class III device the failure of which would be reasonably likely to have serious adverse health consequences or which is intended to be:

(1) implanted in the human body for more than one year; or
(2) a life sustaining or life supporting device used outside a device user facility".

Post-market surveillance under Section 522 of the FD&C Act enables the FDA to obtain additional safety and effectiveness data for a device after it has been cleared through a 510(k) or approved through a PMA, Humanitarian Device Exemption (HDE), or Product Development Protocol (PDP) process, when it is necessary to protect the public health. Post-market surveillance is not a substitute for obtaining the necessary pre-market information to support 510(k) clearance or PMA, HDE or PDP approval.

The FDA decides when post-market surveillance is necessary, what the process is for notifying and involving the manufacturer, what different types of post-market surveillance tools may be appropriate, how the manufacturer should conduct and report post-market surveillance and how the FDA will review and follow up on orders for post-market surveillance [37].

The FDA;s current guidance document *Post-Market Surveillance under Section 522 of the Federal Food, Drug and Cosmetic Act*, published in 2006, provides some examples of situations that may raise post-market questions, during both pre-market and post-market periods, including the following:

- New or expanded conditions of use for existing devices;
- Significant changes in device characteristics (technology);
- Longer-term follow-up or evaluation of rare events; and
- Public health concern(s) resulting from reported or suspected problems in marketed devices.

In 2011 the FDA has issued a new draft of this guidance document, which, once finalized, will replace the 2006 version. Among others, the new draft guidance has an updated list of types of post-market surveillance – with definitions – that may be used to address the public health question [38].

6.4.2.2 Medical Device Reporting

The Medical Device Reporting (MDR) tool is one of the post-market surveillance tools the FDA uses to monitor device safety and performance. The MDR regulation 21 CFR 803 defines the statutory requirements for manufacturers, importers and device user facilities (hospital, ambulatory surgical facility, nursing home, outpatient diagnostic facility or outpatient treatment facility, which is not a physician's office) to report device-related serious adverse events and other product problems to the FDA [39].

The definition of MDR-reportable events is similar with the definition of reportable incidents in the EU. An event must be reported to the FDA within the timelines provided in Table 6.15 if the device marketed by the manufacturer:

(1) May have caused or contributed to a death or serious injury; or
(2) Has malfunctioned and this device or a similar device marketed by the manufacturer would be likely to cause or contribute to a death or serious injury, if the malfunction were to recur.

The current FDA guidance document *Medical Device Reporting for Manufacturers*, published in 1997, provides definitions and details on reporting and record-keeping requirements applicable to manufacturers of medical devices for certain device-related adverse events [41].

Table 6.15 Timelines for reporting incidents in the United States

Reporter	Reportable incident	To whom	Timeline
Manufacturer	Death, serious injuries and malfunctions	FDA	Within **30 calendar days** of becoming aware
Manufacturer	Events designated by the FDA, events that require remedial action to prevent unreasonable risk of substantial harm to the public health	FDA	Within **5 work days** of becoming aware
Importer	Deaths, serious injuries	FDA, manufacturer	Within **30 calendar days** of becoming aware
Importer	Malfunctions	Manufacturer	Within **30 calendar days** of becoming aware
User facility	Device-related death	FDA, manufacturer	Within **10 work days** of becoming aware
User facility	Device-related serious injury	Manufacturer; FDA only if manufacturer unknown	Within **10 work days** of becoming aware
User facility	Annual summary of death and serious injury reports	FDA	January 1 for the preceding year

Source: FDA [40]

In 2013 the FDA issued a new draft of this guidance document, which, once finalized, will replace the 1997 version. The new draft contains more details and clarification regarding manufacturer reporting requirements [42].

6.4.2.3 Medical device recalls

Corrective actions required to address a problem with a medical device that violates FDA law include product recalls. A recall is required when a medical device is defective or poses a risk to health or both. The following types of actions may be considered recalls:

- Inspecting the device for problems
- Repairing the device
- Adjusting settings on the device

- Re-labelling the device
- Destroying the device
- Notifying patients of a problem
- Monitoring patients for health issues

The FDA's enforcement policy is defined in 21 CFR Part 7 [43]. According to 21 CFR §7.3(g), "Recall means a firm's removal or correction of a marketed product that the FDA considers to be in violation of the laws it administers and against which the agency would initiate legal action, e.g., seizure". A company (manufacturer, distributor or other responsible party) whose medical devices violate FDA law needs to recall the device and notify the FDA.

A recall is either a correction or a removal, depending on where the action takes place:

- *Correction* – addresses a problem with a medical device in the place where it is used or sold; or
- *Removal* – addresses a problem with a medical device by removing it from where it is used or sold.

According to 21 CFR Part 806 [44]:

- *Correction* means the repair, modification, adjustment, re-labelling, destruction or inspection (including patient monitoring) of a device without its physical removal from its point of use to some other location.
- *Removal* means the physical removal of a device from its point of use to some other location for repair, modification, adjustment, re-labelling, destruction or inspection.

Recall does not include a market withdrawal, stock recovery or routine servicing; these are defined as follows:

- *Market withdrawal* means a firm's removal or correction of a distributed product that involves a minor violation that would not be subject to legal action by the FDA or that involves no violation, for example, normal stock rotation practices, routine equipment adjustments and repairs, etc.
- *Stock recovery* means a firm's removal or correction of a product that has not been marketed or that has not left the direct control of the firm, that is, the product is located on

premises owned by, or under the control of, the firm and no portion of the lot has been released for sale or use.

- *Routine servicing* means any regularly scheduled maintenance of a device, including the replacement of parts at the end of their normal life expectancy, for example, calibration, replacement of batteries and responses to normal wear and tear. Repairs of an unexpected nature, replacement of parts earlier than their normal life expectancy or identical repairs or replacements of multiple units of a device are not routine servicing.

Recalls are classified according to the relative degree of health hazard presented by the product being recalled:

- Class I – a situation in which there is a reasonable probability that the use of, or exposure to, a violative product will cause serious adverse health consequences or death;
- Class II – a situation in which use of, or exposure to, a violative product may cause temporary or medically reversible adverse health consequences or where the probability of serious adverse health consequences is remote; and
- Class III – a situation in which use of, or exposure to, a violative product is not likely to cause adverse health consequences.

The depth of recall, any public warning and the effectiveness of checks will have to be defined in the recall strategy.

Depending on the degree of hazard and extent of distribution, the *depth of recall* may be applied at a:

- Consumer or user level, including any intermediate wholesale or retail level;
- Retail level, including any intermediate wholesale level; or
- Wholesale level.

A *public warning* should be sent out when it is necessary to alert the public that the product being recalled presents a serious hazard to health. It can be issued either as a general public warning through the general news media – national or local – or through specialized news media – professional or trade press, specific segments of the population such as physicians, hospitals, etc.

Effectiveness checks are required to verify that all consignees (at the recall depth specified in the recall strategy) have received notification about the recall and have taken appropriate action. The manufacturer may contact consignees by personal visits, telephone calls, letters or a combination thereof. The level of effectiveness checks should be also specified in the recall strategy:

- Level A – 100% of the total number of consignees to be contacted;
- Level B – a percentage of the total number of consignees to be contacted, determined on a case-by-case basis, but greater than 10% and less than 100% of the total number of consignees;
- Level C – 10% of the total number of consignees to be contacted;
- Level D – 2% of the total number of consignees to be contacted; or
- Level E – no effectiveness checks.

The FDA guidance document *Product Recalls, Including Removals and Corrections*, issued in 2003, provides details on preparing and submitting recalls notifications to the FDA and public notifications in situations where a product may pose a significant public health risk [45].

In 2014 the FDA has also published the guidance document titled *Distinguishing Medical Device Recalls from Medical Device Enhancements.* This guidance emphasizes the key factor in distinguishing a medical device recall from an enhancement, that is, the existence of a violation of the FD&C Act or associated regulations enforced by the FDA. According to this guidance, a device enhancement is (1) a change to improve the performance or quality of a device that is (2) *not* a change to remedy a violation of the FD&C Act or associated regulations enforced by the FDA. Device enhancements include changes designed to better meet the needs of the user, changes to make the device easier to manufacture, changes to improve a non-violative device's safety or performance and changes to the appearance of the device that do not affect its use [46].

6.4.3 *Australian Statutory Requirements*

6.4.3.1 Post-marketing system

In Australia, Regulations require that manufacturers of a kind of device establish and keep up to date a post-market monitoring, reporting and corrective action system. These requirements are defined in Schedule 3 of conformity assessment procedures of the Regulations:

- Part 1 Full quality assurance procedures, Section 1.4;
- Part 3 Verification procedures, Section 3.4;
- Part 4 Production quality assurance procedures, Section 4.4;
- Part 5 Product quality assurance procedures, Section 5.4;
- Part 6 Declaration of conformity, Section 6.5;
- Part 6A Procedures applying only to certain classes of in-house IVD medical devices, Section 1.4; and
- Part 7 procedures for medical devices used for a special purpose, Sections 7.2 (6) and 7.5 (3) and (4).

Under the post-market surveillance system the manufacturer is required to:

(a) Systematically review experience gained in the post-production phase in relations to medical devices of that kind; and
(b) Implement appropriate means to apply any necessary corrective action in relation to the design or production of such devices; and
(c) Notify the TGA, as soon as practicable after becoming aware of:

  - Information about any malfunction or deterioration in the characteristics or performance of the kind of device; any inadequacy in the design, production, labelling, instructions for use or advertising materials of the kind of device; or any use in accordance with, or contrary to, the use intended by the manufacturer of the kind of device; and
  - Information related to any technical or medical reason for a malfunction or deterioration of a kind mentioned in the previous point that has led the manufacturer to take steps to recover devices of that kind that have been distributed.

6.4.3.2 Vigilance

Section 5.7 of the Regulations (Section 41FN of the Act on conditions applying to devices included onto the *Australian Register for Therapeutic Goods* [ARTG]) defines the actions required to be undertaken by the TGA and the sponsor and/or manufacturer after any party becomes aware of an adverse event. Failure to report adverse events represents a breach of conditions for inclusions onto the ARTG, which may lead to suspension or cancellation of the entry from the ARTG, as well as constituting a criminal offence and/or resulting in a civil penalty.

An adverse event is an event that leads to death, a serious injury or serious deterioration of health to a patient, user or other person, including a life-threatening illness or injury, a permanent impairment of a body function, a permanent damage to a body structure or a condition necessitating medical or surgical intervention to prevent permanent impairment of a body function or permanent damage to a body structure.

An adverse event is reportable to the TGA if these three reporting criteria are met:

- An adverse event has occurred.
- The manufacturer's medical device is associated with the adverse event.
- The event led or might lead to (a so-called near-adverse event) death or serious injury or might lead to death or serious injury if it were to occur again.

The manufacturer and sponsor must inform the TGA of all reportable adverse events within the statutory time frames provided in Table 6.16. Details about the format and content of adverse event reports are provided on the TGA's website [47].

Additional detailed information on post-market vigilance and monitoring requirements are provided in Section 22 of the ARGMD guidance [48].

6.4.3.3 Recalls, suspensions, cancellations and tampering

Actions taken during the course of post-marketing surveillance include the following:

Table 6.16 Timelines for reporting incidents in Australia

Reporter	Reportable incident	To whom	Timeline
Manufacturer/Australian Sponsor	Serious public health threat	TGA	Within **48 hours** of becoming aware
Manufacturer/Australian Sponsor	Death or serious injury	TGA	Within **10 days** of becoming aware
Manufacturer/Australian Sponsor	Near-adverse event	TGA	Within **30 days** of becoming aware

- Take corrective actions and preventive actions (CAPAs) under the manufacturer's QMS.
- Inform the users of the device.
- Make corrections to the device.
- Remove the device from the market.

Medical devices in violation of the Regulations may be subject of a recall. Such situations arise, for instance, when the medical device does not meet the Essential Principles (EPs), conformity assessment procedures have not been applied to the medical device, the medical device has been illegally supplied, the medical device has been cancelled or suspended from the ARTG or therapeutic goods have been or could possibly be subject to actual or potential tampering.

There are three types of recall actions:

- *Correction*, which may involve temporary removal from the market or from use, for example, repair, modification, adjustment or re-labelling of a medical device, which may take place at the user's premises or any other agreed location;
- *Permanent removal* of deficient medical devices from the market or from use; and
- *Hazard alert*, which is information issued to healthcare professionals about issues or deficiencies relating to an implanted medical device or biological product and advice about the ongoing management of patients.

Actions that are not considered to be a recall include:

- *Safety alert* – intended to provide information on safe use of devices, as distinct from a recall action, which addresses product deficiencies. Safety alerts are issued to provide additional advice to healthcare professionals in situations where the use of the device, although meeting all specifications and therapeutic indications, could present an unreasonable risk of substantial harm if certain specified precautions or advice are not observed – for example, specific precautions about the longevity of an implanted medical device.
- *Product notification* – issue of precautionary information about a device in a situation that is unlikely to involve significant adverse health consequences.
- *Product withdrawal* – the sponsor's removal from supply or use of devices for reasons not related to their quality, safety or performance.
- *Product recovery* – the sponsor recovers devices that have been manufactured or imported but not yet supplied to the market – for example, recovery of devices in a warehouse.
- *User information* – generally conducted by the sponsor in response to issues with the use of a medical device; it includes in-house sessions, seminars and improved educational materials such as posters.

Recalls are classified according to the health hazard presented by the device being recalled:

- Class I (urgent, safety related) – product deficiency is potentially life threatening or could cause a serious risk to health.
- Class II (urgent, safety related) – product deficiency could cause illness or injury or result in mistreatment, but the recovery of the patient is likely.
- Class III (routine, non-safety-related) – product deficiency may not pose a significant hazard to health, but action may be initiated for other reasons, for example, quality-related issues.

There are four levels of recalls in Australia:

- *Wholesale* – includes wholesalers and state/territory purchasing authorities;
- *Hospital* – includes nursing homes and institutions, hospital pharmacists, ambulance services, blood and tissue banks and laboratories, as well as wholesale, as appropriate;
- *Retail* – includes retail pharmacists, medical, dental and other healthcare professionals, as well as wholesale and hospital, as appropriate; and
- *Consumer* – includes patients and consumers, as well as wholesale, hospital and retail levels, as appropriate.

Additional detailed information on post-market vigilance and monitoring requirements are provided in Section 23 of the ARGMD guidance [49].

6.4.4 *Canadian Statutory Requirements*

6.4.4.1 Complaint handling

In Canada, the requirements to establish and implement a complaint handling system are defined in Sections 57 and 58 of the Medical Devices Regulations. Manufacturers, importers and distributors are required to maintain records of consumer complaints and reported problems relating to the safety and performance of medical devices and any corrective actions taken in response to the reported problems.

Furthermore, manufacturers, importers and distributors must establish and implement documented procedures for CAPAs, including the effective and timely investigation of reported problems and recalls of medical devices.

Health Canada's *Guidance on Investigation of Reported Medical Device Problems* provides detailed directions for establishing an effective procedure for investigation of reported problems [50].

6.4.4.2 Mandatory problem reporting

Requirements for reporting serious adverse events are defined in Sections 59, 60 and 61 of the Medical Devices Regulations.

Manufacturers and importers must submit to Health Canada's reports of problems involving medical devices.

Incidents are reportable if they meet the following criteria:

- An incident has occurred within or outside Canada.
- The device contributed to the incident, either through a device failure or through a deterioration of its effectiveness or an inadequacy of its labelling or instructions for use. In assessing the link between the device and the incident, the reporter should take into account:
  - The opinion, based on available information, from a health professional;
  - Information concerning previous, similar incidents;
  - Complaint trends; and
  - Any other information held by the reporter.
- The incident led to one of the following outcomes:
  - Death of a patient, user or other person;
  - Serious deterioration in health of a patient, user or other person (a life-threatening disease, disorder or abnormal physical state, the permanent impairment of a body function or permanent damage to a body structure or a condition that necessitates an unexpected medical or surgical intervention to prevent such a disease, disorder or abnormal physical state or permanent impairment or damage); and
  - Potential for death or serious deterioration in health of a patient, user or other person ("near incidents").

The manufacturer and importer must inform Health Canada of all reportable incidents, within the statutory time frames provided in Table 6.17. Details about the format and content of incident reports are provided on Health Canada's website [51].

Additional details are provided in Health Canada's guidance document *Mandatory Problem Reporting for Medical Devices* [52].

Table 6.17 Timelines for reporting incidents in Canada

Reporter	Reportable incident	To whom	Timelines
Manufacturer/Canadian Importer	Death of a patient, user or other person	Health Canada	Within **10 calendar days** of becoming aware
Manufacturer/Canadian Importer	Serious deterioration in health of a patient, user or other person	Health Canada	Within **10 calendar days** of becoming aware
Manufacturer/Canadian Importer	Near incident	Health Canada	Within **30 calendar days** of becoming aware

6.4.4.3 Recall of medical devices

According to Canadian Medical Devices Regulations a recall means any action taken by the manufacturer, importer or distributor of the device to recall or correct the device or to notify its owners and users of its defectiveness or potential defectiveness after becoming aware that the device:

(a) May be hazardous to health;
(b) May fail to conform to any claim made by the manufacturer or importer relating to its effectiveness, benefits, performance characteristics or safety; or
(c) May not meet the requirements of the Medical Devices Regulations.

Sections 64 and 65 of the Medical Devices Regulations define the actions that must be taken by manufacturers and importers in the event of a recall. A recall may include:

- The removal of the medical device from the market and its consignees;
- An on-site correction of the medical device;
- An advisory concerning a problem or potential problem with instructions to work around the problem until an on-site correction can be implemented;
- The supply of revised labelling related to corrective action; or
- The supply of instructions to stop using the medical device and destroy remaining units in stock.

A recall does not include a stock recovery, that is, the removal or correction of a device that has not been distributed or that has not left the direct control of the company.

There are four levels of recall in Canada:

- General public (consumers and patients);
- Retail;
- Users (healthcare facilities, healthcare professionals); and
- Distributors/importers.

The effectiveness checks are the same as those defined by the FDA in the United States:

- Level A – 100% of consignees to be contacted;
- Level B – a percentage of the total number of consignees to be contacted to be determined on a case-by-case basis but greater than 10% and less than 100% of the total number of consignees;
- Level C – 10% or less of the total number of consignees to be contacted; percentage to be determined on a case-by-case basis; or
- Level D – no effectiveness checks.

Further details are provided in Health Canada's *Guide to Recall of Medical Devices* [53].

6.4.5 *Japanese Statutory Requirements*

The Ministry of Health, Labor and Welfare (MHLW) Ministerial Ordinance No. 135 of 2004 sets out the Good Vigilance Practice (GVP) requirements that Marketing Authorization Holders (MAHs) must comply with. The GVP requirements cover the collection of safety management information (information required for the safe and effective use of a device) and the implementation of safety assurance duties (collection and review of safety management information and resulting actions, referred to as safety assurance measures) (12 pp. 131–148).

Sources of safety management information include, but are not limited to:

- Product complaints (including reports of product malfunctions, side effects, infections) received from patients and healthcare professionals;
- Servicing and repairs reports; and
- Notifications and advisory notices issued by regulatory agencies, industry associations and other organizations.

The Quality Manager is responsible for the gathering and processing of quality-related feedback. The Safety Manager is responsible for gathering and processing of the safety-related feedback, as well as for reporting of product-related serious adverse events to the PMDA within statutory time frames (see Table 6.18). The appointment of a Quality Manager and a Safety Manager is an organizational requirement for a MAH or a Designated Marketing Authorization Holder (DMAH) (see also Section 5.1.1.5, "Japanese Designated Marketing Authorization Holder").

Article 253 of the Enforcement Regulations stipulates that adverse events must be reported within 15 or 30 days, depending on their criticality (severity of hazard) and predictability (whether they are anticipated or not).

The following events are considered critical:

(1) Death;
(2) Disability;
(3) Any events possibly leading to death or disability;
(4) Any case that requires hospitalization for treatment or prolongs the duration of hospitalization (serious injury);
(5) Any other serious cases involving items (1) through (4) above; and
(6) Any congenital disease or anomaly in the offspring of a treated patient.

Unanticipated adverse events refer to events that have not been identified in the instructions for use, for example, under warnings and precautions, or events with a rate of occurrence higher than originally predicted.

Based on Tables 12-2, 12-3 and 12-4 in *Fundamentals of Japanese Regulatory Affairs* [12]

Table 6.18 Timelines for reporting incidents in Japan

Reporter	Reportable incident	To whom	Timeline
	Reports on medical device malfunctions		
Safety Manager	Critical severity, unanticipated occurrence Critical severity, anticipated occurrence, other than those for which the anticipated rate of occurrence is exceeded	PMDA	Within **30 days** of becoming aware
Safety Manager	Critical severity, anticipated occurrence for which anticipated rate of occurrence is exceeded	PMDA	Within **15 days** of becoming aware + periodic reports for domestic incidents
Safety Manager	Non-critical, unanticipated occurrence of domestic events	PMDA	Periodic reports
	Reports on side effects related to medical devices		
Safety Manager	Death – all domestic incidents Death – unanticipated occurrence of foreign incidents Death – anticipated occurrence of foreign incidents for which anticipated rate of occurrence is exceeded	PMDA	Within **15 days** of becoming aware
Safety Manager	Death – anticipated occurrence of foreign incidents, other than those for which anticipated rate of occurrence is exceeded	PMDA	Within **30 days** of becoming aware
Safety Manager	Serious injury – unanticipated occurrence Serious injury – anticipated occurrence for which anticipated rate of occurrence is exceeded	PMDA	Within **15 days** of becoming aware + periodic reports for domestic incidents with predicted rate of occurrence

(Contd.)

Table 6.18 (*Contd.*)

Reporter	Reportable incident	To whom	Timeline
Safety Manager	Serious injury – anticipated occurrence, other than those for which anticipated rate of occurrence is exceeded	PMDA	Within **30 days** of becoming aware
Safety Manager	Serious injury – anticipated occurrence, other than those for which anticipated rate of occurrence is exceeded and that may lead to increased rate of infections due to the use of medical device	PMDA	Within **15 days** of becoming aware
Safety Manager	Non-critical, unanticipated occurrence of domestic events		Periodic reports
	Reports on infections related to medical devices		
Safety Manager	All critical events, both domestic and foreign, anticipated and unanticipated occurrence	PMDA	Within **15 days** of becoming aware
	Non-critical, unanticipated occurrence of domestic events		

Table 6.19 Reporting of serious adverse events in Singapore

Reportable incident	Timeline
Serious threat to public health	Within **48 hours** of becoming aware
Death or a serious deterioration in the state of health of a patient, a user of the medical device or any other person	Within **10 days** of becoming aware
Events a recurrence of which might lead to the death or a serious deterioration in the state of health of a patient, a user of the medical device or any other person	Within **30 days** of becoming aware

Source: Singapore Health Sciences Authority [56]

Corrective actions required to address a problem with a medical device include product recalls and related safety management information. A recall may involve the complete retrieval of the product from the market or the repair of the device.

Detailed guidelines assisting manufacturers with the implementation of post-market surveillance requirements can be obtained from the Japan Federation of Medical Devices Association [54] and the Japan Pharmaceutical Manufacturers Association [55].

6.4.6 *Emerging Markets' Statutory Requirements*

At the time of going to print post-market surveillance regulations are being developed and put in place in emerging markets. Some, like Singapore, which has adopted the ASEAN MDD, follow the European model for vigilance (see Table 6.19). Others, like China, are using elements of medical device reporting regulations in established markets to develop their own (see Table 6.20).

Table 6.20 Reporting of serious adverse events in China [31]

Reportable incident	Timeline
Death	Within **5 working days** of becoming aware
Serious injury or possibly leading to serious injury or death	Within **15 days** of becoming aware

Details on serious adverse events reporting, field safety corrective actions, including recalls, and field safety notifications are being made available as developed from the official websites of the Regulatory Authorities.

6.5 Product Obsolescence

Obsolescence is part of the normal product life cycle. New products using the latest technology gradually replace older generations of devices. However, before a product is discontinued a manufacturer must take into consideration regulatory aspects as well as ensure appropriate support to patients and other users.

For example, when obsoleting old models of external controllers used for driving active implantables, the manufacturer must ensure that the new or upgraded controllers are compatible with the version of active implantable devices already implanted – in other words, they are backward-compatible with the implants of existing patients. Manufacturers may need to continue to provide spare parts and servicing for devices being discontinued for a number of years.

The obsolescence of a medical device needs to be carefully timed, especially in jurisdictions where annual licence fees are charged to maintain the regulatory approvals. If a manufacturer wishes to cancel a product certification or registration (e.g., in the EU or Australia) the notification of cancellation to the agency should by timed before the next annual fees invoicing cycle to avoid charges for another full year but not before the last devices are being placed on the market to avoid distributing devices without a valid approval.

Also, a manufacturer may decide to discontinue an old device and cancel its regulatory approval in one market but continue to distribute it in other markets. In this case, any claims or markings indicating an "approved" status in the market where it is being discontinued will have to be removed. For example, if a manufacturer cancels the European approval but continues to distribute his or her product in the United States (assuming it has a valid FDA approval), the CE marking, which indicates compliance with the EU regulations must be removed from the device labels and user instructions. Furthermore, if the manufacturer distributes the device in emerging markets relying on Certificates of Free Sale (CFS) issued on the basis of a valid CE marking approval, he or she must consider what implications the cancellation will have in these markets.

6.6 Quality Management System

6.6.1 *Organizational Structure and Business Processes*

At the core of an effective, efficient and compliant QMS are its business processes. The ISO 13485:2009 standard states that "any activity that receives inputs and converts them to outputs can be considered as a process. For an organization to function effectively, it has to identify and manage numerous linked processes" (ISO 13485:2009, Section 0.2, Process approach).

Typically a medical device company would encompass the following main business functions (listed in no particular order) that interact with each other in a network of interconnected processes:

- Research and technology – invention and innovation, new technology and new product ideas;
- Marketing – market research, product definition, product launch and product management throughout the product life cycle;
- D&D – development of new product ideas from proof of concept through to mass production, including maintenance (product changes) of existing products;
- Manufacturing and logistics – production and product distribution to warehouses in the target markets;
- Communications – generation of product labelling, including translations (labels, instructions for use, product training materials, websites, brochures, product launch campaigns and other marketing materials) and corporate communications (media releases and announcements);
- Sales – forecast and execution of sales transactions;
- Customer support – first point of contact for customer feedback (e.g., call centre), servicing and repairs;

- Regulatory – marketing authorizations in target markets and compliance with regulations applicable to medical device;
- Clinical – planning and execution of clinical investigations and ongoing clinical evaluation of existing products;
- Quality assurance – definition and ongoing management of regulated processes in compliance with medical device regulations;
- Finance – financial planning and reporting and accounting operations;
- Legal – compliance with corporate law and protection of company's intellectual property (IP registration, IP law suits);
- Human resources – employee recruitment, training and development and performance management;
- Operations – corporate infrastructure, including IT systems; and
- Management – corporate leadership and business risk management.

An effective QMS needs a well-defined structure with clearly mapped business processes, including the roles and responsibilities of each business function. Each business process needs to identify the process steps (actions), the inputs and outputs and the various functions' responsibilities. Processes must be described in procedures and work instructions to ensure consistent implementation. The records generated represent the evidence that a process has been followed, as described.

6.6.2 *QMS Documentation*

The QMS documentation is usually structured like a pyramid, with high-level documents with wider coverage and low level of detail at the top and low-level documents with limited coverage and high level of detail at the bottom (see Fig. 6.11).

The Quality Manual is at the top of the QMS pyramid, providing an overview of the organization, including company size and geographical locations, high-level organizational charts, main business processes and functional responsibilities.

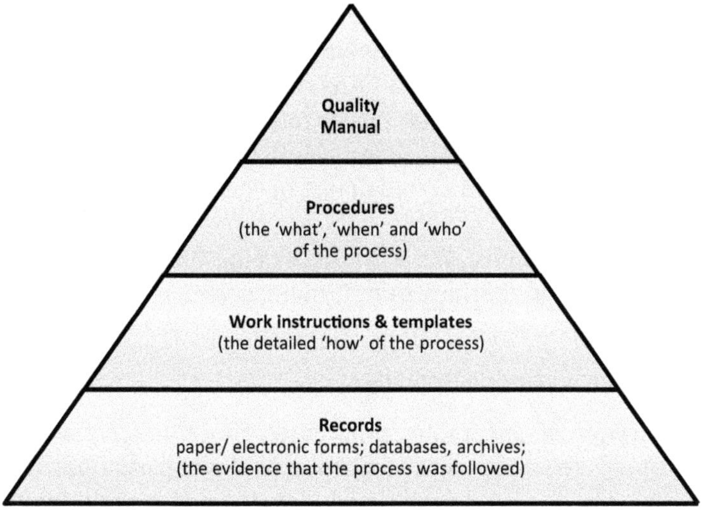

Figure 6.11 Typical hierarchical structure of QMS documentation.

On the next level down are the procedures, each describing a main business process – what the main actions or process steps are, the process inputs and outputs, including records to be generated, and where the record are stored (the "what"); the timing, timelines and/or correct order of actions (the "when"); and the roles and responsibilities within functions involved in the process steps (the "who"). A flowchart with "swim lanes" is a good way of representing a business process.

On the next level down are work instructions and templates describing in detail how the process is implemented (the "how"), for instance, how to use the company's electronic document management system (EDMS) to review and approve (or reject) a draft engineering document as part of the D&D process or the steps that an operator on the production line must follow to correctly assemble a particular product.

Records include the filled-in, dated and signed-off forms, the populated electronic databases and the Design History Files (DHFs), Device Master Records (DMRs) and Device History Records (DHRs) of products. They are very important because Regulatory Authorities and Conformity Assessment Bodies (CABs) check them to determine whether the company followed its own procedures and whether the quality system complies with regulatory requirements. Records are the evidence that CABs refer to when they raise non-conformities during quality system audits and cite deficiencies related to product safety and effectiveness. The locations for storing and archiving regulated records must be identified in the relevant procedures.

Some common mistakes when developing QMS documentation include situations like those described hereafter.

6.6.2.1 The vocational training

The purpose of generating procedures, work instructions and templates is to ensure consistency across the organization, not to teach people how to do their jobs. For instance, procedures that regurgitate entire regulatory guidelines do not add any value to the QMS and would require revising every time guidelines are updated. Important information, however, such as statutory timelines for reporting adverse events can and should be reproduced, for instance, in a table in the relevant procedures covering clinical trials, vigilance and post-market surveillance.

Another example is a procedure dedicated to design reviews that launches into elaborate discussions in the passive voice: "Detailed design reviews may be conducted locally (within the design or project team) for individual components, sub-assemblies and parts. Detailed design reviews should be considered part of the day to day normal interface between engineers and if done properly will make the larger design reviews quicker and more efficient, with fewer risks and unknowns. Engineers from different disciplines should proactively engage in detailed design reviews." These sorts of statements belong more in a training program for design engineers than a QMS procedure.

More appropriate and useful perhaps would be to include this paragraph in a procedure covering the end-to-end D&D process: "Design reviews are specific to configuration of the design at a certain point in time. The project team may hold design reviews on specifications, analyses, design documentation, validation protocols, validation results, etc., as appropriate for the project. The project

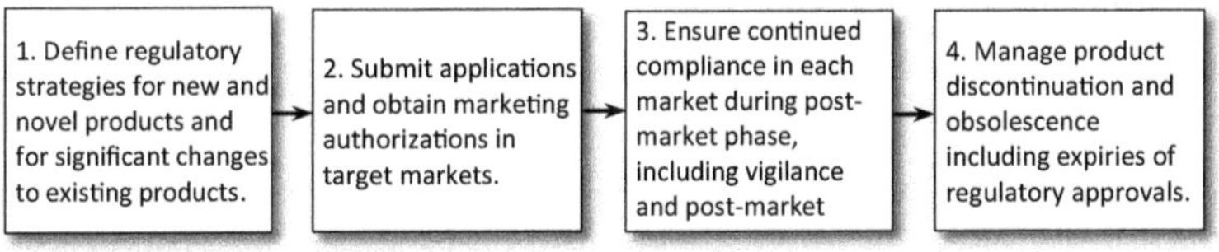

Figure 6.12 Steps in the regulatory end-to-end process.

plan must define the minimum required design reviews. At least one design review is required but can be combined with a phase review."

6.6.2.2 The labyrinth

A labyrinth of QMS documents ensues when processes and process steps are fragmented to the nth degree. For example, the regulatory end-to-end process is comprised of four major steps or sub-processes, as shown below (Fig. 6.12).

Depending on the size and complexity of an organization, this process can be described in one procedure covering the end-to-end regulatory process; it can be split into four procedures – one for each regulatory sub-process; or it can be "absorbed" in procedures covering the pre- and post-market business processes – D&D (pre-market); marketing authorizations; production, distribution and customer support (post-market); and product end of life. Details such as the maintenance of the regulatory submissions repository would be covered in related work instructions.

Fragmenting each sub-process further into many separate procedures creates a maze of documents cross-referencing each other. Take, for instance, this example where a mid-size medical device company generated separate procedures for individual process steps. There was one separate procedure just for checking whether product certificates are about to expire and another separate procedure for setting up a management meeting to decide which products should be re-certified and which not. These are two steps in a sub-process that could have been easily covered in one or two paragraphs of a single procedure.

The total number of QMS documents in this company ballooned to over 100 policies, procedures and work instructions, which made it increasingly confusing and difficult for employees to "see the woods for the trees". It also required a great deal of maintenance just to keep cross-references up to date and to keep employees' training records up to date each time QMS documents were revised. The complexity had a negative effect, not just on efficiency, but also on compliance, because it created more opportunities for mistakes. It opened though a few job opportunities for paper shufflers.

6.6.2.3 The band aid

The band aid is perhaps one of the most often encountered situations. Without a clear and comprehensive map of processes and procedures as a starting point, procedures are generated more or less willy-nilly, usually as a knee-jerk reaction to an audit non-conformance. Procedures written to quickly fill a gap may seem like a good idea at the time, but this method of documenting a QMS creates all sorts of problems – duplications and contradictions, leaving other gaps unaddressed.

This is, for instance, how a company ended up with a "Risk Class Determination Procedure", a "Software PMA Supplement Procedure" and another "Procedure for Preparing PMA Supplements". It would have probably been more effective to (1) include a paragraph on risk class determination, including references to the applicable regulatory guidelines, in the relevant pre-market procedure, and (2) include a paragraph or two on applicable regulatory actions required for significant changes, including references to the applicable regulatory guidelines, in the relevant post-market procedure.

6.6.3 *QMS Performance*

The performance of the QMS must be measured against pre-determined quality objectives and regulatory requirements. Performance data consists of feedback from various sources such as non-conformities, findings and recommendations raised during quality system audits, product non-conformance reports (NCRs) raised via process controls, customer complaints, returned devices and surveys.

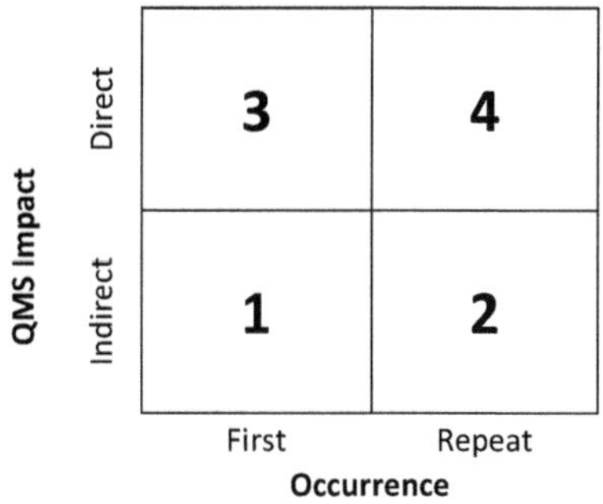

Figure 6.13 Non-conformity grading matrix. *Source*: GHTF [57].

Examples of quality objectives that would require ongoing analysis and reporting during regular quality management reviews include:

- Product reliability and other product metrics expressed in statistical limits (failure and malfunction rates, return rates, service and repair metrics, production yield);
- Timeliness of addressing customer complaints;
- Timelines of completing analysis of returned devices;
- Timeliness and effectiveness of addressing non-conformities;
- Timeliness of submitting statutory adverse events reports and field notifications to Regulatory Authorities;
- Adherence to internal audit plan and supplier audit plan; and
- Market access metrics (timeliness of obtaining regulatory and reimbursement approvals).

Non-conformities raised during quality system audits are graded according to their occurrence and impact on the QMS, as shown in Fig. 6.13, which is reproduced from the Global Harmonization Taskforce (GHTF) guidance *Quality management system – Medical devices – Nonconformity grading system for regulatory purposes and information exchange* [57].

The *y* axis of the grading matrix represents the *QMS impact* on medical device safety and performance. Non-conformities are assigned a score of 3 if they have a direct impact or a score of 1 if they have an indirect impact, as defined hereafter:

- *Indirect QMS impact*: ISO 13485:2009, Clauses 4.1 through 6.3 are seen as enablers (making it possible or feasible) for the QMS processes to operate. These clauses are therefore considered to have indirect influence on medical device safety and performance.
- *Direct QMS impact*: ISO 13485:2009, Clauses 6.4 through 8.5 are seen as having direct influence on design and manufacturing controls. These clauses are therefore considered to have direct influence on medical device safety and performance.

The *x* axis of the grading matrix represents the *occurrence* of the non-conformity. Non-conformities cited to the same QMS third-level sub-clause ("X.X.X") of ISO 13485:2009, even if not identical, are considered repeat and the grade increases by 1, as defined hereafter:

- *First*: The first category addresses non-conformities in a particular "X.X.X" sub-clause identified for the first time. The "first time" is defined as not observed in the two previous QMS audits that evaluated the same sub-clause.
- *Repeat*: The second category addresses non-conformities that have been identified within either of two previous QMS audits that evaluated the same "X.X.X" sub-clause. Such non-conformities pose an increased risk because it indicates that a corrective action has not been adequately taken or implemented.

Audit non-conformities with a score of 1 usually require a correction only to *eliminate the symptom*. Those with a score of 2, 3 or 4 would typically require a CAPA to *eliminate the root cause*.

Product-related non-conformities (NCRs) are raised when manufactured units fail quality control inspections and testing during production or as a result of customer complaints and returned devices. Depending on the level of risk (determined as the combination between the severity of harm and the frequency of occurrence of that harm), product-related non-conformities either may be accepted via a concession, addressed by a correction (repair, rework or adjustment), or may require a CAPA.

Product malfunctions and failures must be captured, investigated, categorized and trended. Failure rates must remain within the acceptable limits according to the state of the art. Information about what is acceptable is typically collected from scientific literature and from databases of reported adverse events maintained by Regulatory Authorities. If the incidence of any failure modes increases and starts trending above the acceptable limits, a CAPA must be raised to investigate and eliminate the root cause. The GHTF guidance document *Manufacturer's Trend Reporting of Adverse Events* provides an example of establishing basic trending parameters (baseline, threshold and time interval) and identifying a significant increase in observed occurrence [58].

In addition, any unanticipated, new hazards and failure modes that haven't been previously identified must be fed back into the risk management process (refer to Section 2.5, "Risk Management").

Customer complaints involving serious adverse events must be reported to the relevant authorities in accordance with the vigilance and adverse event–reporting regulations in each jurisdiction where the product is being used. In certain circumstances the product may have to be recalled from the market. A simplified representation of the ongoing process for QMS monitoring and improvement is shown in Fig. 6.14.

Additional details on QMS process improvement can be found in the following GHTF guidance documents:

- *Implementation of risk management principles and activities within a Quality Management System* [59];
- *Quality management system – Medical Devices – Guidance on corrective action and preventive action and related QMS processes* [60]; and
- *Quality management system – Medical Devices – Guidance on the Control of products and Services Obtained from Suppliers* [61].

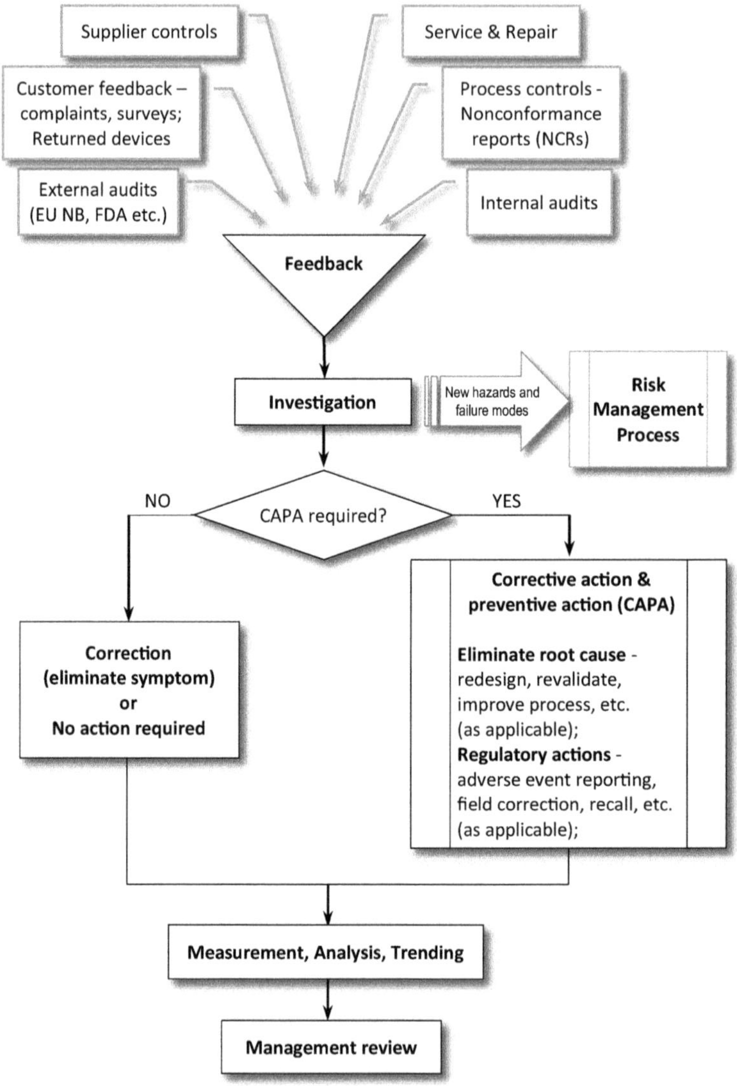

Figure 6.14 Ongoing QMS performance monitoring and improvement process: simplified representation.

6.6.4 *Preparing for External Audits*

Manufacturers of medical devices and IVDs requiring the involvement of a CAB prior to placing the products on the market are subject to initial and follow-up quality system audits. Organizations need to prepare carefully for external audits to minimize delays to approvals and avoid unnecessary rework.

At least two or three months before an external audit the manufacturer should check that the QMS documentation is up to date, that employees' job descriptions and training status are current and that relevant records can be easily retrieved.

The quality assurance department should organize an "audit backroom" manned with key subject matter experts who can quickly answer questions and find the documentation that may be requested by the auditor. Some companies have a "scribe" and "runners" in the audit room. Runners are there to relate questions and requests for documents from the audit room to the backroom and bring the requested documents back to the audit room. The scribe types the questions and answers on his or her laptop, which are then projected in the backroom. In this way the backroom always knows what is happening in the audit room and starts preparing answers and documents for the runners to take back to the audit room.

People with responsibilities in a business process should be prepared to answer questions related to the process and the records generated from the process. Responses should be factual and point, wherever possible, to the relevant sections in a document – procedure, work instruction, technical specification, protocol or report – to ensure that different people being asked the same or similar question provide consistent answers.

If the person being asked questions by the auditor does not understand the question, he or she should refrain from making assumptions and should ask for clarifications. If he or she doesn't know the answer to a question, he or she should just say "I am not the best person to answer that" or "I will organize the information for you". He or she should never speculate or assume ("I think", "I believe", "I guess").

Each answer should ask the question and only the question, without digressing, chit-chatting or volunteering additional information.

Above all, each answer must be truthful. Nothing derails an audit more than getting caught for making false, misleading or deceptive statements.

6.7 Regulatory Systems and Processes

6.7.1 *Product Regulatory Status Database*

Companies with a large product portfolio and a global reach need to find ways to manage the information on product regulatory status and to notify stakeholders - manufacturing and logistics, quality assurance, D&D, marketing, sales, etc. – when the product regulatory status changes in key markets.

The current regulatory status of a company's products represents essential information. Accessing it should be a straightforward exercise. Instead, all too often it becomes a task that takes too much time and resources to execute. Information on the worldwide regulatory status of company's products is captured in spreadsheets and other non-validated systems and communicated to stakeholders across the business on an ad hoc basis using emails, PowerPoint presentations and phone calls, with little or no global product information readily available that is validated and up to date.

If a growing company already develops or distributes more than 15–20 products globally, then perhaps it is time to consider establishing a global Product Regulatory Status Database. Some of the benefits of implementing such a system are:

- Use of a single, validated source of truth to access complete, accurate and current information about the regulatory status of all products, in all markets;
- Implementation of a well-defined, consistent process to trace product regulatory status information and notify stakeholders when the status changes; and
- Significant reduction in the time and effort required to access information about product regulatory status in all markets and thus optimization of use of resources.

Product information

- product family
- product model designation
- product short description
- GMDN code
- catalog number
- (production) part number
- legal manufacturer (responsible for the final QC release)
- critical suppliers

Regulatory status information

- "in development" - this status is applied by default to each country/ single market for new products still in development;
- "submitted" - this status is aplied to each country/ single market where an application for marketing authorization has been submitted; link status to application cover letter/ form held in the Regulatory Submissions Repository;
- "approved/ registered" - this status is applied to each country/ single market where the product has marketing authorization; link status to certificate/ registration/ letter of approval (where applicable);
- "withdrawn" - this status is applied to each country/ single market where the aplication has been withdrawn (prior approval);
- "discontinued/ obsolete" - this status is applied to each country/ single market where the product has been discontinued or the product registration/ certification has expired;

Geographical information

- list of countries/ single markets

Figure 6.15 Example of information captured and tracked in the Product Regulatory Status Database.

An example of the sort of information that a company might want to capture and track in the database is shown in Fig. 6.15.

Important functionalities for a Product Regulatory Status Database include, but are not limited to, the following:

- Automated notifications to subscribed stakeholders when the regulatory status has changed in a country/single market; for approved/registered status includes information on validity period, if applicable;
- Automated reminders starting six months before a product registration/certificate is due to expire, if applicable;
- Search and navigation capabilities that enables different search criteria requirements (e.g., per product, per regulatory status, per country/single market);
- Report-generating capabilities for extracting information related to products, regulatory status and country/single market; and

- Ability to link regulatory documents such as certificates, registrations, approval letters, etc., stored in the Regulatory Submissions Repository.

6.7.2 *Regulatory and Business Process KPIs*

The effectiveness of a medical device company's business processes is often reflected in that company's ability to obtain regulatory approvals relatively fast and without too many rounds of questions and answers with the assessing authorities. The Product Regulatory Status Database can be used to collect process data at critical steps in the regulatory process and put in place key performance indicators (KPIs) for the company's regulatory performance, for instance, "Obtain regulatory approvals within four months from receiving the first round of questions, and after no more than two rounds of questions and answers".

The following data should be recorded for process KPI measurements:

- Date of submission – planned and actual;
- Time elapsed between the receipt of a round of questions/deficiencies and the submission of responses to that round of questions/deficiencies;
- Date of approval;
- Overall time elapsed between application and approval; and
- Total number of iterations with the assessing authority (rounds of questions and answers) for the same submission.

By measuring milestones in the regulatory process (see Fig. 6.16), a manufacturer can identify the pain points and outliers in the business processes (design controls, process controls, etc.) and implement targeted CAPAs.

Certain timelines, such as waiting for the assessing authority to complete the review, are independent of manufacturers' processes and outside their influence; hence they should be factored in when measuring the regulatory process timelines.

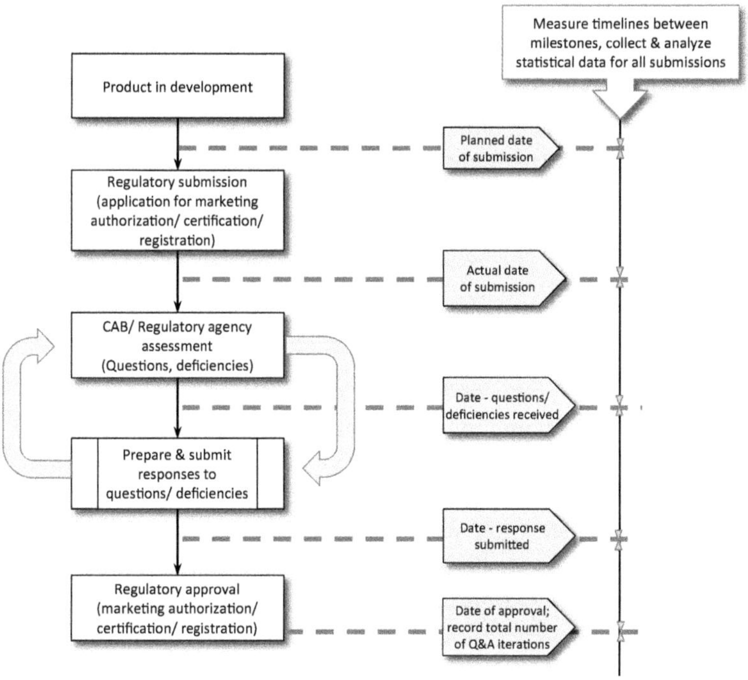

Figure 6.16 Measuring the performance of business processes using milestones in the regulatory process.

6.8 Case Study: Square Peg in a Round Hole

To improve efficiency in handling an increasing volume of changes in the post-market phase, a growing medical device company decided to switch from the existing paper-based change management process to an electronic system. The manufacturer selected Cool Breeze (not an actual brand), an off-the-shelf software program that boasted to have "increased speed and efficiency of document reviews and change control" for companies in the aircraft and automotive manufacturing industries.

The company implemented the Cool Breeze "out of the box" change process, which involved the following steps:

(1) Change request
Anyone in the company could raise a change request. Once a change request was put through the system, a unique change request tracking number (CR#) was assigned for traceability purposes.
(2) Selection of full-track or fast-track process
A D&D engineer with the administrator role in Cool Breeze would assess the change request and select whether it should be processed via a full-track or a fast-track review and approval process.
(3) Change request review and approval (full-track)
The change request would be circulated for review and approval, including to the relevant regulatory professional. The aim of the change request was to obtain approval for resources to be allocated so that work on the change (documentation, V&V) can start, hence the change request did not have detailed, comprehensive supporting information (risk analysis, completed V&V) attached to it.
(4) Change note review and approval (full-track)
Another D&D or manufacturing engineer would be assigned to create a change note and related change tasks (revised specifications, V&V, etc.). The change note and its attached change tasks would be assigned a unique change note tracking number (CN#) and then circulated for review and approval, including to the relevant regulatory professional.
(5) Change implementation
Approved change notes and their associated change tasks would proceed to implementation.
(6) Fast-track changes
Changes assessed by the Cool Breeze administrator as being fast-track would proceed directly to change implementation.

Soon enough problems started to surface, such as:

- A very high volume of change requests were being put through the system due to a lack of adequate planning and triaging. Conflicting or duplicating change requests were being put through the system. Many changes lingered unaddressed for months or even years in the system. This resulted in more, not less, bureaucracy and administrative burden compared to the previous paper-based system.

- Some change requests were bundled in a change note; others were addressed by change tasks spread across a number of change notes; although CR#s were linked to CN#s, there was no clear traceability of what was actually changing and no clear evidence that product configuration still met requirements.
- In some instances (deadlines pressure) originators of change requests would reverse-engineer the change description so that it would fit the fast-track criteria and thus result in speedy implementation without the required scrutiny. This would potentially cause serious regulatory non-compliance.
- The initial fast-track criteria had been defined without input from the regulatory function.
- The change management procedure stated that the approval of the change request represented an "approval of the change" rather than an authorization for allocating resources to start working on the change. This resulted in stakeholders across the business to consider the change note as a mere notification of an already approved change.
- The change management process did not make provision for multiple regulatory submissions and approvals in various target markets. To compensate for this deficiency, implementation of significant changes would be put on manual hold and wait for approval in the country with the strictest regulatory regime (United States). Only after approval that took the longest was obtained, the manual hold would be lifted and the change implemented in all markets.

This is an example of how quickly good intentions can result in bad outcomes. Bending internal business processes and implementing laborious workarounds to fit an off-the-shelf software tool, which was not designed for medical device companies in the first place, created more problems than solving them.

In doing so, the company broke a cardinal rule when switching from a manual to an automated change management process; this rule says that you should *map the correct business process first*, and then select, and if necessary customize, the appropriate software tool. The software tool needs to fit the business process and not the other way around. Automating a poorly defined and/or non-compliant process will only amplify and exacerbate its deficiencies.

6.9 Concluding Summary

Chapter 6 discusses some of the important aspects that affect regulatory compliance in the post-market phase:

- Planning and execution of a product launch, ensuring that marketing claims align with approved labelling, and observing the rules applicable to product advertising;
- A translation procedure for product documentation such as instructions for use and promotional material;
- Regulatory requirements for assessing changes in the post-market phase and determining whether changes are significant (requiring approval prior implementation) or not;
- Change controls, change management process, configuration management and examples of how a medical device manufacturer might implement them;
- Considerations for defining a regulatory strategy in the post-market phase;
- Statutory requirements for post-market surveillance – post-market clinical follow-up, vigilance/serious adverse events reporting and recalls;
- Things to consider when obsoleting a product;
- QMS documentation and processes – examples of QMS KPIs, QMS auditing and performance measurement; and
- Regulatory systems and processes – examples of information captured and tracked in a Product Regulatory Status Database and how it can be used to measure timelines between regulatory milestones to drive performance improvement for business processes.

References

1. European Commission. Directive 2005/29/EC concerning unfair business-to-consumer commercial practices in the internal market. *eur-lex.europa.eu.* [Online] May 11, 2005. [Cited: December 1, 2014.] http://eur-lex.europa.eu/legal-content/en/ALL/?uri=CELEX:32005L0029.
2. European Commission. Unfair commercial practices. *ec.europa.eu.* [Online] June 30, 2014. [Cited: December 1, 2014.] http://ec.europa.eu/justice/consumer-marketing/unfair-trade/unfair-practices/index_en.htm.
3. European Commission. Directive 2006/114/EC concerning misleading and comparative advertising. *eur-lex.europa.eu.* [Online] December 12, 2006. [Cited: December 1, 2014.] http://eur-lex.europa.eu/legal-content/en/ALL/?uri=CELEX:32006L0114.
4. European Commission. Misleading advertising. *ec.europa.eu.* [Online] July 16, 2013. [Cited: December 1, 2014.] http://ec.europa.eu/justice/consumer-marketing/unfair-trade/false-advertising/index_en.htm.
5. Food and Drug Administration. Device Labeling. *www.fda.gov.* [Online] June 30, 2014. [Cited: December 1, 2014.] http://www.fda.gov/MedicalDevices/DeviceRegulationandGuidance/Overview/DeviceLabeling/ucm2005422.htm.
6. Food and Drug Administration. False or Misleading Labeling. *www.fda.gov.* [Online] July 30, 2014. [Cited: December 1, 2014.] http://www.fda.gov/MedicalDevices/DeviceRegulationandGuidance/Overview/DeviceLabeling/GeneralDeviceLabelingRequirements/ucm052190.htm.
7. Food and Drug Administration. Inspections, Compliance, Enforcement and Criminal. *www.fda.gov.* [Online] August 16, 2012. [Cited: December 1, 2014.] Examples of false labeling include:.
8. Therapeutic Goods Administration. Regulation of therapeutic goods advertising in Australia. *www.tga.gov.au.* [Online] April 8, 2011. [Cited: December 1, 2014.] https://www.tga.gov.au/regulation-therapeutic-goods-advertising-australia.
9. Therapeutic Goods Administration. Advertising therapeutic goods. *www.tga.gov.au.* [Online] October 28, 2014. [Cited: December 1, 2014.] https://www.tga.gov.au/advertising-therapeutic-goods.
10. Therapeutic Goods Administration. Regulatory compliance framework. *www.tga.gov.au.* [Online] June 27, 2013. [Cited: December 1, 2014.] https://www.tga.gov.au/regulatory-compliance-framework.

11. Health Canada. Regulatory Requirements for Advertising – Policies and Guidance Documents. *www.hc-sc.gc.ca.* [Online] September 16, 2014. [Cited: December 1, 2014.] http://www.hc-sc.gc.ca/dhp-mps/advert-publicit/pol/index-eng.php.
12. Regulatory Affairs Professionals Society. *Fundamentals of Japanese Regulatory Affairs, First Edition.* Rockville, MD 20852 : Regulatory Affairs Professionals Society, 2010.
13. Baker & McKenzie. Promoting Medical products Globally – Handbook of Pharma and MedTech Compliance – Japan. *www.bakermckenzie.com.* [Online] 2012. [Cited: December 1, 2014.] http://www.bakermckenzie.com/files/Uploads/Documents/Global%20Pharmaceuticals/Japan.pdf.
14. European Commission. Countries. *europa.eu.* [Online] [Cited: December 1, 2014.] http://europa.eu/about-eu/countries/index_en.htm.
15. EFTA. The EFTA States. *www.efta.int.* [Online] [Cited: December 1, 2014.] http://www.efta.int/about-efta/the-efta-states.
16. European Commission. New version of the "Blue Guide" on the implementation of EU product rules. *ec.europa.eu.* [Online] February 28, 2014. [Cited: December 1, 2014.] http://ec.europa.eu/enterprise/newsroom/cf/itemdetail.cfm?item_id=7326.
17. European Commission. Interpretative document of the Commisions's services – Placing on the market of medical devices. *ec.europa.eu.* [Online] November 16, 2010. [Cited: December 1, 2014.] http://ec.europa.eu/health/medical-devices/files/guide-stds-directives/placing_on_the_market_en.pdf.
18. Food and Drug Administration. 21 CFR Part 820 Quality System Regulation – Section 820.184 Device History Record. *www.accessdata.fda.gov.* [Online] September 1, 2014. [Cited: October 3, 2014.] http://www.accessdata.fda.gov/scripts/cdrh/cfdocs/cfcfr/CFRSearch.cfm?fr=820.184.
19. NB-MED. Recommendation 2.5.2/Rec2 Reporting of design changes and changes of the quality system. *www.team-nb.org.* [Online] November 2008. [Cited: November 18, 2014.] http://www.team-nb.org/documents/2011/Approved_NB-MED_2_5_2_rec_2_november_2008.pdf.
20. NBOG. BPG 2014-3 Guidance for manufacturers and Notified Bodies on reporting of design changes and changes of the quality system. *www.nbog.eu.* [Online] November 2014. [Cited: November 18, 2014.] http://www.nbog.eu/resources/NBOG_BPG_2014_3.pdf.
21. Food and Drug Administration. Deciding When to Submit a 510(k) for a Change to an Existing Device (K97-1). *www.fda.gov.* [Online]

January 10, 1997. [Cited: November 18, 2014.] http://www.fda.gov/MedicalDevices/DeviceRegulationandGuidance/GuidanceDocuments/ucm080235.htm.

22. Food and Drug Administration. How To Prepare A Special 510(k). *www.fda.gov.* [Online] October 10, 2014. [Cited: November 18, 2014.] http://www.fda.gov/MedicalDevices/DeviceRegulationandGuidance/HowtoMarketYourDevice/PremarketSubmissions/PremarketNotification510k/ucm134573.htm.
23. Food and Drug Administration. PMA Supplements and Amendments. *www.fda.gov.* [Online] September 5, 2014. [Cited: November 18, 2014.] http://www.fda.gov/MedicalDevices/DeviceRegulationandGuidance/HowtoMarketYourDevice/PremarketSubmissions/Premarket ApprovalPMA/ucm050467.htm.
24. Food and Drug Administration. Real-Time Premarket Approval Application (PMA) Supplements. *www.fda.gov.* [Online] April 28, 2006. [Cited: November 18, 2014.] http://www.fda.gov/MedicalDevices/DeviceRegulationandGuidance/GuidanceDocuments/ucm089602.htm.
25. Food and Drug Administration. 30-Day Notices, 135-Day Premarket Approval (PMA) Supplements and 75-Day Humanitarian Device Exemption (HDE) Supplements for Manufacturing Method or Process Changes. *www.fda.gov.* [Online] April 13, 2011. [Cited: November 18, 2014.] http://www.fda.gov/MedicalDevices/DeviceRegulationandGuidance/GuidanceDocuments/ucm080192.htm.
26. Food and Drug Administration. Supplements to Approved Applications for Class III Medical Devices: Use of Published Literature, Use of Previously Submitted Materials, and Priority Review. *www.fda.gov.* [Online] May 20, 1998. [Cited: November 18, 2014.] http://www.fda.gov/MedicalDevices/DeviceRegulationandGuidance/GuidanceDocuments/ucm080183.htm.
27. Health Canada. Guidance for the Interpretation of Significant Change of a Medical Device. *www.hc-sc.gc.ca.* [Online] January 20, 2011. [Cited: November 18, 2014.] http://www.hc-sc.gc.ca/dhp-mps/md-im/applic-demande/guide-ld/signchng_modimportante-eng.php#a27.
28. Xiao, L. Guide for Australian medical technology companies seeking to engage in China (First edition – draft). *www.ausbiotech.org.* [Online] [Cited: November 18, 2014.] www.ausbiotech.org/data/downloads/V9_Draft%20China%20Guide.docx.
29. Health Sciences Authority. GN-02: Guidance on Licensing for Manufacturers, Importers and Wholesalers of Medical Devices.

www.hsa.gov.sg. [Online] December 2014. [Cited: December 1, 2014.] http://www.hsa.gov.sg/content/dam/HSA/HPRG/Medical_Devices/Overview_Framework_Policies/Guidances_for_Medical_Device_Registration/GN-02-R3%20Guidance_on_Licensing_for_Manufacturers_Importers_and_Wholesalers_of_Medical_Devices.pdf.

30. Food and Drug Administration. Design Control Guidance for Medical Device Manufacturers, Section I. Design Changes. *www.fda.gov.* [Online] March 11, 1997. [Cited: November 18, 2014.] http://www.fda.gov/MedicalDevices/DeviceRegulationandGuidance/GuidanceDocuments/ucm070627.htm#_Toc382720791.
31. Food and Drug Administration. Medical Device Recall Report FY2003 to FY2012. *www.fda.gov.* [Online] [Cited: November 18, 2014.] http://www.fda.gov/downloads/AboutFDA/CentersOffices/OfficeofMedicalProductsandTobacco/CDRH/CDRHTransparency/UCM388442.pdf.
32. Food and Drug Administration. General Principles of Software Validation. *www.fda.gov.* [Online] January 11, 2002. [Cited: November 18, 2014.] http://www.fda.gov/medicaldevices/deviceregulationand guidance/guidancedocuments/ucm085281.htm.
33. Institute of Configuration Management. What Is Configuration Management (CM)? *icmhq.com.* [Online] 2013. [Cited: December 1, 2014.] http://icmhq.com/cmii-configuration_management/.
34. Global Harmonization Taskforce. GHTF study group 2 – Post-market surveillance/vigilance. *www.imdrf.org.* [Online] [Cited: November 18, 2014.] http://www.imdrf.org/documents/doc-ghtf-sg2.asp.
35. European Commission. MEDDEV 2.12/1 Medical Devices Vigilance System. *ec.europa.eu.* [Online] January 2013. [Cited: November 18, 2014.] http://ec.europa.eu/health/medical-devices/files/meddev/2_12_1_ol_en.pdf.
36. European Commission. MEDDEV 2.12/2 Postmarket Clinical Follow-Up Studies. *ec.europa.eu.* [Online] January 2012. [Cited: September 22, 2014.] http://ec.europa.eu/health/medical-devices/files/meddev/2_12_2_ol_en.pdf.
37. Food and Drug Administration. Postmarket Surveillance Under Section 522 of the Federal Food, Drug and Cosmetic Act. *www.fda.gov.* [Online] April 25, 2006. [Cited: September 22, 2014.] http://www.fda.gov/medicaldevices/deviceregulationandguidance/guidancedocuments/ucm072517.htm.
38. Food and Drug Administration. Draft Guidance for Industry and Food and Drug Administration Staff – Postmarket Surveillance Un-

der Section 522 of the Federal Food, Drug and Cosmetic Act. *www.fda.gov.* [Online] August 16, 2011. [Cited: November 18, 2014.] http://www.fda.gov/medicaldevices/deviceregulationandguidance/guidancedocuments/ucm268064.htm.

39. Food and Drug Administration. 21 CFR Part 803 Medical Device Reporting. *www.accessdata.fda.gov.* [Online] September 1, 2014. [Cited: November 18, 2014.] http://www.accessdata.fda.gov/scripts/cdrh/cfdocs/cfcfr/CFRsearch.cfm?CFRPart=803.
40. Food and Drug Administration. Mandatory Reporting Requirements: Manufacturers, Importers and Device User Facilities. *www.fda.gov.* [Online] September 10, 2014. [Cited: November 18, 2014.] http://www.fda.gov/MedicalDevices/DeviceRegulationandGuidance/PostmarketRequirements/ReportingAdverseEvents/ucm2005737.htm.
41. Food and Drug Administration. Medical Device Reporting for Manufacturers. *www.fda.gov.* [Online] March 1997. [Cited: November 18, 2014.] http://www.fda.gov/medicaldevices/deviceregulationandguidance/guidancedocuments/ucm094529.htm.
42. Food and Drug Administration. Draft Guidance for Industry and Food and Drug Administration Staff – Medical Device Reporting for Manufacturers. *www.fda.gov.* [Online] July 9, 2013. [Cited: November 18, 2014.] http://www.fda.gov/MedicalDevices/DeviceRegulationandGuidance/GuidanceDocuments/ucm359130.htm.
43. Food and Drug Administration. 21 CFR Part 7 Enforcement Policy. *www.accessdata.fda.gov.* [Online] September 1, 2014. [Cited: November 18, 2014.] http://www.accessdata.fda.gov/scripts/cdrh/cfdocs/cfcfr/CFRSearch.cfm?CFRPart=7.
44. Food and Drug Administration. 21 CFR Part 806 – Medical Devices: Reports of Corrections and Removals. *www.accessdata.fda.gov.* [Online] September 1, 2014. [Cited: November 18, 2014.] http://www.accessdata.fda.gov/scripts/cdrh/cfdocs/cfcfr/CFRSearch.cfm?fr=806.2.
45. Food and Drug Administration. Product Recalls, Including Removals and Corrections. *www.fda.gov.* [Online] November 3, 2003. [Cited: November 18, 2014.] http://www.fda.gov/safety/recalls/industryguidance/ucm129259.htm.
46. Food and Drug Administration. Distinguishing Medical Device Recalls from Medical Device Enhancements. *www.fda.gov.* [Online] October 15, 2014. [Cited: November 18, 2014.] http://www.fda.gov/downloads/medicaldevices/deviceregulationandguidance/guidancedocuments/ucm418469.pdf.

47. Therapeutic Goods Administration. Reporting problems. *www.tga.gov.au.* [Online] November 14, 2014. [Cited: November 18, 2014.] http://www.tga.gov.au/reporting-problems.
48. Therapeutic Goods Administration. Australian regulatory guidelines for medical devices (ARGMD) – Section 22. Post-market vigilance and monitoring requirements. *www.tga.gov.au.* [Online] May 2011. [Cited: November 18, 2014.] https://www.tga.gov.au/sites/default/files/devices-argmd-01.pdf.
49. Therapeutic Goods Administration. Australian regulatory guidelines for medical devices (ARGMD) – Section 23. Recalls, suspensions, cancellations, and tampering of medical devices. *www.tga.gov.au.* [Online] May 2011. [Cited: November 18, 2014.] https://www.tga.gov.au/sites/default/files/devices-argmd-01.pdf.
50. Health Canada. Guidance on Investigation of Reported Medical Device Problems (GUI-0065). *www.hc-sc.gc.ca.* [Online] March 25, 2011. [Cited: November 18, 2014.] http://www.hc-sc.gc.ca/dhp-mps/compli-conform/prob-report-rapport/gui-0065_md-im_problem_doc-eng.php.
51. Health Canada. Problem Reporting. *www.hc-sc.gc.ca.* [Online] October 29, 2013. [Cited: November 18, 2014.] http://www.hc-sc.gc.ca/dhp-mps/compli-conform/prob-report-rapport/index-eng.php.
52. Health Canada. Guidance Document for Mandatory Problem Reporting for Medical Devices. *www.hc-sc.gc.ca.* [Online] October 3, 2011. [Cited: November 18, 2014.] http://www.hc-sc.gc.ca/dhp-mps/pubs/medeff/_guide/2011-devices-materiaux/index-eng.php.
53. Health Canada. Guide to Recall of Medical Devices (GUI-0054). *www.hc-sc.gc.ca.* [Online] March 25, 2011. [Cited: November 18, 2014.] http://www.hc-sc.gc.ca/dhp-mps/compli-conform/prob-report-rapport/gui-0054_recall-retrait-doc-eng.php#def31.
54. JFMDA. JFMDA. *www.jfmda.gr.jp.* [Online] http://www.jfmda.gr.jp/e/.
55. JPMA. JPMA. *www.jpma.or.jp.* [Online] http://www.jpma.or.jp/english/.
56. Health Sciences Authority. GN-05: Guidance on the Reporting of Adverse Events for Medical Devices. *www.hsa.gov.sg.* [Online] September 2013. [Cited: November 18, 2014.] http://www.hsa.gov.sg/content/dam/HSA/HPRG/Medical_Devices/Overview_Framework_Policies/Guidances_for_Medical_Device_Registration/GN-05-R2_Guidance%20on%20the%20Reporting%20of%20Adverse%20Events%20for%20Medical%20Devices.pdf.
57. Global Harmonization Taskforce. GHTF SG3/N19:2012 Nonconformity grading systen for regulatory purposes and information ex-

change. *www.imdrf.org.* [Online] November 2, 2012. [Cited: November 18, 2014.] http://www.imdrf.org/docs/ghtf/final/sg3/technical-docs/ghtf-sg3-n19-2012-nonconformity-grading-121102.pdf.

58. Global Harmonization Taskforce. GHTF/SG2/N36R7:2003 Manufacturer's trend reporting of adbverse events. *www.imdrf.org.* [Online] January 2003. [Cited: November 18, 2014.] http://www.imdrf.org/docs/ghtf/final/sg2/technical-docs/ghtf-sg2-n36r7-2003-manufacturer-trend-reporting-adverse-event-030101.pdf.
59. Global Harmonization Taskforce. GHTF SG3/N15R8 Implementation of risk management principles and activities within a quality management system. *www.imdrf.org.* [Online] May 20, 2005. [Cited: November 18, 2014.] http://www.imdrf.org/docs/ghtf/final/sg3/technical-docs/ghtf-sg3-n15r8-risk-management-principles-qms-050520.pdf.
60. Global Harmonization Taskforce. GHTF SG3/N18:2010 Quality management system – Medical devices – Guidance on corrective action and preventive action and related QMS processes. *www.imdrf.org.* [Online] November 4, 2010. [Cited: November 18, 2014.] http://www.imdrf.org/docs/ghtf/final/sg3/technical-docs/ghtf-sg3-n18-2010-qms-guidance-on-corrective-preventative-action-101104.pdf.
61. Global Harmonization Taskforce. GHTF SG3/N17:2008 Quality management system – Medical devices – Guidance on the control of products and services obtained from suppliers. *www.imdrf.org.* [Online] December 11, 2008. [Cited: November 18, 2014.] http://www.imdrf.org/docs/ghtf/final/sg3/technical-docs/ghtf-sg3-n17-guidance-on-quality-management-system-081211.pdf.

List of Abbreviations

AHRQ	Agency for Healthcare Research and Quality
AI	Additional Information
AIDC	automatic identification and data capture
AIMD	active implantable medical device
AIMDD	Active Implantable Medical Device Directive
AMDD	ASEAN Medical Devices Directive
ANSI	American National Standards Institute
ANVISA	Agência Nacional de Vigilância Sanitária
APAC	Asia Pacific
ARGMD	*Australian Regulatory Guidelines for Medical Devices*
ASEAN	Association of Southeast Asian NationS
BBP	benzyl butyl phthalate
BGTD	Biologics Genetic Therapies Directorate
BOM	bill of materials
BOO	bill of operations
BRH	Brazil Registration Holder
BSE	bovine spongiform encephalopathy
CA	Competent Authority
CAB	Conformity Assessment Body
CAPA	corrective action and preventive action
CASO	conformity assessment standards orders
CBER	Center for Biologics Evaluation and Research
CD	compact disc
CDER	Center for Drug Evaluation and Research
CDRH	Center of Devices and Radiological Health
CE	Conformité Européenne
CEPS	Comité Economique des Produits de Santé

CFDA	China Food and Drug Administration
CFR	*Code of Federal Regulations*
CFS	Certificates of Free Sale
CJD	Creutzfeldt–Jakob disease
CMDCAS	Canadian Medical Devices Conformity Assessment System
CMDE	Centre for Medical Device Evaluation
CMS	Centers for Medicare & Medicaid Services
CMV	cytomegalovirus
CoA	Certificate of Analysis
CSDT	Common Submission Dossier Template
CTN	Clinical Trial Notification
CTX	Clinical Trial Exemption
CWD	chronic wasting disease
D&D	design and development
DBP	dibutyl phthalate
DCC	Document Control Center
DEHP	bis(2-ethylhexyl)phthalate
DFMEA	design failure modes and effects analysis
DHF	Design History File
DHR	Device History Record
DI	Device Identifier
DMAH	Designated Marketing Authorization Holder
DMR	Device Master Record
DoC	Declaration of Conformity
DoE	Design of Experiments
DOU	*Diário Oficial da União*
DPC	Diagnosis Procedure Combinations
DRG	Diagnostic Related Group
DVD	digital video disc
eBS	eBusiness Services
EC	European Commission
EDMS	electronic document management system
EDQM	European Directorate for the Quality of Medicines and Healthcare
EEA	European Economic Area
ELISA	enzyme-linked immunosorbent assay
EMA	European Medicines Agency

EMC	electromagnetic compatibility
EN	European Norms
EP	Essential Principle
EPA	Environmental Protection Agency
ES	Essential Requirement
EtO	ethylene oxide
EU	European Union
FD&C Act	Food, Drug, and Cosmetic Act
FDA	Food and Drug Administration
FIH	first-in-human
FMA	Foreign Manufacturer Accreditation
FMEA	failure mode and effects analysis
FSCA	field safety corrective action
FSN	field safety notice
FURLS	FDA Unified Registration and Listing Systems
G-BA	Gemeinsamer Bundesausschuss
GCP	Good Clinical Practice
GDPMDS	Good Distribution Practice for Medical Devices
GGP	Good Guidance Practice
GHTF	Global Harmonization Taskforce
GLP	Good Laboratory Practice
GMP	Good Manufacturing Practice
GQP	Good Quality Practice
GUDID	Global Unique Device Identification Database
GVP	Good Vigilance Practice
HAS	Haute Autorité de Santé
HAS	Health Sciences Authority
HC	Health Canada
HDE	humanitarian-device exemption
HIBCC	Health Industry Business Communications Council
HIRA	Health Insurance Review and Assessment Services
HIV	human immunodeficiency virus
HL7	Health Level Seven
HLA	human leukocyte antigen
HREC	Human Research Ethics Committee

HRI	human-readable interpretation
HTA	Health Technology Assessment
HTLV	human T-lymphotropic virus
HUD	humanitarian-use device
IAF	International Accreditation Forum
ICCBBA	International Council for Commonality in Blood Banking Automation
IDE	investigational-device exemption
IEC	International Electrotechnical Commission
IFA	immunofluorescence assay
IFU	instruction for use
IMDRF	International Medical Device Regulatory Forum
INMETRO	National Institute of Metrology, Quality and Technology
IQ	installation qualification
IQWiG	Institute for Quality and Efficiency in Health Care
IRB	institutional review board
ISO	International Organization for Standardization
ISTA	International Safe Transit Association
IUO	Investigational Use Only
IVD	in vitro diagnostics
IVDD	In Vitro Diagnostics Directive
JIS	Japanese Industrial Standards
JMDN	Japanese Medical Device Nomenclature
J-PAL	Japanese Pharmaceutical Affairs Law
KOL	key opinion leader
KPI	key performance indicator
LCD	Local Coverage Determination
LoC	level of concern
LPPR	Liste des Produits et Prestations Remboursables
MAH	Marketing Authorization Holder
MAUDE	Manufacturer and User Facility Device Experience
MD	medical device
MDALL	Medical Device Active Licence Listing
MDD	Medical Devices Directive
MDEL	Medical Device Establishment Licence

MDL	Medical Device Licence
MDR	Medical Device Reporting
MDSO	medical device standards orders
MDUFMA	Medical Device User Fee and Modernization Act
MEDDEV	Medical Devices
MHLW	Ministry of Health, Labor and Welfare
MLA	Multilateral Agreement
MOH	Ministry of Health
MRA	Mutual Recognition Agreement
MRI	magnetic resonance imaging
Nando	New Approach Notified and Designated Organizations
NB-MED	Notified Bodies Medical Devices
NBOG BPG	Notified Body Operations Group Best Practice Guides
NCD	National Coverage Determination
NCR	non-conformance report
NDRC	National Development and Reform Commission
NHI	National Health Insurance
NHMRC	National Health and Medical Research Council
NIH	National Institutes of Health
NSE	not substantially equivalent
OCP	Office of Combination Products
OJ	operational qualification
OK	*Official Journal of the European Union*
OTC	over-the-counter
PBB	polybrominated biphenyl
PBDE	polybrominated diphenyl ether
PBR	Payment-by-Result
PFMEA	process failure modes and effects analysis
PI	Production Identifier
PIP	Poly Implant Prothèse
PMA	Premarket Approval
PMCF	Post-Market Clinical Follow-Up
PMD Act	Pharmaceutical and Medical Devices Act
PMDA	Pharmaceuticals and Medical Devices Agency
PMP	Project Management Plan
PQ	process qualification

PSA	prostate-specific antigen
PVC	polyvinyl chloride
QA	quality assurance
QC	quality control
QMS	quality management system
QoS	quality of service
QSIT	*Quality System Inspection Technique*
QSR	quality system regulation
R&TTE	Radio and Telecommunications Terminal Equipment
RA	Regulatory Authority
RCB	Registered Certification Body
RED	Radio Equipment Directive
RF	radio frequency
RFID	radio frequency identification
RPS	Regulated Product Submission
RTA	Refuse to Accept
RTR	real-time review
RUO	Research Use Only
RUSP	ready-to-use software product
SAE	serious adverse event
SAL	sterility assurance level
SaMD	software as a medical device
SAS	special access scheme
SCENIHR	Scientific Committee of Emerging and Newly Identified Health Risks
SFDA	State Food and Drug Administration
SMDR	*Singapore Medical Device Register*
SPL	Structured Product Label
SRD	short-range device
SSED	Summary of Safety and Effectiveness Data
STD	sexually transmitted disease
STED	Summary Technical Documentation
TFEU	Treaty on the Functioning of the European Union
TGA	Therapeutic Goods Administration
TPD	Therapeutic Products Directorate
TRF	Test Report form
TSE	transmissible spongiform encephalopathy

UDI	Unique Device Identifier
UDID	UDI Database
UEN	Unique Entity Number
UNCAM	Union Nationale des Caisses d'Assurance Maladie
UPI	Unique Product Identifier
V&V	verification and validation
VAD	ventricular assist device
vCJD	variant Creutzfeldt–Jakob disease
WEEE	Waste of Electrical and Electronic Equipment
WHO	World Health Organization
WIPO	World Intellectual Property Organization
WMA	World Medical Association
WTO	World Trade Organization
XML	extensible markup language

Index

For Product Safety Concerns and Information please contact our EU
representative GPSR@taylorandfrancis.com
Taylor & Francis Verlag GmbH, Kaufingerstraße 24, 80331 München, Germany

www.ingramcontent.com/pod-product-compliance
Ingram Content Group UK Ltd.
Pitfield, Milton Keynes, MK11 3LW, UK
UKHW022200190926
475702UK00003B/125

* 9 7 8 9 8 1 4 6 6 9 1 0 8 *